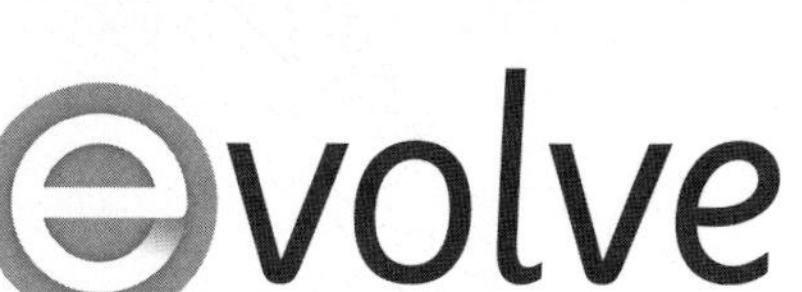

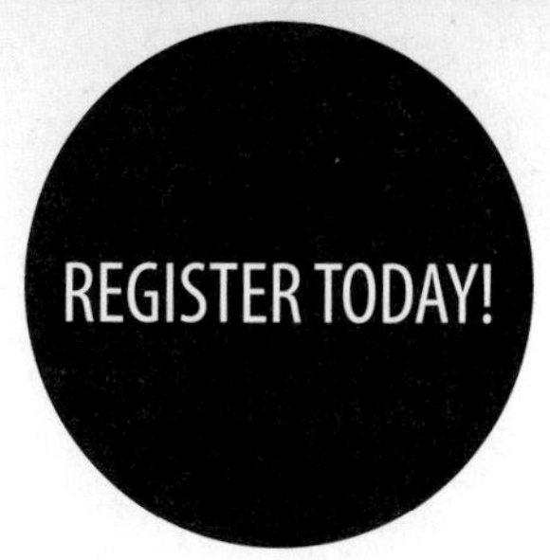

To access your Student Resources, visit:

http://evolve.elsevier.com/Buck/practicekit/

Evolve Student Learning Resources for Buck: Practice Kit for Medical Front Office Skills offers the following features

- **Audio Files**
  These MP3 files contain medical dictation files for transcription and telephone messages.
- **Forms Library and Task Documents**
  For your convenience, the forms from Appendix 4 are also included electronically along with documents needed to complete certain Tasks.
- **Medisoft Base Data**
  This data, combined with your Medisoft CD, will allow you to create your South Padre Medical Office.
- **ABHES and CAAHEP Skill Checks**
  Skill checks evaluate student progress and list the CAAHEP and ABHES competencies that are fulfilled by completing each Task.
- **Patient Directory**
  As a helpful resource, a comprehensive list of all patients included in this kit is provided.
- **Software Instructions and Tips**
  Detailed instructions for installing and using Medisoft and Practice Partner.
- **Content Updates**
  Continually updated information to provide the latest content updates on relevant issues for this kit.

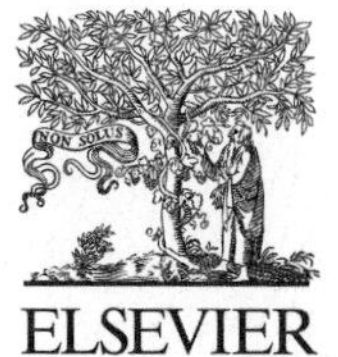

STUDENT MANUAL WITH DAILY TASKS

PRACTICE KIT FOR

MEDICAL FRONT OFFICE SKILLS

From Practice to Application

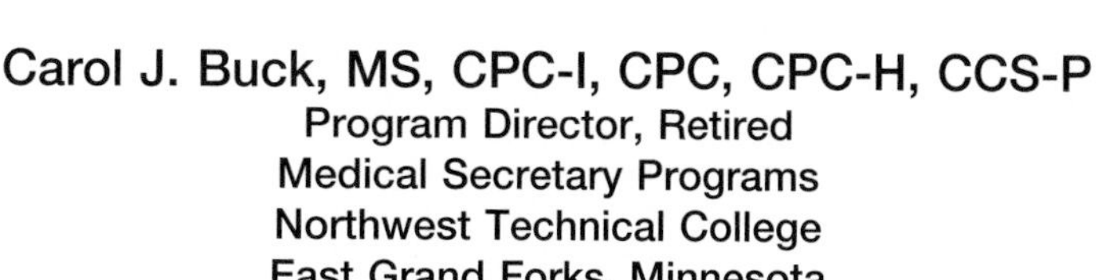

Carol J. Buck, MS, CPC-I, CPC, CPC-H, CCS-P
Program Director, Retired
Medical Secretary Programs
Northwest Technical College
East Grand Forks, Minnesota

Technical Collaborator
Jacqueline Klitz Grass, MA, CPC
Coding Specialist
Grand Forks, North Dakota

Competency Developer
Lyn O'Neal, RMA
Co-Chair and Instructor
Allied Health Department
Skagit Valley College
Mount Vernon, Washington

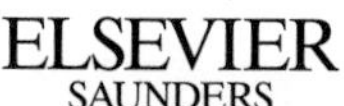

THIRD EDITION

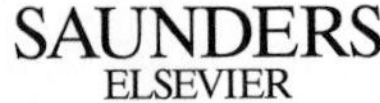

3251 Riverport Lane
St. Louis, Missouri 63043

STUDENT MANUAL WITH DAILY TASKS FOR PRACTICE KIT FOR MEDICAL FRONT OFFICE SKILLS, THIRD EDITION PART NUMBER 9996077616

NOTE: *Current Procedural Terminology, 2010,* was used in updating this text.

Notices

Knowledge and best practice in this field are constantly changing. As new research and experience broaden our understanding, changes in research methods, professional practices, or medical treatment may become necessary.

Practitioners and researchers must always rely on their own experience and knowledge in evaluating and using any information, methods, compounds, or experiments described herein. In using such information or methods they should be mindful of their own safety and the safety of others, including parties for whom they have a professional responsibility.

With respect to any drug or pharmaceutical products identified, readers are advised to check the most current information provided (i) on procedures featured or (ii) by the manufacturer of each product to be administered, to verify the recommended dose or formula, the method and duration of administration, and contraindications. It is the responsibility of practitioners, relying on their own experience and knowledge of their patients, to make diagnoses, to determine dosages and the best treatment for each individual patient, and to take all appropriate safety precautions.

To the fullest extent of the law, neither the Publisher nor the authors, contributors, or editors, assume any liability for any injury and/or damage to persons or property as a matter of products liability, negligence or otherwise, or from any use or operation of any methods, products, instructions, or ideas contained in the material herein.

To the fullest extent of the law, neither the Publisher nor the authors, contributors, or editors, assume any liability for any injury and/or damage to persons or property as a matter of products liability, negligence or otherwise, or from any use or operation of any methods, products, instructions, or ideas contained in the material herein.

Publisher: Michael S. Ledbetter
Associate Developmental Editors: Jennifer Boudreau, Jamie Augustine
Publishing Services Manager: Pat Joiner-Myers
Designer: Kim Denando

Printed in the United States of America

Last digit is the print number: 9 8 7 6 5 4 3 2 1

This work is dedicated to students who approach every new project with enthusiasm and determination to do their best.

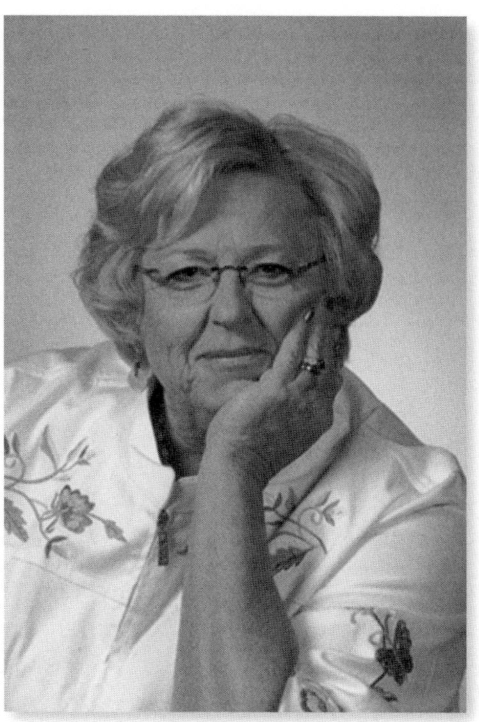

Carol J. Buck

Reviewers

Mary M. Broussard, CPC, CMRS
Department Chair, Medical Coding and Billing Program
Remington College
Shreveport, Louisiana

Robin Kern, RN, BSN
Medical Assisting Program Director
Moultrie Technical College
Moultrie, Georgia

Denice Klassen, RN, BSN
Instructor, Medical Assistant Program
Wichita Area Technical College
Wichita, Kansas

Tammy Lucas, CPC, CPC-I, CPMA
Allied Health Instructor
Remington College
Shreveport, Louisiana

Helen Spain, MSEd
Coordinator, Medical Office Administration
Instructor, Office Systems Technology
Wake Technical Community College
Raleigh, North Carolina

Preface

The hub of the modern medical office is the computer. Practice management is accomplished by means of computer software designed to process and store medical records, appointments, billing, and numerous other medical office tasks. Many health care facilities are now paperless and others are in varying stages of transition to become paperless. There are, however, facilities that remain papered offices. The extent to which you will utilize a computer to accomplish your daily tasks will be determined by the facility in which you are employed, but regardless of the extent of the use of the computer, you will need to be familiar with a wide range of tasks that are standard in the medical office. For example, medical dictation may be transcribed and stored in electronic medium or printed on paper to be filed into the medical record. Either way, you need to be able to transcribe medical dictation, no matter what the terminal storage. The learning is what is important in the process, not whether the task is performed with or without a computer. To enhance your familiarity with all types of office settings and to give you the option of how to complete the tasks, many tasks may be accomplished using either a paper or computer approach, depending on your instructor's preference.

No matter which approach you use to complete the tasks in this packet, you will learn how to accomplish many of the basic medical office tasks and better prepare yourself to begin your new career in a medical setting.

Success is the sum of small efforts, repeated day in and day out.
—Robert Collier

Contents

DAY **NINE**

DAY **TEN**

Appendices

Supplies, *221*

Introduction

Learning Objectives

Upon completion of this Practice Kit, you should be able to:

1. Demonstrate basic knowledge of confidentiality and HIPAA regulations.
2. Prepare the appointment schedule for appointment scheduling.
3. Schedule patient appointments according to office rules based on patient need, facility availability, and physician preference.
4. Schedule inpatient and outpatient admissions and procedures.
5. Prepare a daily Patient List.
6. File medical records.
7. Complete daily bank deposit ticket.
8. Reconcile a bank statement.
9. Post entries on a daysheet.
10. Perform accounts receivable procedures.
11. Perform accounts payable procedures.
12. Prepare monthly patient bills.
13. Perform collection procedures.
14. Establish a petty cash fund.
15. Post adjustments.
16. Process a credit balance.
17. Process refunds.
18. Post nonsufficient fund checks.
19. Post collection agency payments.
20. Obtain preauthorization for procedures.
21. Obtain managed care referrals and precertifications.
22. Apply the correct procedural and diagnosis codes for services provided.
23. Prepare an insurance claim form for Medicare, Medicaid, managed care carrier, and private health insurance carrier.
24. Use a fee schedule to correctly calculate payment for services.
25. Record a variety of telephone messages left on an answering machine.
26. Set up and maintain patient files.
27. Prepare draft documents for your supervisor's review.
28. Demonstrate understanding of risk management procedures.
29. Perform inventory of equipment.
30. Perform routine maintenance of administrative equipment.
31. Key documents from your supervisor's drafts.
32. Transcribe dictation from several people consisting of medical documents and general correspondence.
33. Use computer software to maintain systems.
34. Perform installation of Practice Partner software.
35. Manipulate data using Dashboard functions.
36. Demonstrate understanding of the EHR.
37. Exhibit ability to obtain information from the EHR.

Contents of the Practice Kit

The Practice Kit packet contains the following items:

- Student Manual with Daily Tasks (1)
- Patient Appointment Schedules (20)
- File Folders (36)
- File Labels (60: 30 preprinted; 30 plain)
- Check Register (1)
- Companion Evolve site (1) with phone messages and dictation files, Forms Library, Medisoft base data, and Patient Directory
- Medisoft Advanced Version 16 Software CD (1)
- Practice Partner Version 9.3.2 Software CD (1)

Student Manual with Daily Tasks

The *Student Manual with Daily Tasks* provides you with directions for each of the tasks that you will be completing during your internship, along with reference materials and forms. The Supplies section of this manual contains many of the forms that you will be using while completing the various tasks. First, read through the information presented in "Your Internship Tasks" on p. xvii.

PATIENT APPOINTMENT SCHEDULES

You will be scheduling the patient appointments on several days of your internship. Appendix 2 (p. 163) contains directions to guide you in the appointment-scheduling process.

FILE FOLDERS

This packet contains 36 file folders that you will use when establishing patient medical records and general supplies files.

FILE LABELS

Contained within this packet are two sheets of file labels (30 preprinted labels, 30 blank labels) that you will use to prepare patient medical records and general supplies files. On the job you would print labels using the computer; however, these labels have been prepared for you.

TASK TOOLS

The tasks in this practice kit contain instructions and supplies for both a paper-based office management system and a software-based office management system. The kit can be completed using the paper-based system or in conjunction with the Medisoft software. **It is not recommended that you switch systems from one task to another because each task builds upon another.** For example, a task requires that you schedule Mr. Jones for a patient visit in the next available appointment period. You schedule this visit using the paper-based system. The next task may require that you schedule Mr. Smith for a patient visit. If for this task you choose to use the software to schedule the appointment, you may have scheduled both patients during the same time period because these systems cannot exchange this information.

Look for this symbol when you are to complete a task using paper supplies,

and this symbol when you may complete a task using a computer.

COMPANION EVOLVE SITE

The **companion** Evolve site contains a patient directory, base data for Medisoft (to create the South Padre office), audio files, and the actual forms necessary to complete the tasks. This Forms Library is also provided in Appendix 4 at the back of this text. Please note that not all of these forms are intended to be completed electronically. They are simply provided on the Evolve site for convenience.

The following forms are located in the Forms Library in Appendix 4 and on the Evolve site:

- Check No. 999
- CMS-1500 Health Insurance Claim
- Continuation
- Deposit Ticket
- History and Physical Examination, South Padre Medical Center
- Interoffice Memo, South Padre Medical Center
- Journal of Daily Charges and Payments
- Letterhead, South Padre Medical Center
- Telephone Quiz Answer Sheet
- Patient Information
- Petty Cash Journal
- Phone Record
- Referral
- Request for Inpatient Consultation
- Request for Preauthorization for Surgery
- Statement
- Subsequent Findings
- Superbill
- Surgical Request and Information
- Patient Health History
- Operative Report, South Padre Hospital

For the software to work correctly, you must change the date on your computer to April 7, 2008. You do this by double clicking the time display on the bar at the lower right of the computer screen. When you double click the time display, a dialog box opens that allows you to reset the date. Reset the month to "April," the day to "7," the year to "2008," and you can leave the time as displayed. Now, your computer will keep time from the initial date of April 7, 2008.

On some of the forms that are completed electronically, a second page. is sometimes necessary. In this instance, the second page will be automatically formatted, with the patient name (last name, first name, middle initial) in the upper left-hand corner.

To save a form that you have completed electronically, use the "Save As" feature on your computer and title the document with the task number and patient name, if applicable. Remember to save the document to a location on your computer that you can easily access in the future.

AUDIO FILES ON EVOLVE SITE

The **audio** portion of the Evolve site contains medical dictation files for transcription and telephone messages. You will be transcribing the information on the Evolve site as directed for specific tasks. These tasks will be identified by the icon appearing next to the task. At the beginning of each item on the recording, the task number will be announced. For example, "This is Day Four, Task 4.1." The end of the transcribed item will also be announced. For example, "This is the end of Day Four, Task 4.1."

The tasks that use the audio will require various forms. These forms are located in the Supplies section (p. 221) of the Student Manual, in the Forms Library in Appendix 4 (p. 197) or on the Evolve site at http://evolve.elsevier.com/Buck/

practicekit/. You will be instructed as to which form(s) to use and the location of the form(s) within the directions for each task.

The following tasks have information dictated onto the Evolve site:

TASK **1.3**	Scheduling Telephone Appointments and Inpatient Consultations
TASK **2.4**	Medical Transcription
TASK **3.2**	Medical Transcription
TASK **4.1**	Telephone Messages and Appointment Schedule
TASK **5.1**	Medical Transcription
TASK **6.3**	Telephone Messages
TASK **7.4**	Telephone Messages
TASK **8.3**	Telephone Messages
TASK **8.4**	Medical Transcription

The following task uses the Internet for a research assignment.

TASK **6.1** Internet Research

MEDISOFT CD

You may use the Medisoft software for scheduling appointments and completing insurance forms and various financial documentations. The **Software Instructions** section of this text contains software operating instructions, including data backup and restoration, which must be done before and immediately after completion of daily assignments.

The following tasks may be completed using the Medisoft software.

TASK **1.2**	Preparing the Schedules
TASK **1.3**	Scheduling Telephone Appointments and Inpatient Consultations
TASK **1.5**	Records Management and Patient List
TASK **2.1**	Patient List
TASK **2.2**	Patient Reception
TASK **2.3**	Scheduling Appointments
TASK **2.5**	Scheduling Emergency or Urgent Appointments
TASK **4.1**	Telephone Messages and Appointment Schedule
TASK **4.3**	Scheduling Appointments
TASK **5.3**	Billing and Banking Procedures
TASK **6.2**	Establishing a Meeting
TASK **6.4**	Scheduling Appointments
TASK **7.3**	Scheduling Nursing Home Services
TASK **7.5**	Scheduling Appointments
TASK **7.6**	Scheduling Surgeries
TASK **7.7**	Medical Records

PRACTICE PARTNER CD

The Practice Partner CD contains electronic health record management software. Days Nine and Ten are dedicated to tasks that guide you through an electronic health record system. Software installation instructions for Practice Partner can be found at the beginning of Day Nine.

Before You Begin

Read Appendix 1, Welcome (p. 161) now and then read Appendix 2, Policies and Procedures (p. 163), which explains the standard operating procedures of the Center. You will be following these Policies and Procedures during your internship. Be certain you complete all items requested in the directions in the Policies and Procedures information.

PRE-TASK **1.1**

Routine Maintenance

SUPPLIES NEEDED:

- 1 file folder (blank)
- 1 file folder label (blank)

You are expected to perform routine maintenance on all administrative equipment that you use while an intern at the Center. At the end of each day, you are to wipe the computer screen with a dry, soft cloth. Never use any type of cleaner on the computer screen because it will damage the screen surface. Use a soft brush to sweep the keyboard at the end of each day. Organize your work and place all papers into the desk drawer at the end of the day and during your breaks. Gladys, medical office assistant, will be your supervisor and will provide you with a key to your desk to be used to lock the desk at the end of the day and on your breaks. Always keep your area clear of patient information that could be seen by others. Clean the top of your desk at the end of each day using the spray cleaner located in the lower right-hand drawer of your desk.

We at the Center understand that each intern's training differs when it comes to use of the various office equipment. Gladys will provide a demonstration on the operation of all equipment you will be using during your internship. Should the equipment malfunction while you are using it, please contact Gladys for any help you require. You have begun your internship at a great time. The practice is just beginning to convert from a paper-based office management system to a computer-based office management system (Medisoft software). Although the paper-based system will be maintained during your internship, occasionally you will be asked to perform tasks that include use of the Medisoft software. You are to complete these tasks only when the Medisoft software is available for that specific task and if your instructor has directed you to use the software feature.

You will find a check-off form in the Supplies section (p. 221) of this Student Manual (labeled "Equipment Maintenance and Desk Security") that is dated for each day of your internship. Enter your name on the form. You are to use this form at the end of each day of your internship to check off that you have performed all necessary maintenance of your equipment and that you have secured your desk. At the end of your internship, you are to turn this form in to Gladys during your internship checkout meeting.

Locate a blank file folder and blank file folder label from your packet. Write "GENERAL" on the file folder label in capital letters and place the label on the file folder. Place the Equipment Maintenance and Desk Security form into the file folder.

Your Internship Tasks

You have completed your review of Appendices 1 (p. 161) and 2 (p. 163) that is required of all new interns and employees. You have completed your "Equipment Maintenance and Desk Security" form (p. 223) and are now ready to begin your work duties. All directions and materials necessary to complete the jobs are included either in the packet, this Student Manual, the Evolve site, or the Medisoft CD. **It is important to complete all tasks in the order presented.**

NOTE: A copy of the CAAHEP (Commission on Accreditation of Allied Health Education Programs) Standards and Guidelines can be obtained at http://www.caahep.org/documents/file/For-Program-Directors/MA2008Standards0209.pdf.

Medisoft Software Instructions

This section will provide you with the information you need to install Medisoft and back up your data. It will also guide you through the process of scheduling patient visits, entering patient demographics, and payment entry, as well as other functions of Medisoft you will need to know to work through this manual.

Part One: Installation and Setup

You will be installing Medisoft on the hard drive of the computer. Once the software is installed, the Medisoft CD will not need to be used. To install Medisoft Advanced Version 16, complete the following instructions:

1. Close all programs that are currently running on your computer.
2. Insert the Medisoft Advanced Version 16 CD in the CD-ROM disc drive. If installation does not start automatically, use the following steps.
3. Click on *Start* button on the lower left corner of your computer screen.
4. When the menu pops up, click on *Run*.
5. Type "D:\AUTORUN.EXE" (where D: = letter of CD/DVD drive) into the *Open:* box and select *OK* as shown in **Figure SI 1-1**.

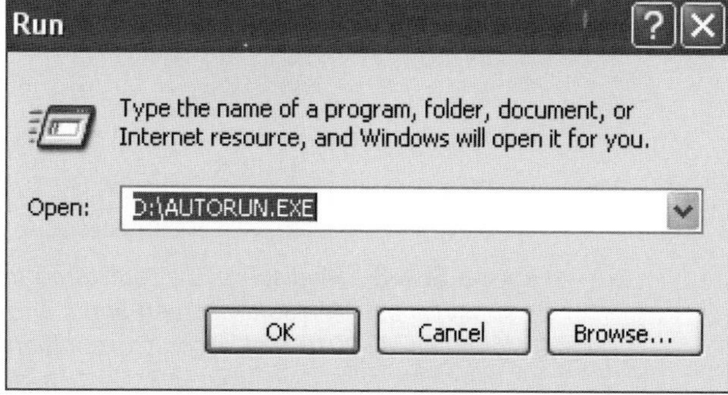

Figure **SI 1-1** *Medisoft® is a registered trademark of McKesson Corporation and/or one of its subsidiaries. Medisoft® screen shots and materials used with the permission of McKesson Corporation. © 2010 McKesson Corporation. All rights reserved.*

6. The IntroDisc window will appear **(Figure SI 1-2)**. Click *Install Medisoft*. The CD should begin installing the demonstration version of the software.

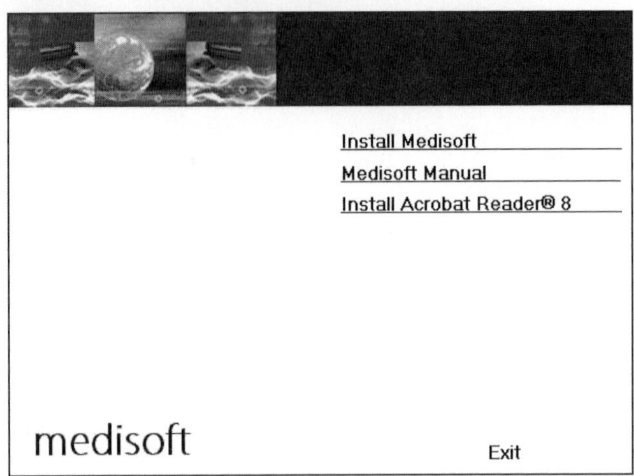

Figure **SI 1-2** *Medisoft® is a registered trademark of McKesson Corporation and/or one of its subsidiaries. Medisoft® screen shots and materials used with the permission of McKesson Corporation. © 2010 McKesson Corporation. All rights reserved.*

7. A Welcome window will appear **(Figure SI 1-3)**. Make sure you have closed all other programs and applications and click *Next*.

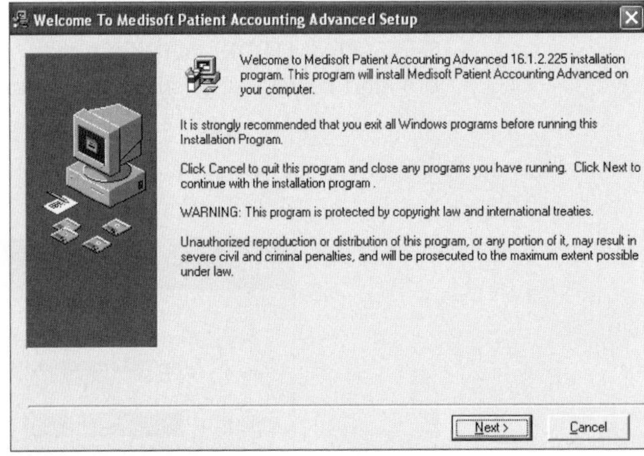

Figure **SI 1-3** *Medisoft® is a registered trademark of McKesson Corporation and/or one of its subsidiaries. Medisoft® screen shots and materials used with the permission of McKesson Corporation. © 2010 McKesson Corporation. All rights reserved.*

8. At the *End User License Agreement* window shown in **Figure SI 1-4**, click *I accept the agreement* and then click *Next*.

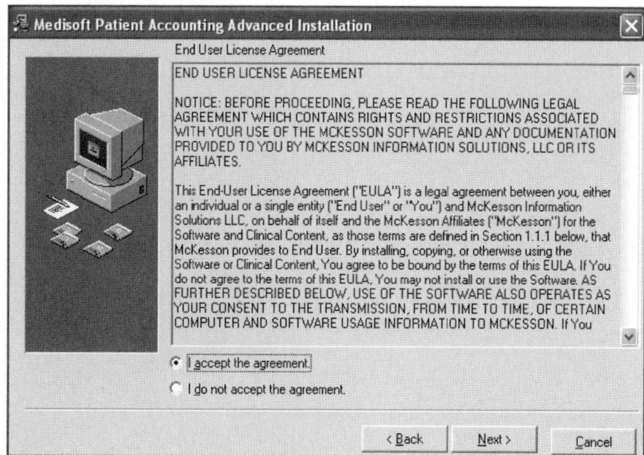

Figure **SI 1-4** *Medisoft® is a registered trademark of McKesson Corporation and/or one of its subsidiaries. Medisoft® screen shots and materials used with the permission of McKesson Corporation. © 2010 McKesson Corporation. All rights reserved.*

9. At the *Subscription Agreement* window **(Figure SI 1-5)**, click *I accept the agreement* and then click *Next*.

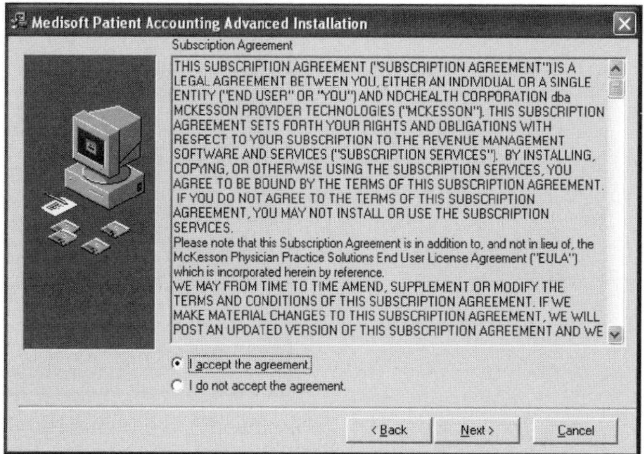

Figure **SI 1-5** *Medisoft® is a registered trademark of McKesson Corporation and/or one of its subsidiaries. Medisoft® screen shots and materials used with the permission of McKesson Corporation. © 2010 McKesson Corporation. All rights reserved.*

MEDISOFT SOFTWARE INSTRUCTIONS

10. At the *Select Destination Directory* window **(Figure SI-6)**, click *Next* to install Medisoft to the directory listed (C:\ProgramFiles\Medisoft DEMO). To select a different destination, use the *Browse* button to locate the desired directory for installation, then click *Next*.

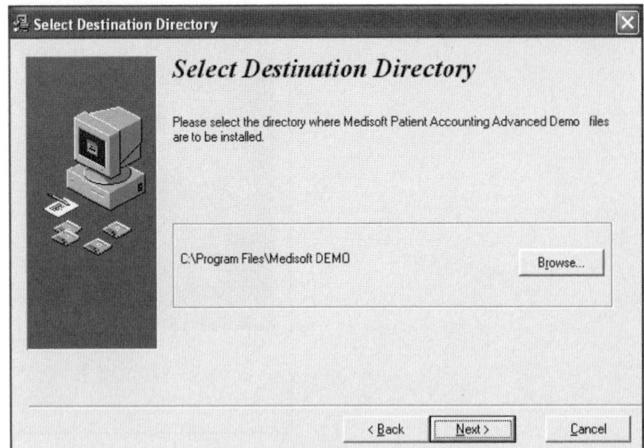

Figure **SI 1-6** *Medisoft® is a registered trademark of McKesson Corporation and/or one of its subsidiaries. Medisoft® screen shots and materials used with the permission of McKesson Corporation. © 2010 McKesson Corporation. All rights reserved.*

11. At the *Ready to Install!* window **(Figure SI 1-7)**, click *Next*. The program will now be written to the hard drive of the computer.

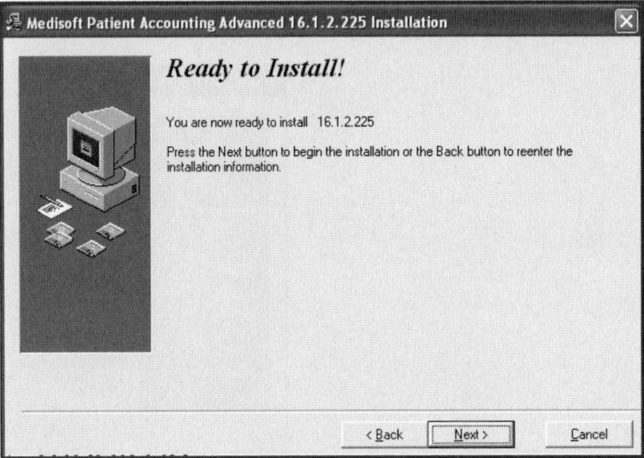

Figure **SI 1-7** *Medisoft® is a registered trademark of McKesson Corporation and/or one of its subsidiaries. Medisoft® screen shots and materials used with the permission of McKesson Corporation. © 2010 McKesson Corporation. All rights reserved.*

12. The *Installing* window appears and tracks the progress of the installation.

13. At the *Installation Completed!* window shown in **Figure SI 1-8**, uncheck the box marked *Launch Medisoft Patient Accounting Demo* and click *Finish.*

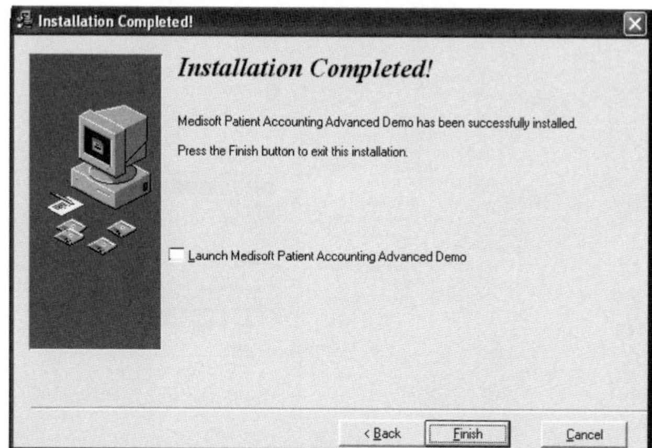

Figure **SI 1-8** *Medisoft® is a registered trademark of McKesson Corporation and/or one of its subsidiaries. Medisoft® screen shots and materials used with the permission of McKesson Corporation. © 2010 McKesson Corporation. All rights reserved.*

You are now finished with the Medisoft CD. Remove it from your CD-ROM drive and prepare to complete the next steps to install the data needed for the class.

Part Two: Adding the South Padre Medical Center Data to the Medisoft Program

1. Log into the companion Evolve site (http://evolve.elsevier.com/Buck/practicekit/).

2. Click on *Course Documents*, then on *Resources*, and then click on the *Base Data* link.

3. Right click on the *Base Data* file and select *Save Target As*, as illustrated in **Figure SI 2-1**.

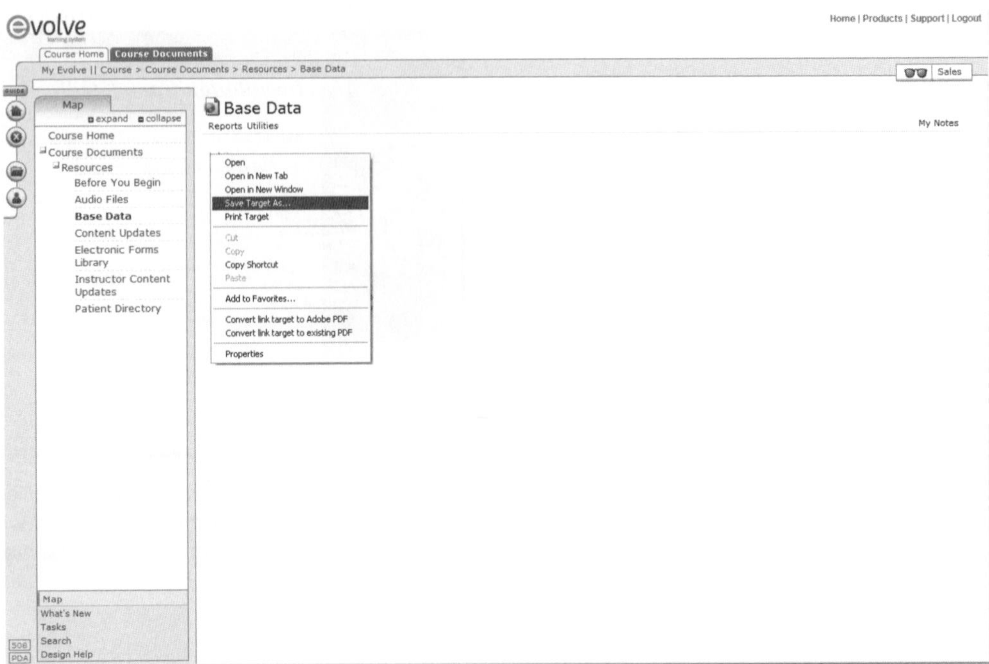

Figure **SI 2-1** *Medisoft® is a registered trademark of McKesson Corporation and/or one of its subsidiaries. Medisoft® screen shots and materials used with the permission of McKesson Corporation. © 2010 McKesson Corporation. All rights reserved.*

4. When the *Save As* window opens, click *My Computer* and search for the (C:) drive **(Figure SI 2-2)**.

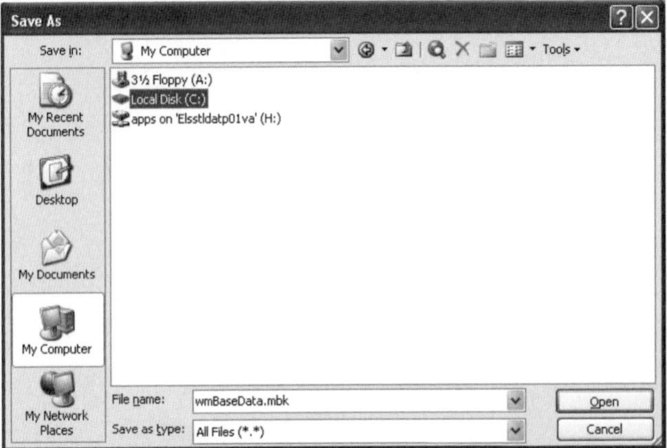

Figure **SI 2-2** *Medisoft® is a registered trademark of McKesson Corporation and/or one of its subsidiaries. Medisoft® screen shots and materials used with the permission of McKesson Corporation. © 2010 McKesson Corporation. All rights reserved.*

5. Double click the (C:) drive and search for the *MediData* folder as demonstrated in **Figure SI 2-3**.

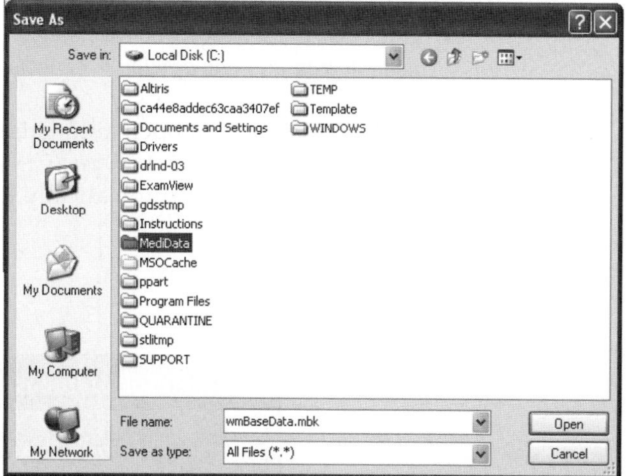

Figure **SI 2-3** *Medisoft® is a registered trademark of McKesson Corporation and/or one of its subsidiaries. Medisoft® screen shots and materials used with the permission of McKesson Corporation. © 2010 McKesson Corporation. All rights reserved.*

6. Double click the *MediData* folder and choose *Save*.

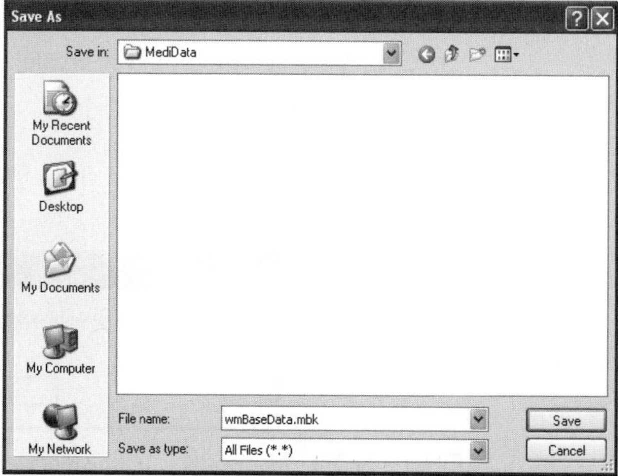

Figure **SI 2-4** *Medisoft® is a registered trademark of McKesson Corporation and/or one of its subsidiaries. Medisoft® screen shots and materials used with the permission of McKesson Corporation. © 2010 McKesson Corporation. All rights reserved.*

7. The *wmBaseData.mbk* file is now loaded into the *MediData* folder.

Part Three: Starting Medisoft Once Installed

After installation of the software, perform the following to begin working in the practice:

1. Click *Start>All Programs>Medisoft>Medisoft Advanced Demo. Also note that there is now an icon on your desktop for Medisoft that can be used.*

2. If Medisoft does not open automatically, the *Find Medisoft Database* window will open as in **Figure SI 3-1**. Type "C:\Medidata" in the window. Click *OK*. (Medisoft may open automatically for some users; if so, proceed to Step 4.)

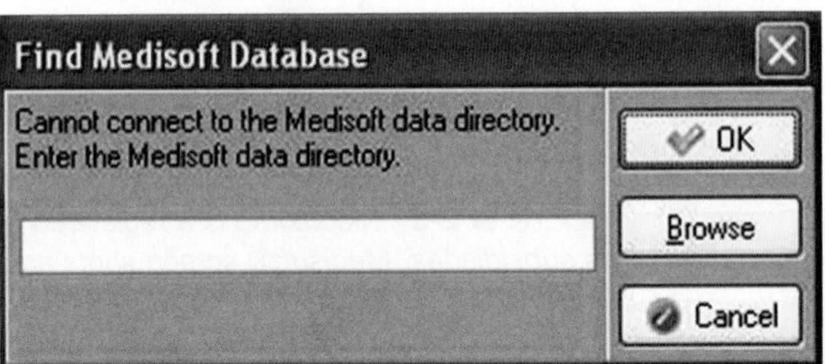

Figure **SI 3-1** *Medisoft® is a registered trademark of McKesson Corporation and/or one of its subsidiaries. Medisoft® screen shots and materials used with the permission of McKesson Corporation. © 2010 McKesson Corporation. All rights reserved.*

3. Click *Yes* when prompted to create a new directory **(Figure SI 3-2)**.

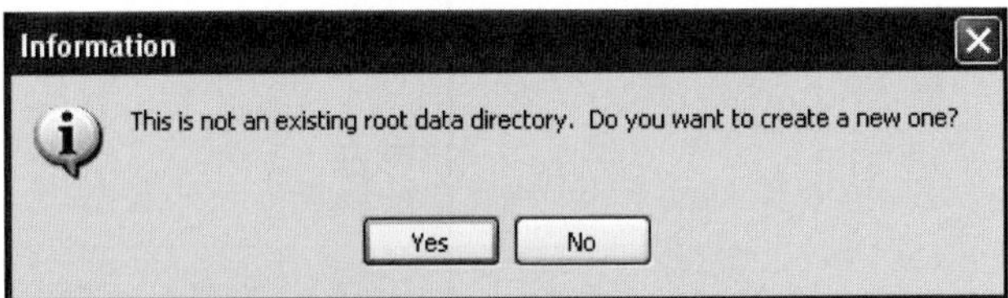

Figure **SI 3-2** *Medisoft® is a registered trademark of McKesson Corporation and/or one of its subsidiaries. Medisoft® screen shots and materials used with the permission of McKesson Corporation. © 2010 McKesson Corporation. All rights reserved.*

4. The main Medisoft window will open. Click *File>Open Practice* as displayed in **Figure SI 3-3**.

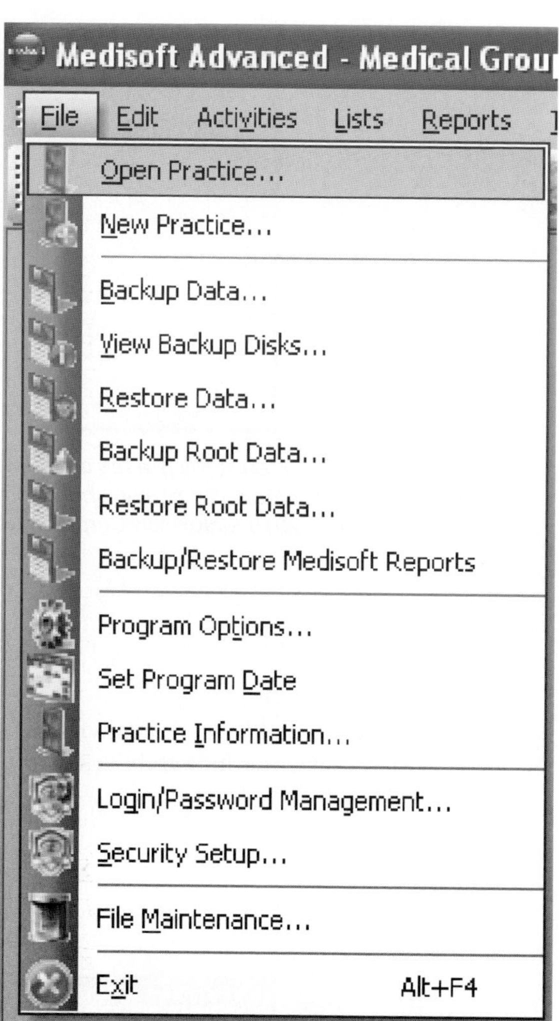

Figure **SI 3-3** *Medisoft® is a registered trademark of McKesson Corporation and/or one of its subsidiaries. Medisoft® screen shots and materials used with the permission of McKesson Corporation. © 2010 McKesson Corporation. All rights reserved.*

MEDISOFT SOFTWARE INSTRUCTIONS

5. The *Open Practice* window will pop up as shown in **Figure SI 3-4**. Click *New*.

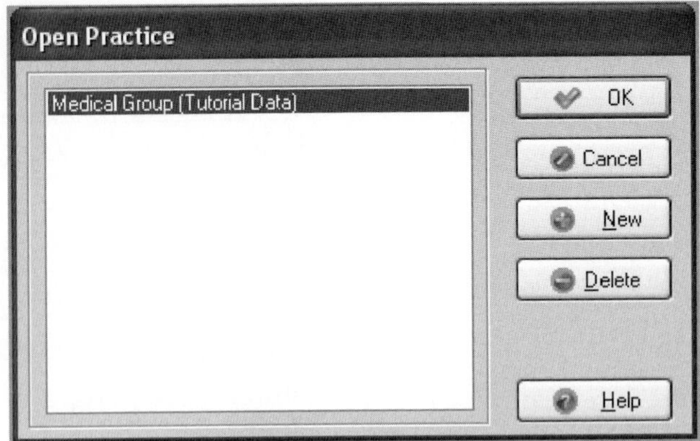

Figure **SI 3-4** *Medisoft® is a registered trademark of McKesson Corporation and/or one of its subsidiaries. Medisoft® screen shots and materials used with the permission of McKesson Corporation. © 2010 McKesson Corporation. All rights reserved.*

6. The *Create a new set of data* window will open. Type "SPMC" for South Padre Medical Center in both boxes as shown in **Figure SI 3-5**. Then click *Create*.

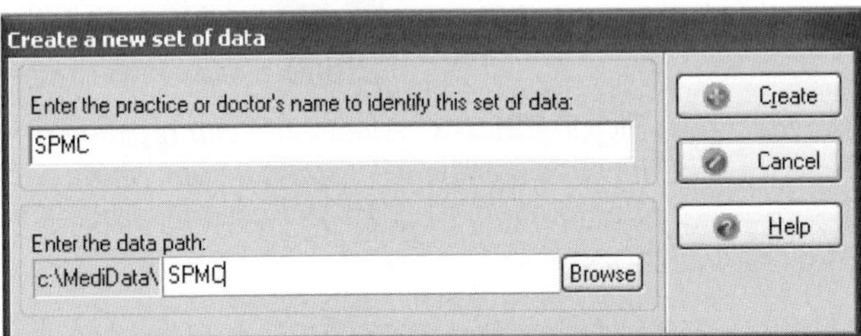

Figure **SI 3-5** *Medisoft® is a registered trademark of McKesson Corporation and/or one of its subsidiaries. Medisoft® screen shots and materials used with the permission of McKesson Corporation. © 2010 McKesson Corporation. All rights reserved.*

7. A *Confirm* window will appear **(Figure SI 3-6)**. Click *Yes*. Medisoft will now create the data for South Padre Medical Center.

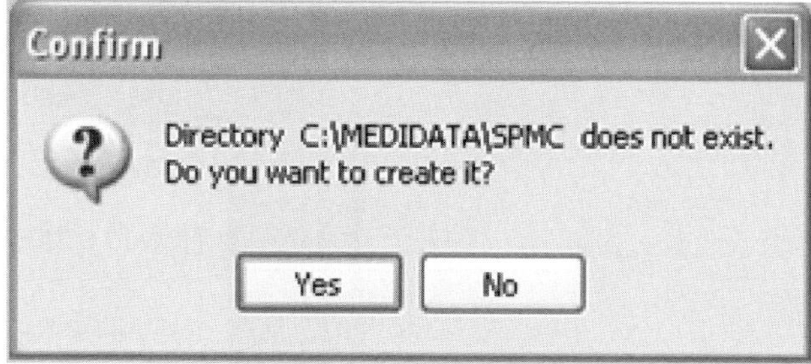
Confirm
Directory C:\MEDIDATA\SPMC does not exist.
Do you want to create it?
Yes
No

Figure **SI 3-6** *Medisoft® is a registered trademark of McKesson Corporation and/or one of its subsidiaries. Medisoft® screen shots and materials used with the permission of McKesson Corporation. © 2010 McKesson Corporation. All rights reserved.*

8. The *Practice Information* window will open as shown in **Figure SI 3-7**. Enter SPMC as the Practice Name and click the *Save* button.

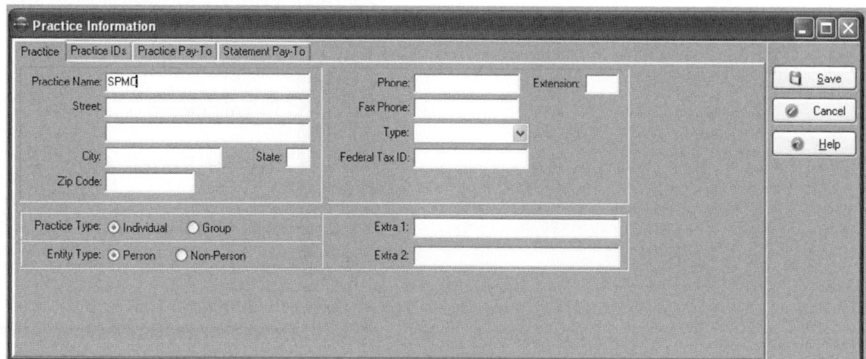

Figure **SI 3-7** *Medisoft® is a registered trademark of McKesson Corporation and/or one of its subsidiaries. Medisoft® screen shots and materials used with the permission of McKesson Corporation. © 2010 McKesson Corporation. All rights reserved.*

9. In order to fully execute the South Padre Medical Center data, you must create a new restore point. Once in the program click *File>Restore Data* as demonstrated in **Figure SI 3-8**.

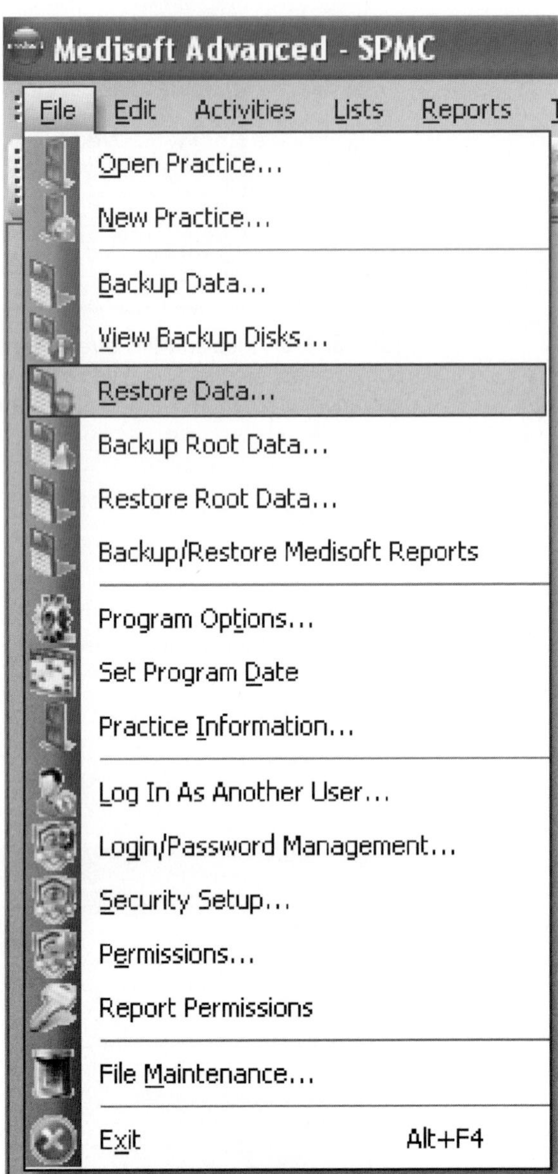

Figure **SI 3-8** *Medisoft® is a registered trademark of McKesson Corporation and/or one of its subsidiaries. Medisoft® screen shots and materials used with the permission of McKesson Corporation. © 2010 McKesson Corporation. All rights reserved.*

10. Click *OK* in the *Warning* window **(Figure SI 3-9)**.

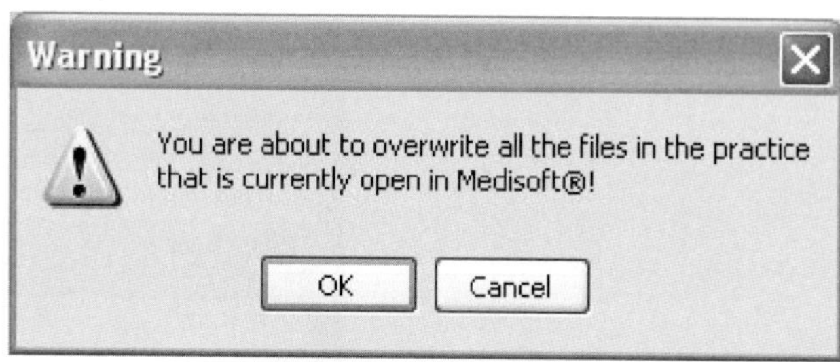

Figure **SI 3-9** *Medisoft® is a registered trademark of McKesson Corporation and/or one of its subsidiaries. Medisoft® screen shots and materials used with the permission of McKesson Corporation. © 2010 McKesson Corporation. All rights reserved.*

11. Using **Figure SI 3-10** as a reference, complete Step 11. In the *Restore* window, under *Backup File Path and Name*, delete the current entry and enter "C:\MediData." The *Existing Backup Files* window will populate with the *wmBaseData.mbk* file. Click on the *wmBaseData.mbk* file to complete the *Backup File Path and Name* field.

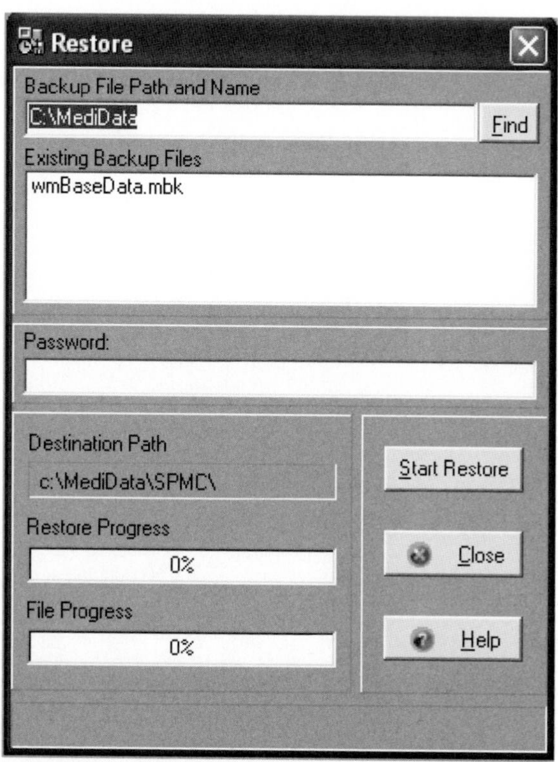

Figure **SI 3-10** *Medisoft® is a registered trademark of McKesson Corporation and/or one of its subsidiaries. Medisoft® screen shots and materials used with the permission of McKesson Corporation. © 2010 McKesson Corporation. All rights reserved.*

MEDISOFT SOFTWARE INSTRUCTIONS

12. Next, click the *Start Restore* button located in the *Restore* window shown in **Figure SI 3-10**. Click *OK* in the confirm window shown in **Figure SI 3-11**.

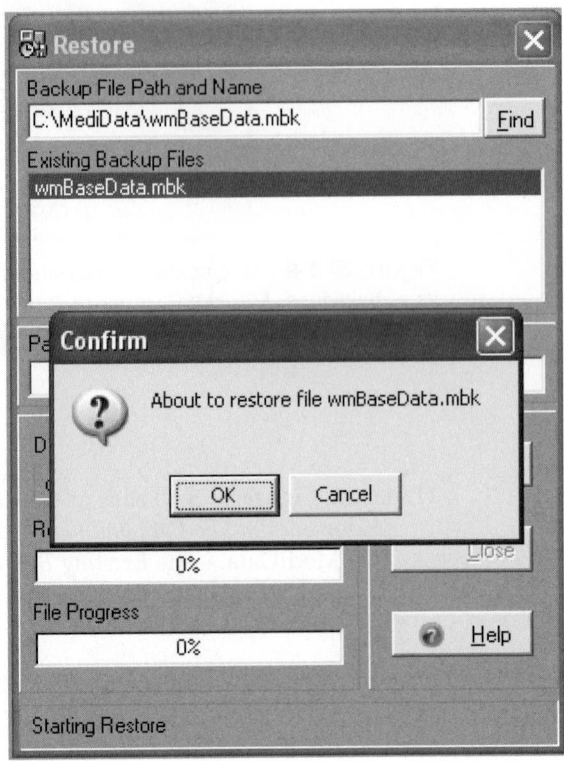

Figure **SI 3-11** *Medisoft® is a registered trademark of McKesson Corporation and/or one of its subsidiaries. Medisoft® screen shots and materials used with the permission of McKesson Corporation. © 2010 McKesson Corporation. All rights reserved.*

13. Once the restoration is complete **(Figure SI 3-12)**, click *OK* in the *Information* window. Click *Close*. Wait a few seconds for the *Log In* screen to open.

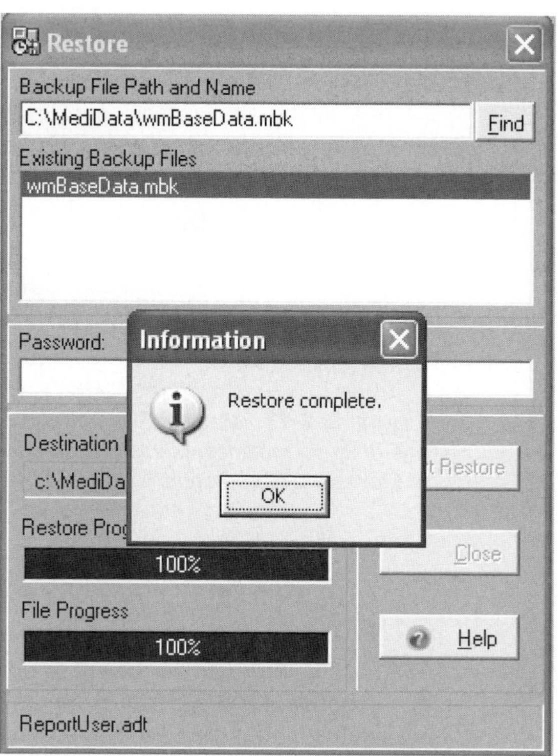

Figure **SI 3-12** *Medisoft® is a registered trademark of McKesson Corporation and/or one of its subsidiaries. Medisoft® screen shots and materials used with the permission of McKesson Corporation. © 2010 McKesson Corporation. All rights reserved.*

MEDISOFT SOFTWARE INSTRUCTIONS

14. You have now added the appropriate providers and patients to the Medisoft program. You will need to sign into the Medisoft program again before beginning the first task of creating a Login Name and Password as illustrated in **Figure SI 3-13**.

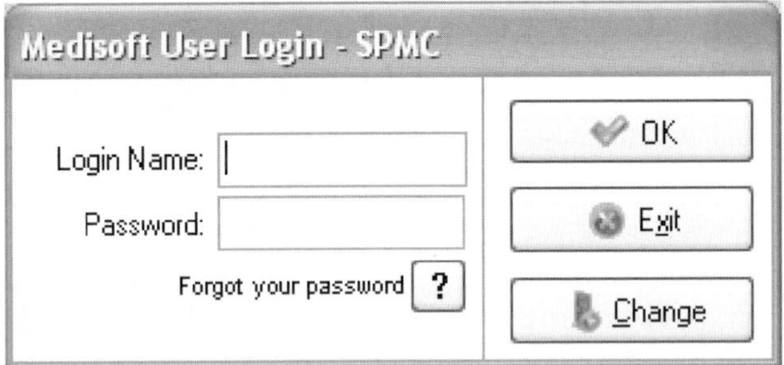

Figure **SI 3-13** *Medisoft® is a registered trademark of McKesson Corporation and/or one of its subsidiaries. Medisoft® screen shots and materials used with the permission of McKesson Corporation. © 2010 McKesson Corporation. All rights reserved.*

15. For this time only, you will log on as Jennifer White, as you will be adding yourself to the Security Setup Users list. Refer to **Figure SI 3-14**. In the Login Name field, enter *JW*. The password is *1*. Click *OK*. You should now be at the *Medisoft Patient Accounting* main screen.

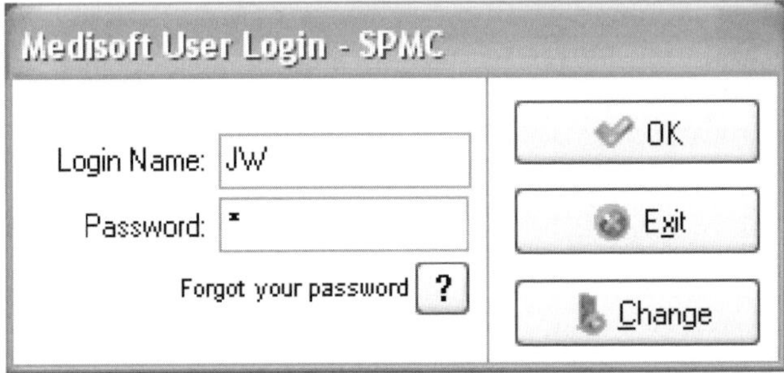

Figure **SI 3-14** *Medisoft® is a registered trademark of McKesson Corporation and/or one of its subsidiaries. Medisoft® screen shots and materials used with the permission of McKesson Corporation. © 2010 McKesson Corporation. All rights reserved.*

16. From the tool bar located at the top of the screen, select *File*. On the drop down menu, click on *Security Setup* **(Figure SI 3-15)**.

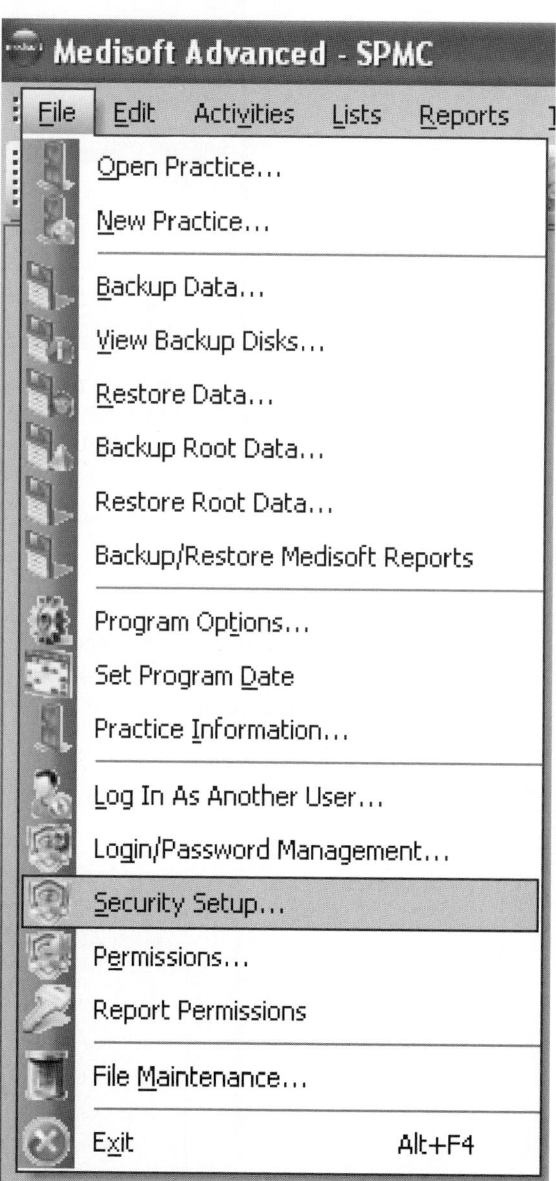

Figure **SI 3-15** *Medisoft® is a registered trademark of McKesson Corporation and/or one of its subsidiaries. Medisoft® screen shots and materials used with the permission of McKesson Corporation. © 2010 McKesson Corporation. All rights reserved.*

MEDISOFT SOFTWARE INSTRUCTIONS

17. In the *Security Setup* window shown in **Figure SI 3-16**, click the *New* button.

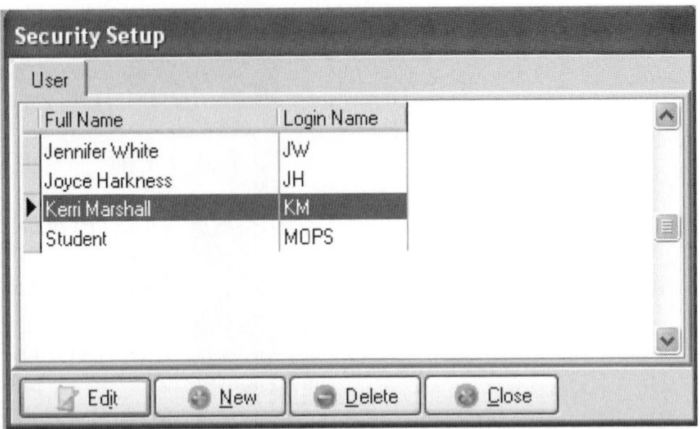

Figure **SI 3-16** *Medisoft® is a registered trademark of McKesson Corporation and/or one of its subsidiaries. Medisoft® screen shots and materials used with the permission of McKesson Corporation. © 2010 McKesson Corporation. All rights reserved.*

18. In the *User Entry* window *Main* tab, enter your first and last initial in the *Login Name* field as demonstrated in **Figure SI 3-17**. Complete the *Full Name* field. Enter a password and reconfirm it. Do not complete the remaining fields or tabs. Click the *Save* button. Use the Tab key to move between fields.

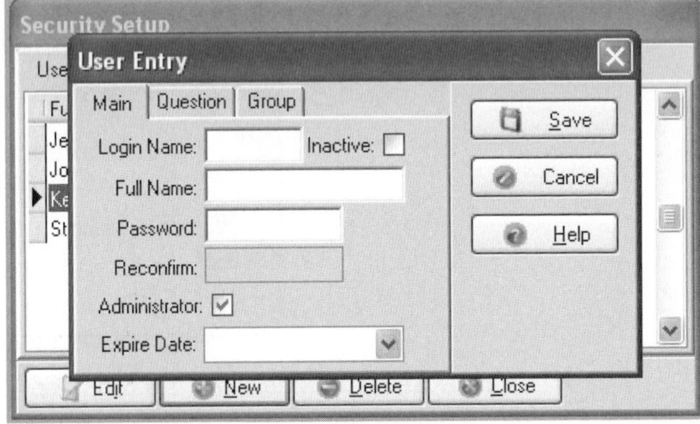

Figure **SI 3-17** *Medisoft® is a registered trademark of McKesson Corporation and/or one of its subsidiaries. Medisoft® screen shots and materials used with the permission of McKesson Corporation. © 2010 McKesson Corporation. All rights reserved.*

19. You should now be returned to the *Security Setup* window **(Figure SI 3-18)**. Verify that you have been added to the *Security Setup Users* list and click the *Close* button located at the bottom of the window. Click *OK* in the *Information* window. A window will appear informing you that you will need to relog on in order for changes to take effect.

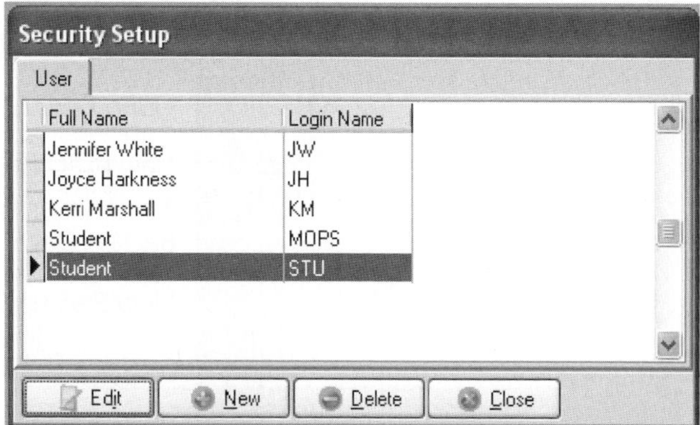

Figure **SI 3-18** *Medisoft® is a registered trademark of McKesson Corporation and/or one of its subsidiaries. Medisoft® screen shots and materials used with the permission of McKesson Corporation. © 2010 McKesson Corporation. All rights reserved.*

MEDISOFT SOFTWARE INSTRUCTIONS

20. You are now at the main screen. Referring to **Figure SI 3-19**, select *File* from the tool bar. From the drop down menu, select *Log In As Another User*. Log in again using your *Login Name* (initials) and *Password*. You need to use this login each time you log on to the Medisoft program.

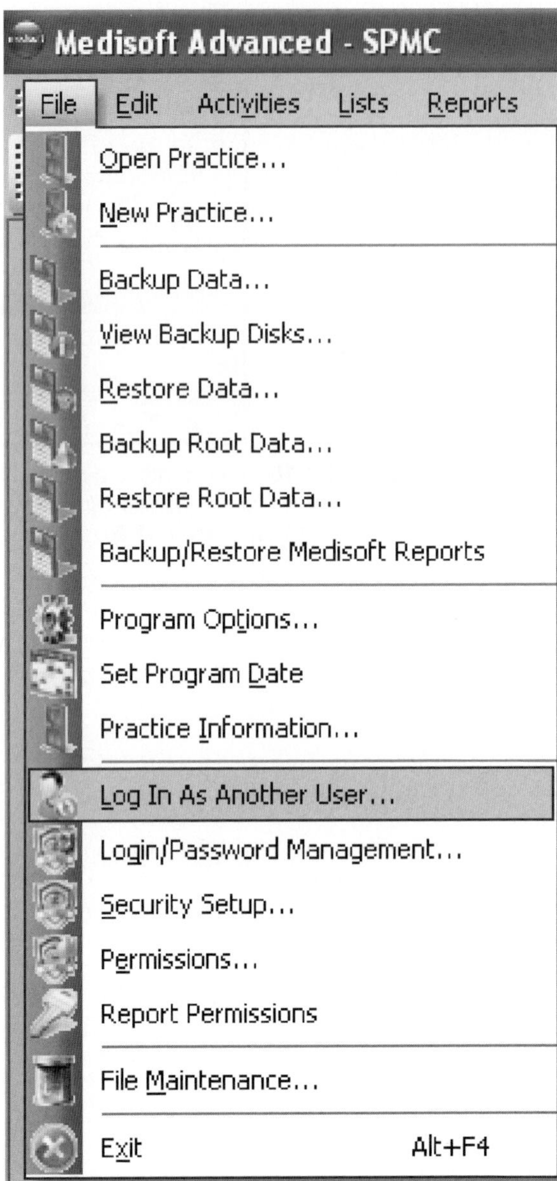

Figure **SI 3-19** *Medisoft® is a registered trademark of McKesson Corporation and/or one of its subsidiaries. Medisoft® screen shots and materials used with the permission of McKesson Corporation. © 2010 McKesson Corporation. All rights reserved.*

21. Now that you have created a Login Name and Password you may proceed to the Data Backup instructions. It is important that you follow these instructions, as they will tell you how to backup the data you create in the Medisoft program. You are now ready to begin using Medisoft!

Part Four: Data Backup

Begin by creating your backup file. While in the Medisoft software main menu screen, click the X located in the top right corner of the screen. In the *Backup Reminder* window **(Figure SI 4-1)** click the *Backup Data Now* button located at the bottom of this window. In the next window, *Backup Warning*, click the *OK* button located in this window **(Figure SI 4-2)**. Now you will create your individual backup file in the backup window **(Figure SI 4-3)**. You will need to know the drive (i.e., A:, C:, D:, or E:) where your storage device is located to begin this step. If you do not have this information you will need to get it now. Do not back up your data to the SPMC folder within the Medidata folder on the C: drive. In the *Destination File Path and Name* window, enter the location of where the backup data is to be stored followed by a back slash and your initials. For example, D:\STU, and click the *Start Backup* button located in the *Backup* window. Write down your backup file path, name, and date saved as you will need this to restore your data later. Once the backup is complete, the Medisoft software program will close. You will need to back up your data after completing your assignments each day before exiting the Medisoft software. Likewise, you will need to restore this data to the Medisoft software before beginning each day's tasks. The steps to restore your data are listed in Part Five: Data Restoration.

MEDISOFT SOFTWARE INSTRUCTIONS

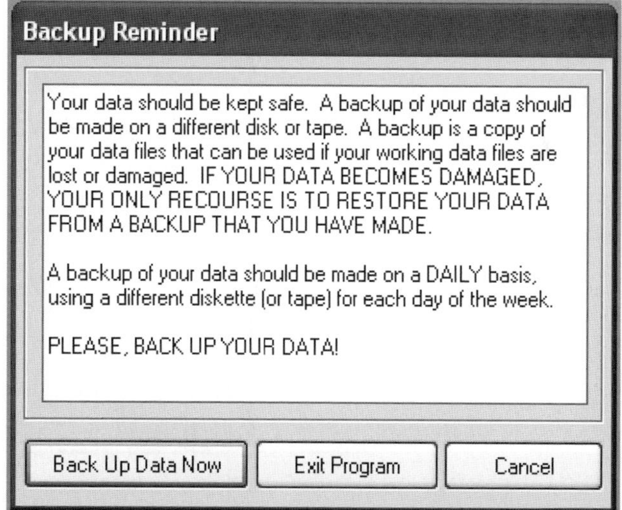

Backup Reminder
Your data should be kept safe. A backup of your data should be made on a different disk or tape. A backup is a copy of your data files that can be used if your working data files are lost or damaged. IF YOUR DATA BECOMES DAMAGED, YOUR ONLY RECOURSE IS TO RESTORE YOUR DATA FROM A BACKUP THAT YOU HAVE MADE.
A backup of your data should be made on a DAILY basis, using a different diskette (or tape) for each day of the week.
PLEASE, BACK UP YOUR DATA!
Back Up Data Now
Exit Program
Cancel

Figure **SI 4-1** *Medisoft® is a registered trademark of McKesson Corporation and/or one of its subsidiaries. Medisoft® screen shots and materials used with the permission of McKesson Corporation. © 2010 McKesson Corporation. All rights reserved.*

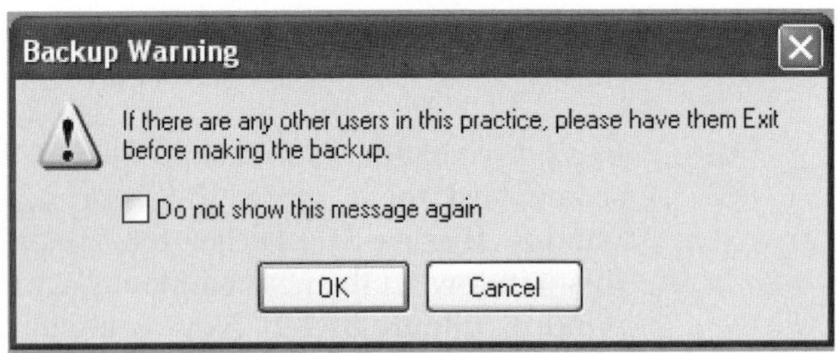
Backup Warning
If there are any other users in this practice, please have them Exit before making the backup.
Do not show this message again
OK
Cancel

Figure **SI 4-2** *Medisoft® is a registered trademark of McKesson Corporation and/or one of its subsidiaries. Medisoft® screen shots and materials used with the permission of McKesson Corporation. © 2010 McKesson Corporation. All rights reserved.*

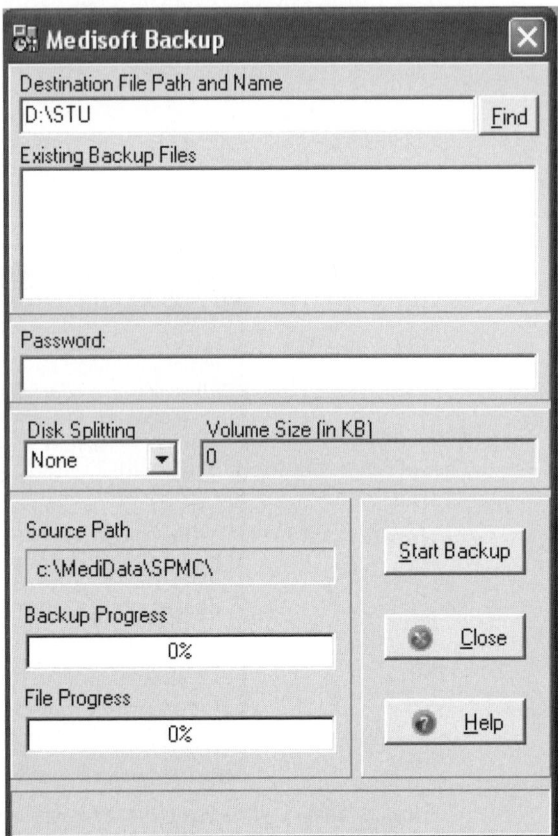

Figure **SI 4-3** *Medisoft® is a registered trademark of McKesson Corporation and/or one of its subsidiaries. Medisoft® screen shots and materials used with the permission of McKesson Corporation. © 2010 McKesson Corporation. All rights reserved.*

Part Five: Data Restoration

In the Medisoft software main menu screen toolbar, select *File*. Next, select *Restore Data* from the drop down menu **(Figure SI 5-1)**. Click *OK* in both *Warning* windows. In the *Restore* window *Backup File Path and Name*, enter your backup file's path and name (i.e., D:\STU) followed by .mbk. The .mbk was attached to your backup file by the software on completion of your first backup. You will need to attach it to your backup file path and name each time you restore your data **(Figure SI 5-2)**. Next, click the desired file from the *Existing Backup Files* and click the *Start Restore* button located in the *Restore* window. Click *OK* in the *Confirm* window. Once the restoration is complete, click *OK* in the *Information* window. You are now ready to begin your daily assignments.

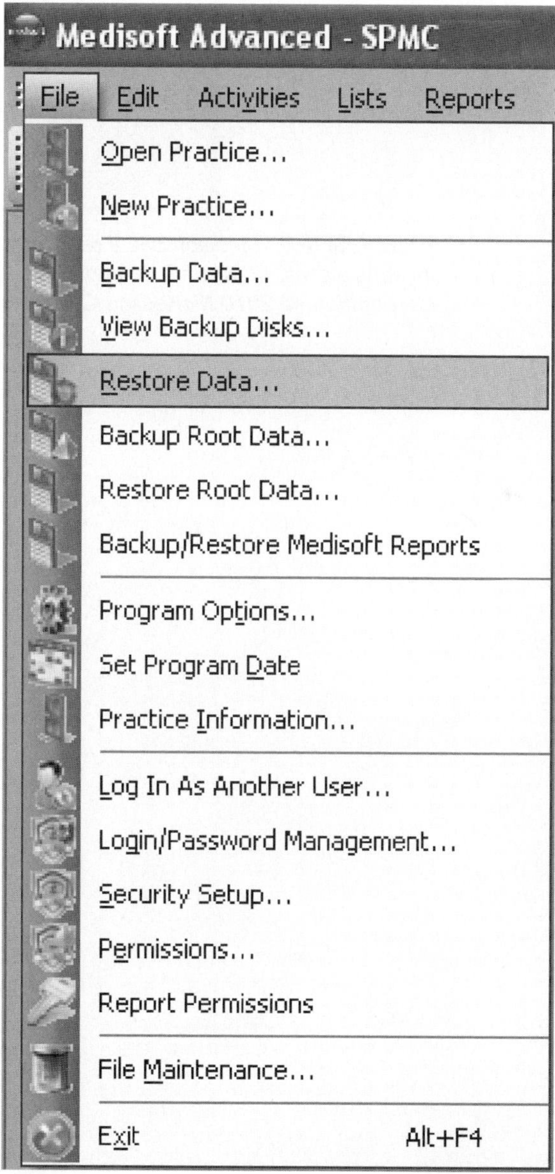

Figure **SI 5-1** *Medisoft® is a registered trademark of McKesson Corporation and/or one of its subsidiaries. Medisoft® screen shots and materials used with the permission of McKesson Corporation. © 2010 McKesson Corporation. All rights reserved.*

MEDISOFT SOFTWARE INSTRUCTIONS

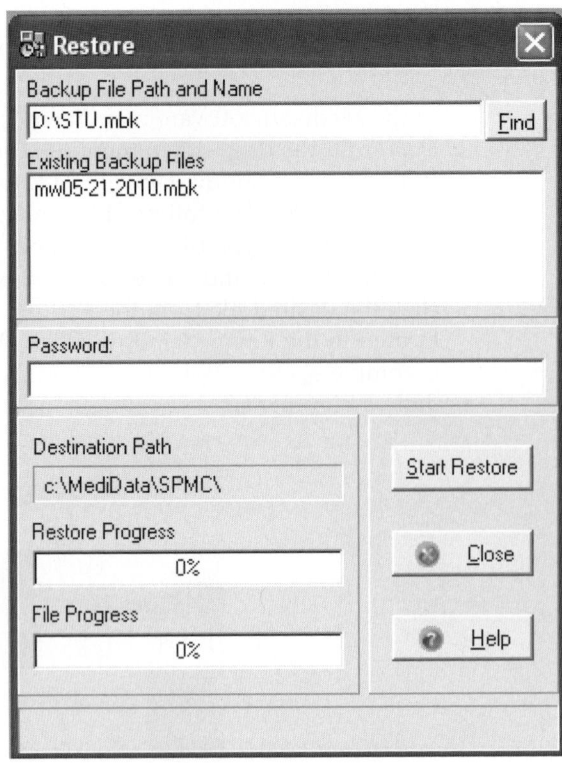

Figure **SI 5-2** *Medisoft® is a registered trademark of McKesson Corporation and/or one of its subsidiaries. Medisoft® screen shots and materials used with the permission of McKesson Corporation. © 2010 McKesson Corporation. All rights reserved.*

Part Six: Scheduling, Patient Entry and Demographics, and Accounting Procedures

From the Main Menu, click on the *Activities* button located on the toolbar at the top of the screen. From the drop down menu, choose *Appointment Book* **(Figure SI 6-1)**. The Appointment Book can also be opened by clicking on the *Appointment Book* (sixth) icon on the icon toolbar **(Figure SI 6-2)**. This will open the *Office Hours* appointment scheduling program **(Figure SI 6-3)**.

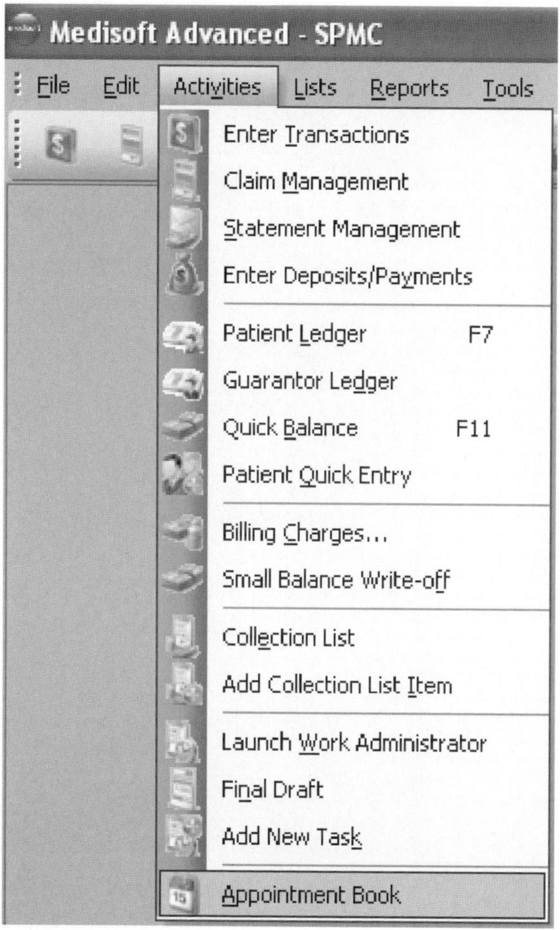

Figure **SI 6-1** *Medisoft® is a registered trademark of McKesson Corporation and/or one of its subsidiaries. Medisoft® screen shots and materials used with the permission of McKesson Corporation. © 2010 McKesson Corporation. All rights reserved.*

MEDISOFT SOFTWARE INSTRUCTIONS

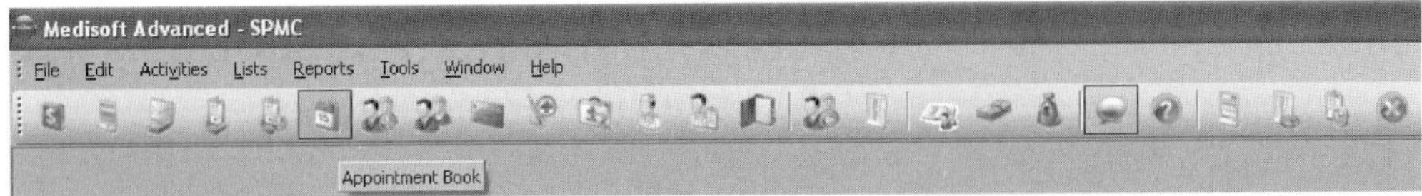

Figure **SI 6-2** *Medisoft® is a registered trademark of McKesson Corporation and/or one of its subsidiaries. Medisoft® screen shots and materials used with the permission of McKesson Corporation. © 2010 McKesson Corporation. All rights reserved.*

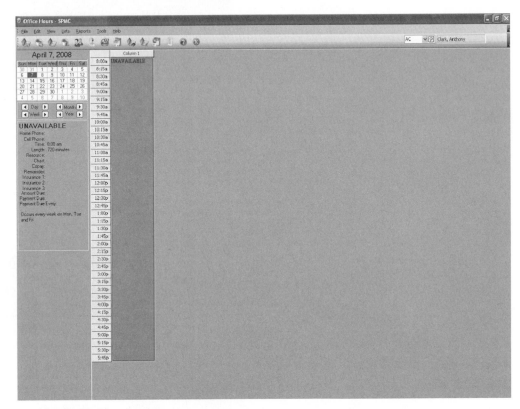

Figure **SI 6-3** *Medisoft® is a registered trademark of McKesson Corporation and/or one of its subsidiaries. Medisoft® screen shots and materials used with the permission of McKesson Corporation. © 2010 McKesson Corporation. All rights reserved.*

To select the physician whose schedule you wish to view/edit, click on the *Search* button (magnifying glass, circled in figure below) beside the information field located on the icon toolbar **(Figure SI 6-4)**.

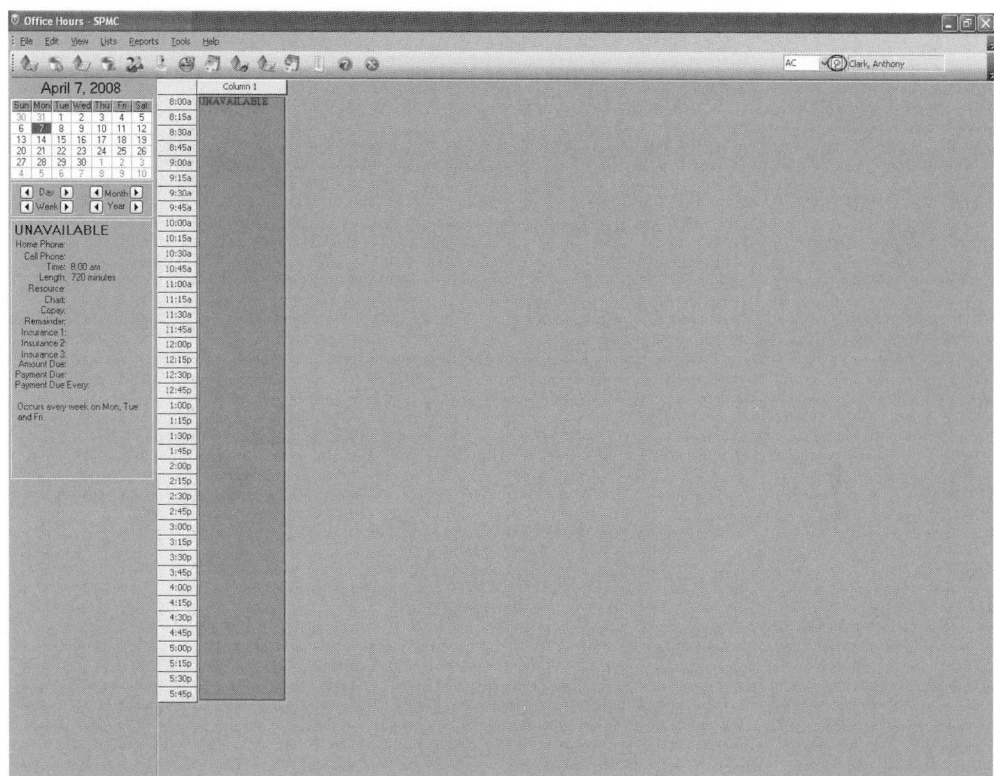

Figure **SI 6-4** *Medisoft® is a registered trademark of McKesson Corporation and/or one of its subsidiaries. Medisoft® screen shots and materials used with the permission of McKesson Corporation. © 2010 McKesson Corporation. All rights reserved.*

From the *Provider Search* window, click on the name of the physician whose schedule you wish to view/edit **(Figure SI 6-5)**. Click the *OK* button located at the bottom of the *Provider Search* window. To change the date of the schedule shown, click on the date in the calendar located to the left of the appointment schedule. Click on the forward or back scroll arrows beside the *Day*, *Week*, *Month*, and *Year* choices located below the calendar to change the calendar to the month needed for scheduling/viewing.

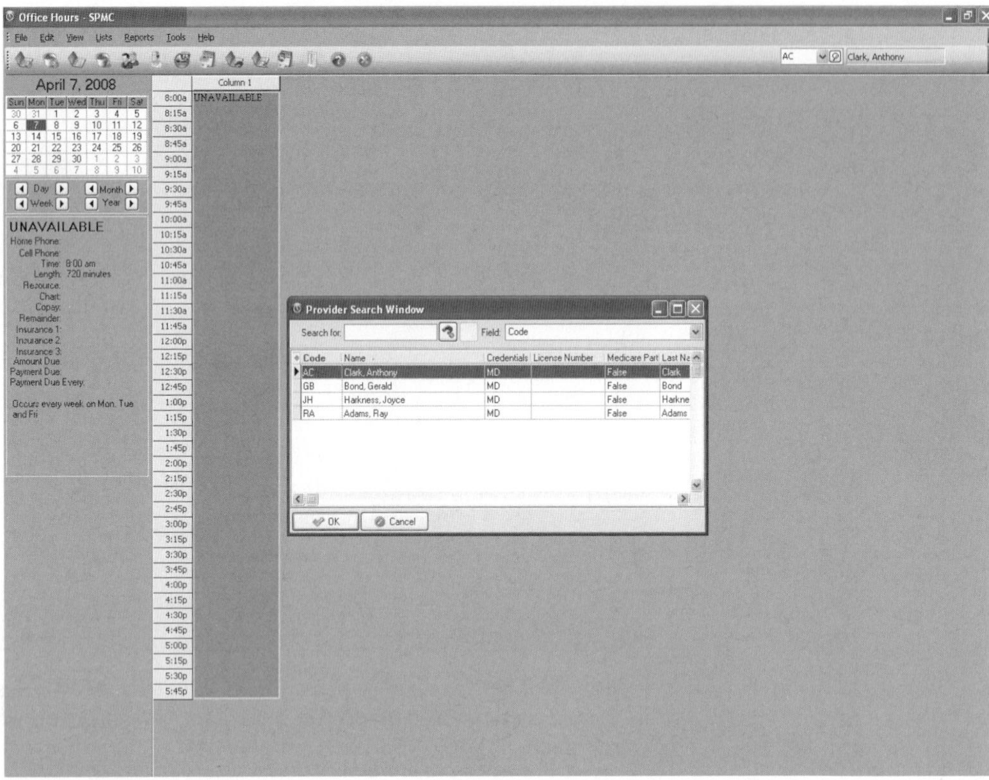

Figure **SI 6-5** *Medisoft® is a registered trademark of McKesson Corporation and/or one of its subsidiaries. Medisoft® screen shots and materials used with the permission of McKesson Corporation. © 2010 McKesson Corporation. All rights reserved.*

A. Matrixing the Calendar/Blocking Time

To block times when the physician is not available for scheduling of patient visits or to indicate times reserved for surgery, a break in the schedule is created. Each break is labeled and highlighted according to the reason for the block. Labels and colors are assigned as follows:

UNAVAILABLE	Red
HOSPITAL ROUNDS	Teal
BOARD MEETING	Fuchsia
LUNCH	Lime
SURGERY	Aqua
MEDICAL SCHOOL	Olive
NURSING HOME VISITS	Purple

Begin by opening the *Provider Search* window. Select the correct physician and the beginning date for which you are matrixing. Once you have the indicated the physician and date, you should begin blocking times during which the physician is unavailable.

Select the correct time slot for the block to begin by clicking on the time's appointment line. With the appointment timeframe highlighted, right click to open scheduling menu. Select and click on *New Break* **(Figure SI 6-6)**. Using the *New Break Entry* window you will provide the information needed to schedule the time blocked **(Figure SI 6-7)**. In the *Description* field enter, in capital letters, the reason for the block from the labels listed above. Once scheduled, this label will appear in the first time slot of the block.

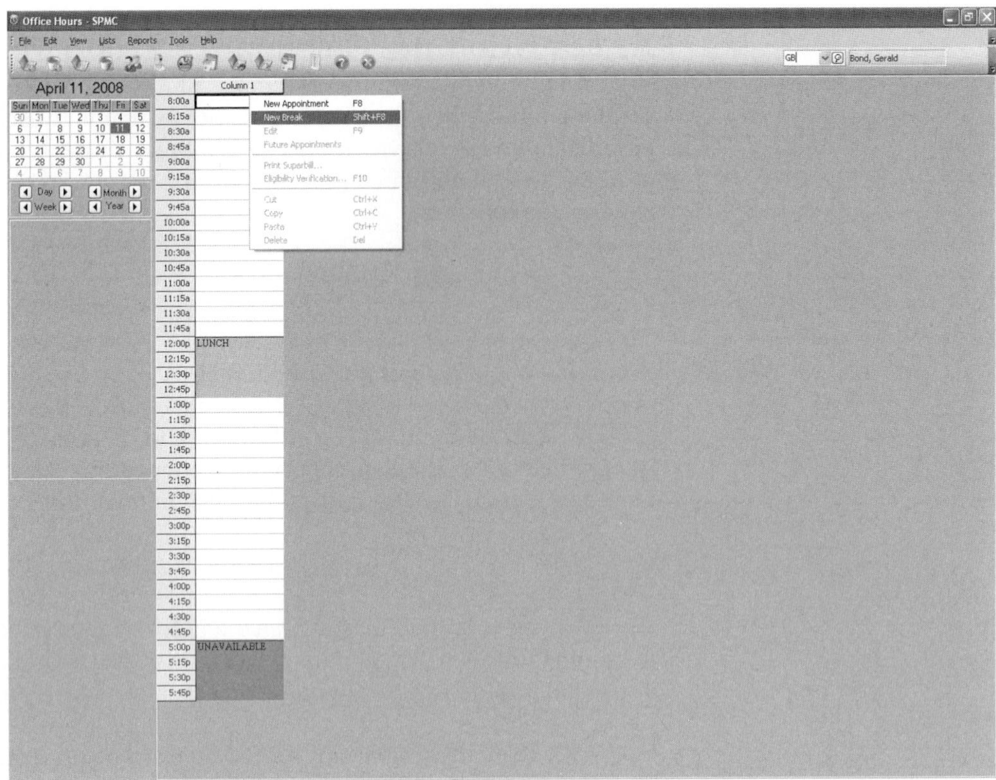

Figure **SI 6-6** *Medisoft® is a registered trademark of McKesson Corporation and/or one of its subsidiaries. Medisoft® screen shots and materials used with the permission of McKesson Corporation. © 2010 McKesson Corporation. All rights reserved.*

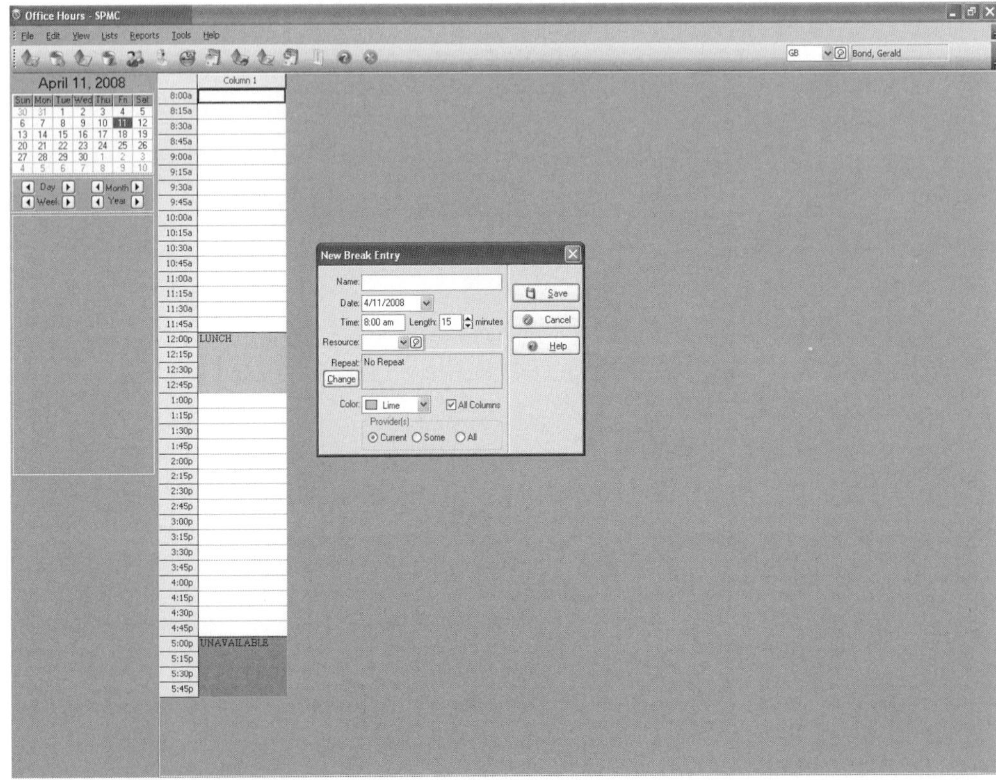

Figure **SI 6-7** *Medisoft® is a registered trademark of McKesson Corporation and/or one of its subsidiaries. Medisoft® screen shots and materials used with the permission of McKesson Corporation. © 2010 McKesson Corporation. All rights reserved.*

Verify that the information in the *Date* and *Time* fields is correct for the scheduling block you are entering. To enter the *Length* of the scheduled block, you may either enter the amount of time needed in the *Length* field or use the up/down arrows located to the right until the amount of time needed appears in the *Length* box. Each time the up/down arrow is used, the time will increase or decrease in increments of 15 minutes. If the block being scheduled is a repeating one (weekly, daily, monthly, or yearly), click on the *Change* button located on the left side of the *New Break Entry* window. In the *Repeat Change* window **(Figure SI 6-8)**, select the frequency for which the break is being scheduled by clicking on the radio button located before either *Daily, Weekly, Monthly*, or *Yearly*. Once the frequency is selected, the *Repeat Change* window will be modified to reflect the frequency interval selected. As you will be scheduling breaks at weekly intervals, you should have selected *Weekly* from the *Repeat Change Frequency* window **(Figure SI 6-9)**. In the modified window indicate the frequency of weeks and days the break is to be repeated. In the *End On* field enter the date for which the repeating break will end. Clicking on the drop down arrow to the right of the *End On* field will open a calendar to assist with this process.

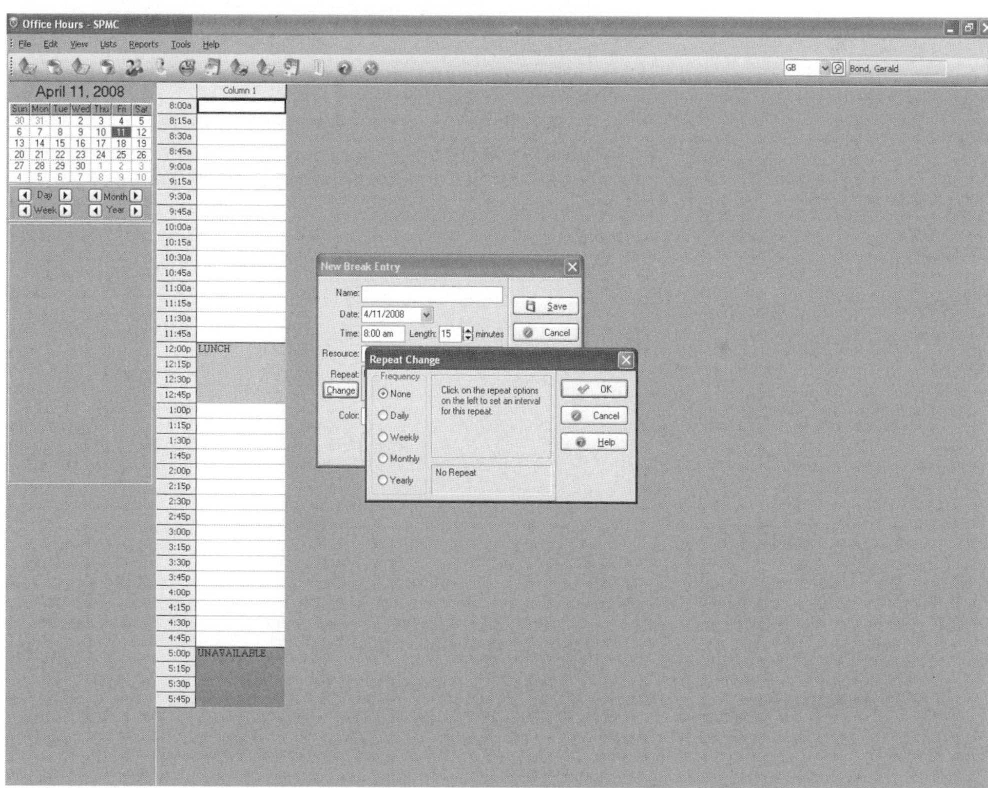

Figure **SI 6-8** *Medisoft® is a registered trademark of McKesson Corporation and/or one of its subsidiaries. Medisoft® screen shots and materials used with the permission of McKesson Corporation. © 2010 McKesson Corporation. All rights reserved.*

MEDISOFT SOFTWARE INSTRUCTIONS

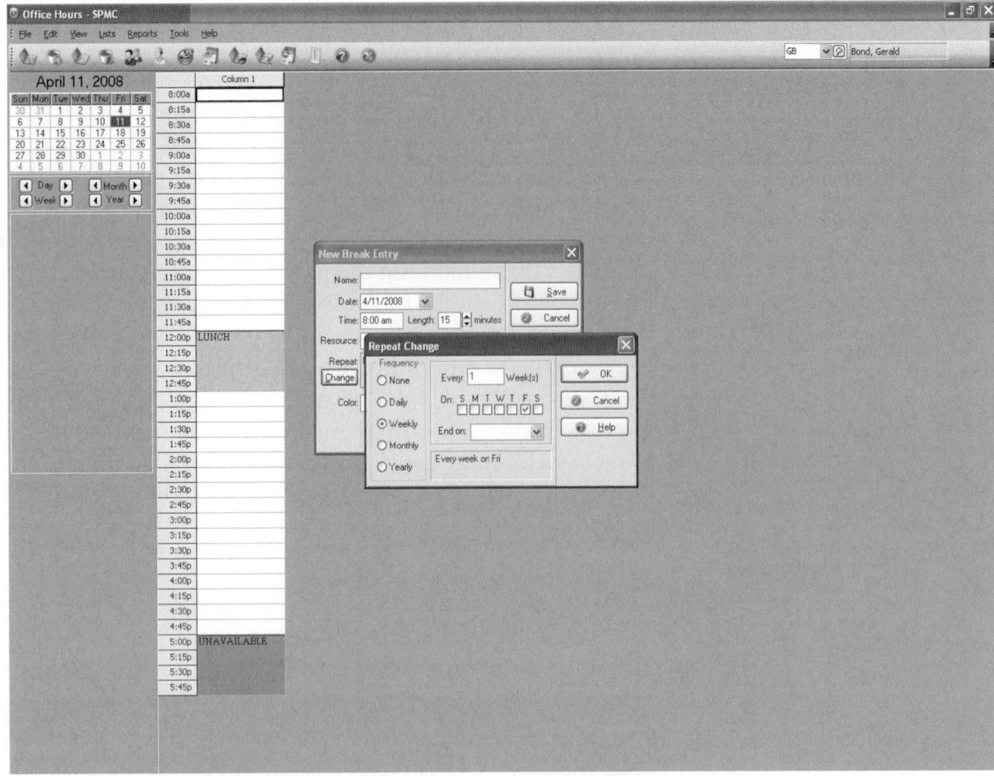

Figure **SI 6-9** *Medisoft® is a registered trademark of McKesson Corporation and/or one of its subsidiaries. Medisoft® screen shots and materials used with the permission of McKesson Corporation. © 2010 McKesson Corporation. All rights reserved.*

From the matrixing list choose the color of the block by clicking the down arrow to view the drop down menu located next to the color window. Click on the appropriate color from the color menu. If not already checked, check the *All Columns* box and the *Current Provider(s)* radio button. After all scheduling block information has been entered and verified to be correct, click the *Save* button located on the right side of the *New Break Entry* window. The blocked time now appears on the physician's schedule.

All blocks except SURGERY time slots are scheduled in this manner. When scheduling blocks for SURGERY, the Label and available surgery times are placed in the time slot before the first available surgery slot **(Figure SI 6-10)**.

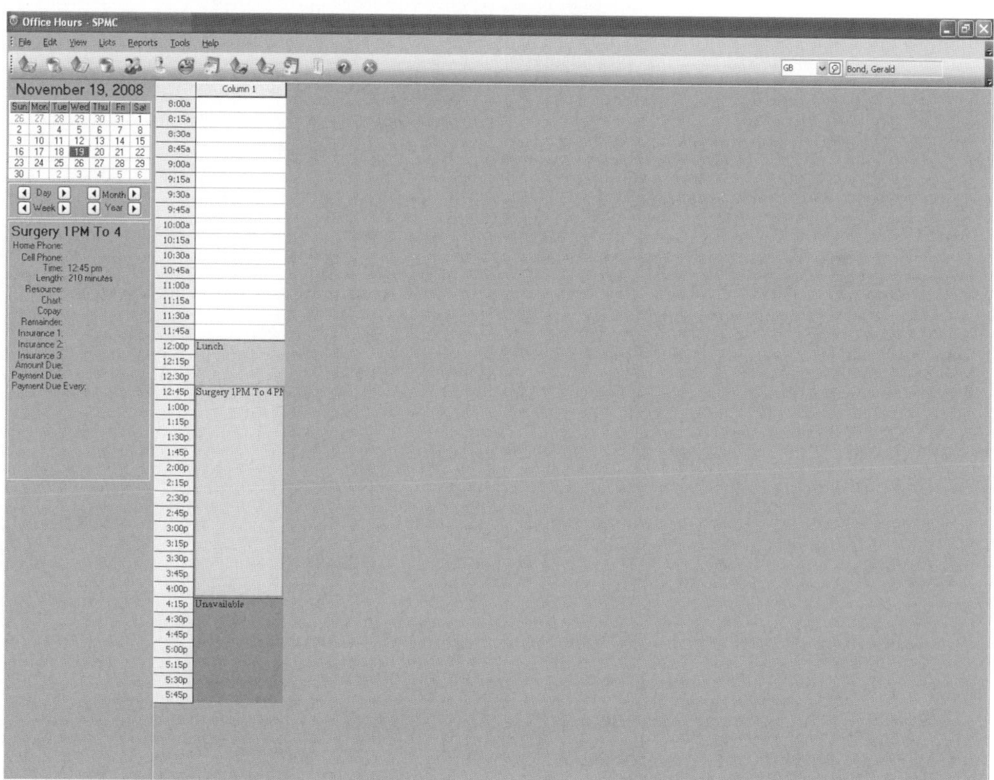

Figure **SI 6-10** *Medisoft® is a registered trademark of McKesson Corporation and/or one of its subsidiaries. Medisoft® screen shots and materials used with the permission of McKesson Corporation. © 2010 McKesson Corporation. All rights reserved.*

B. Scheduling Patient Visits

Begin scheduling office visits from the scheduling window. Select the physician and date needed for scheduling by using the provider search window and calendar. Click on the available time slot for which you are scheduling the appointment. Open the drop down menu and select *New Appointment* **(Figure SI 6-11)** to open the *New Appointment Entry* window **(Figure SI 6-12)**.

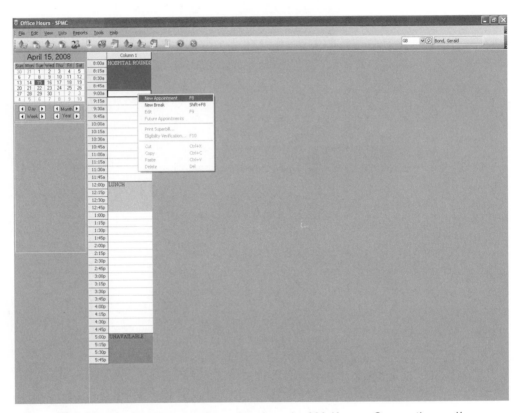

Figure **SI 6-11** *Medisoft® is a registered trademark of McKesson Corporation and/or one of its subsidiaries. Medisoft® screen shots and materials used with the permission of McKesson Corporation. © 2010 McKesson Corporation. All rights reserved.*

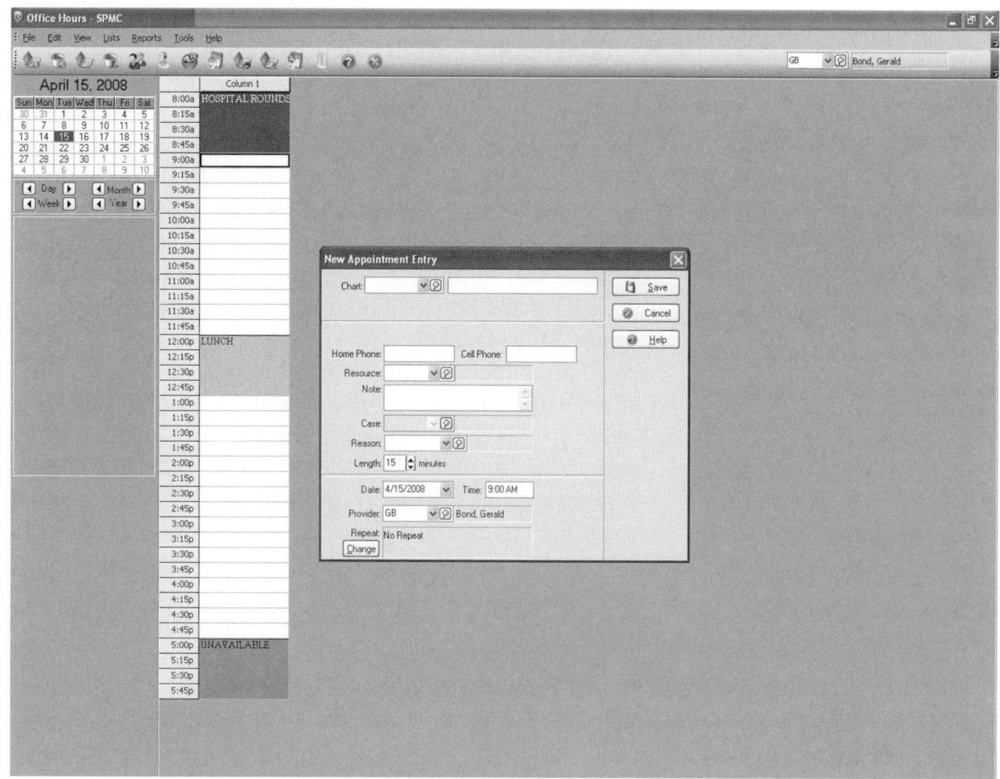

Figure **SI 6-12** *Medisoft® is a registered trademark of McKesson Corporation and/or one of its subsidiaries. Medisoft® screen shots and materials used with the permission of McKesson Corporation. © 2010 McKesson Corporation. All rights reserved.*

SCHEDULING ESTABLISHED PATIENTS

In the *New Appointment Entry* window, use the search button (magnifying glass) located next to the *Chart* field to search for the established patient's information. (This step should also be performed before scheduling a new patient to verify the patient's status as new or established.) In the *Patient Search* window, search for field and enter the patient's last name **(Figure SI 6-13)**. Select the patient from the list by clicking on the patient's name. Click the *OK* button. The patient's name and identification number now populate the *Chart* fields. Using the drop down arrow to the right of the *Resource* field indicate the location in which the patient will be seen **(Figure SI 6-14)**. In the *Note* field enter the reason for the encounter, the referring physician, patient's age (if necessary), and any other information important to this patient's appointment. If the case field is blank, click on the drop down arrow located in this field and select the patient's available case. Next, click on the drop down arrow located in the *Reason* field. Enter the reason for the encounter by selecting it from this list **(Figure SI 6-15)**. The *Length* field will be populated once a reason for the encounter is selected; however, it should be verified for correctness and may be altered by using the up and down arrows in this field. Verify the information in the *Date and Time* and *Provider* fields is correct for the appointment being scheduled. Once you have verified that the information you have entered for this appointment is correct, click the *Save* button. The created appointment now appears on the appointment schedule.

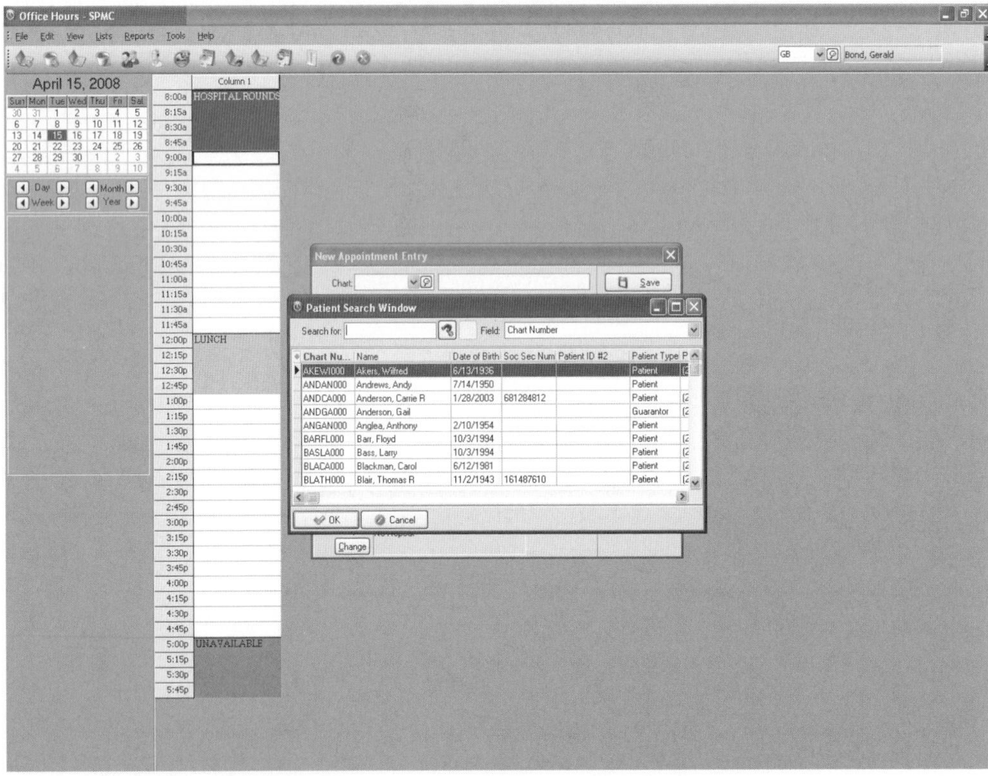

Figure **SI 6-13** *Medisoft® is a registered trademark of McKesson Corporation and/or one of its subsidiaries. Medisoft® screen shots and materials used with the permission of McKesson Corporation. © 2010 McKesson Corporation. All rights reserved.*

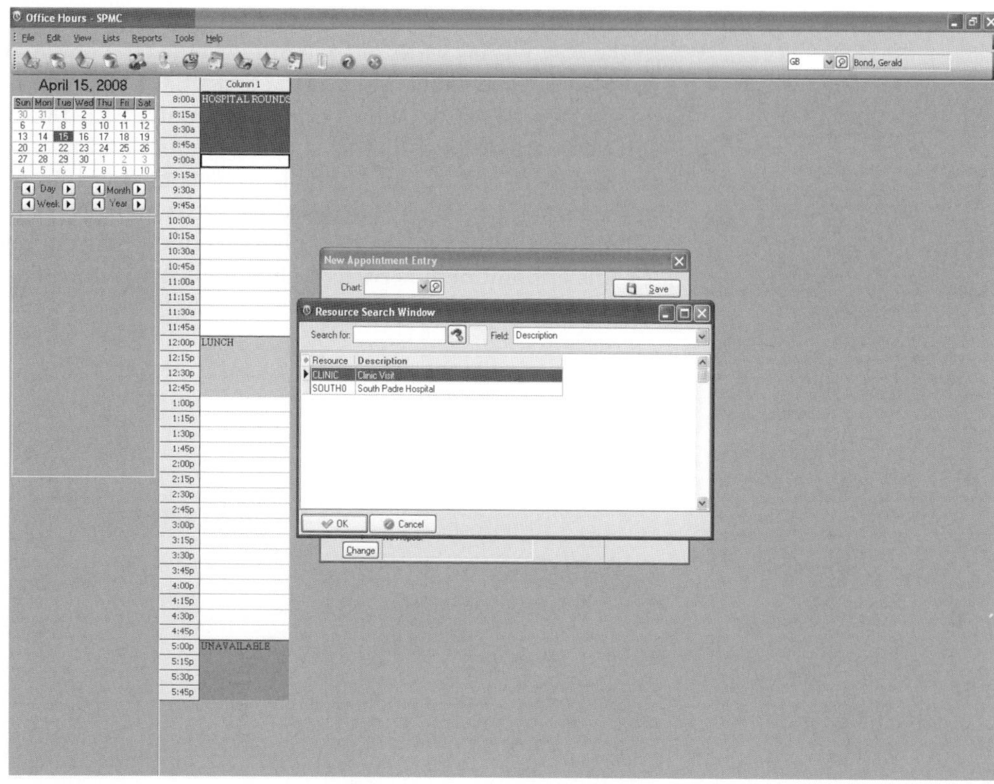

Figure **SI 6-14** *Medisoft® is a registered trademark of McKesson Corporation and/or one of its subsidiaries. Medisoft® screen shots and materials used with the permission of McKesson Corporation. © 2010 McKesson Corporation. All rights reserved.*

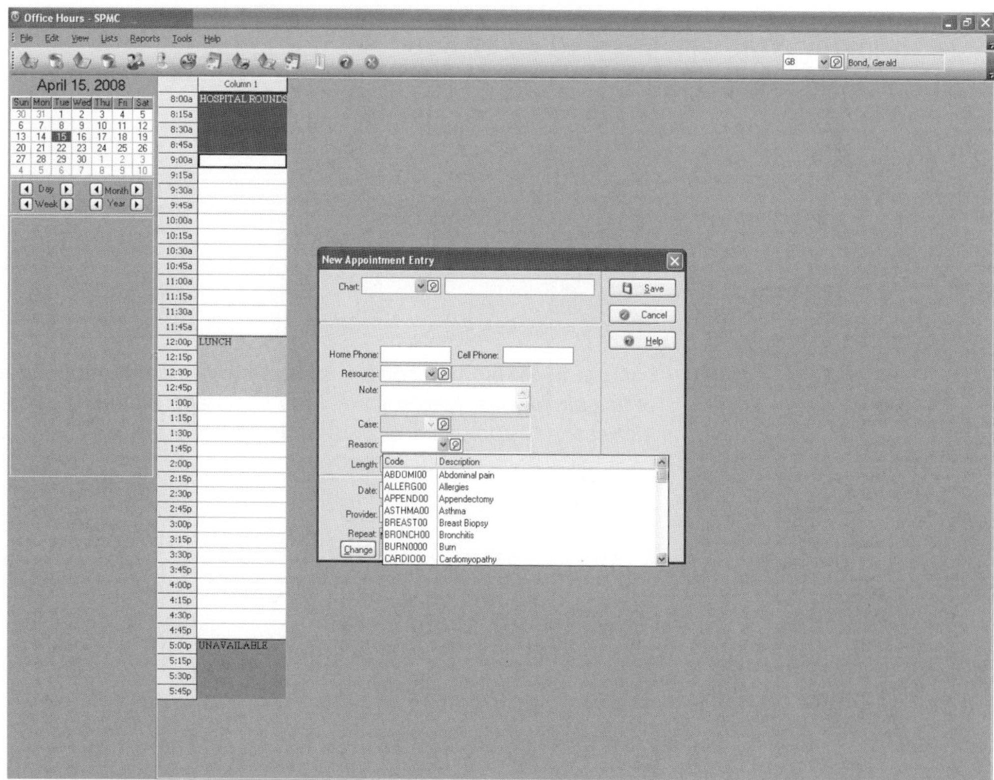

Figure **SI 6-15** *Medisoft® is a registered trademark of McKesson Corporation and/or one of its subsidiaries. Medisoft® screen shots and materials used with the permission of McKesson Corporation. © 2010 McKesson Corporation. All rights reserved.*

SCHEDULING NEW PATIENTS

In the *New Appointment Entry* window, enter the new patient's name (Last, First) in the field located to the right of the *Chart* field. If available, enter the patient's phone number in the *Phone* field in this field **(Figure SI 6-16)**. Do not enter the dashes; the software will do this. As this is a new patient and no case yet exists for this patient, the *Case* field will not be available to be completed. Complete the remaining fields in the same manner as completed for an established patient (see above Scheduling Established Patients). Once you have verified that the information you have entered for this appointment is correct, click the *Save* button. The created appointment now appears on the *Schedule Report*.

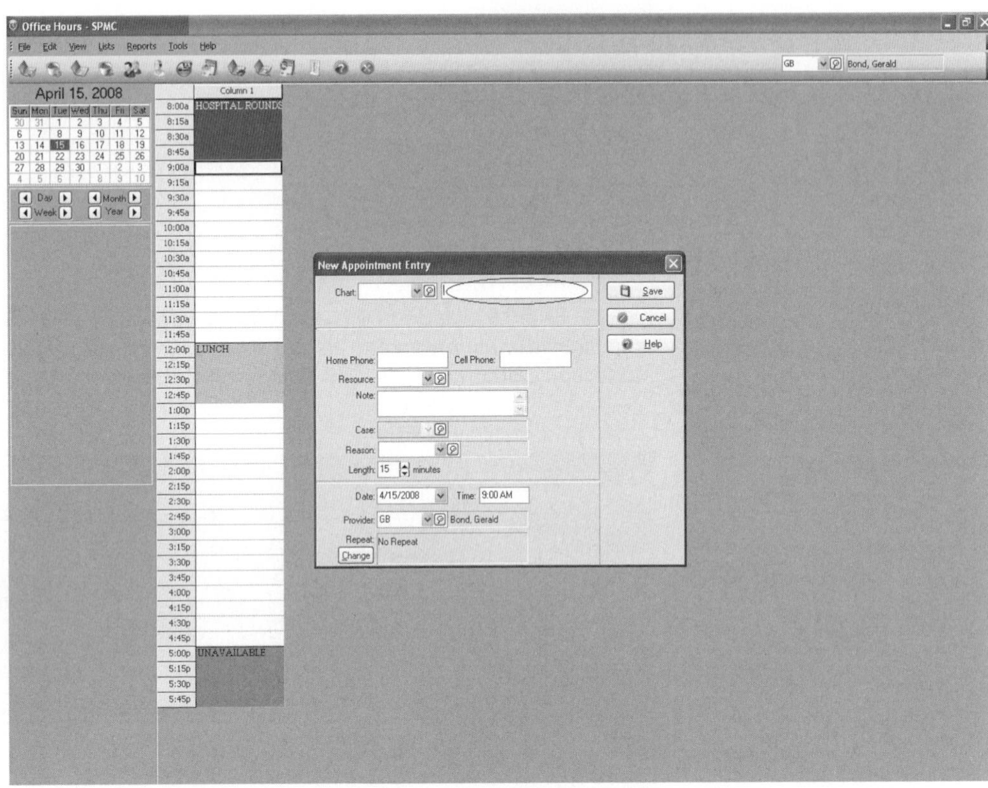

Figure **SI 6-16** *Medisoft® is a registered trademark of McKesson Corporation and/or one of its subsidiaries. Medisoft® screen shots and materials used with the permission of McKesson Corporation. © 2010 McKesson Corporation. All rights reserved.*

C. Editing/Deleting Breaks or Appointments

To reschedule an existing appointment, locate the appointment or break to be rescheduled in the scheduling window. Select the appointment or break by clicking on the patient's name or break description. With the appointment or break highlighted, right click to open the scheduling menu. Select *Edit* from the scheduling menu **(Figure SI 6-17)**. In the *Edit Break* window or *Edit Appointment* window **(Figures SI 6-18** and **SI 6-19)** edit or correct the field in which the error is located. If changing the information in the *Provider* field, be sure to verify that the appointment time to which the break or patient appointment is to be moved is available. Verify that the information is correct and click on the *Save* button.

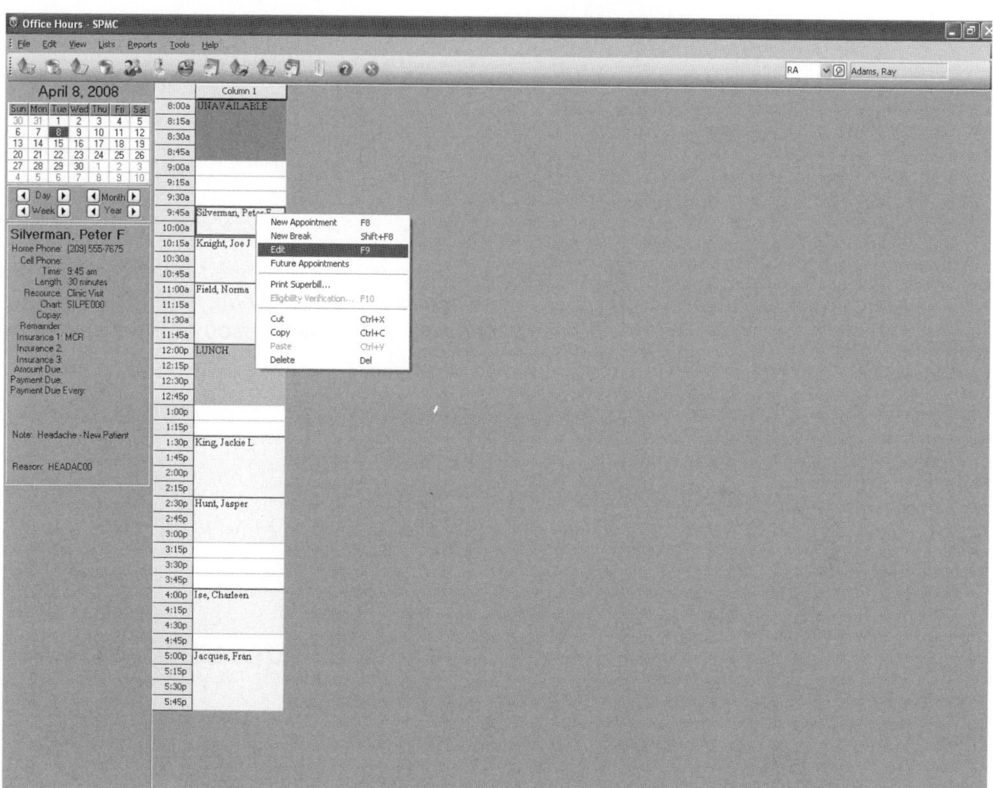

Figure **SI 6-17** *Medisoft® is a registered trademark of McKesson Corporation and/or one of its subsidiaries. Medisoft® screen shots and materials used with the permission of McKesson Corporation. © 2010 McKesson Corporation. All rights reserved.*

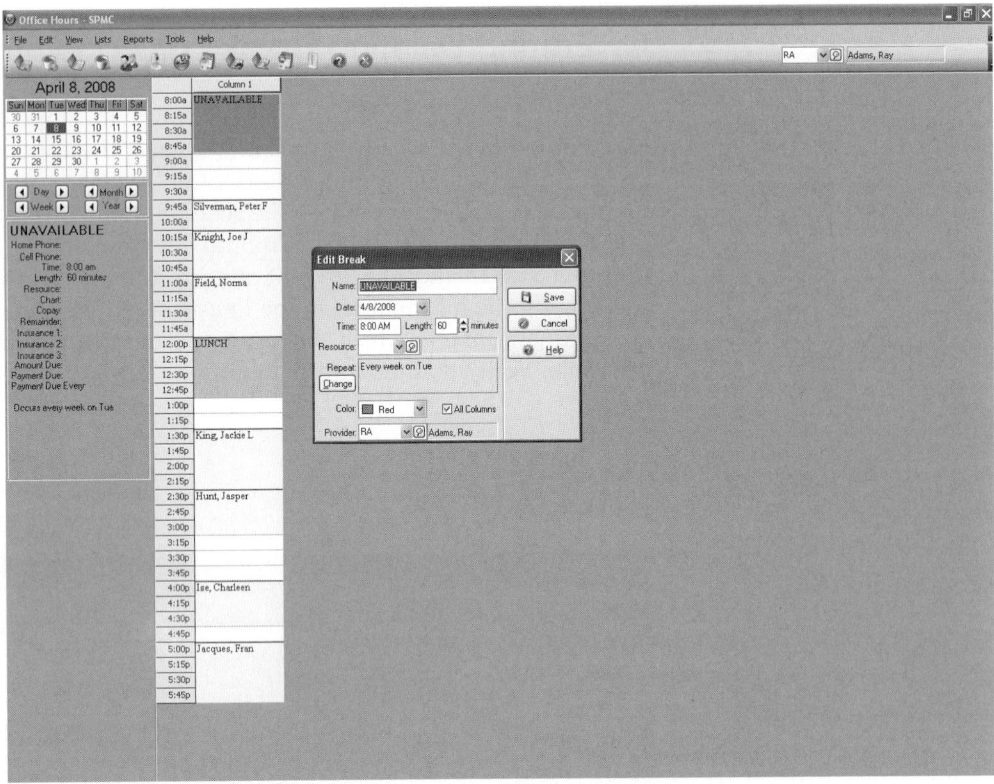

Figure **SI 6-18** *Medisoft® is a registered trademark of McKesson Corporation and/or one of its subsidiaries. Medisoft® screen shots and materials used with the permission of McKesson Corporation. © 2010 McKesson Corporation. All rights reserved.*

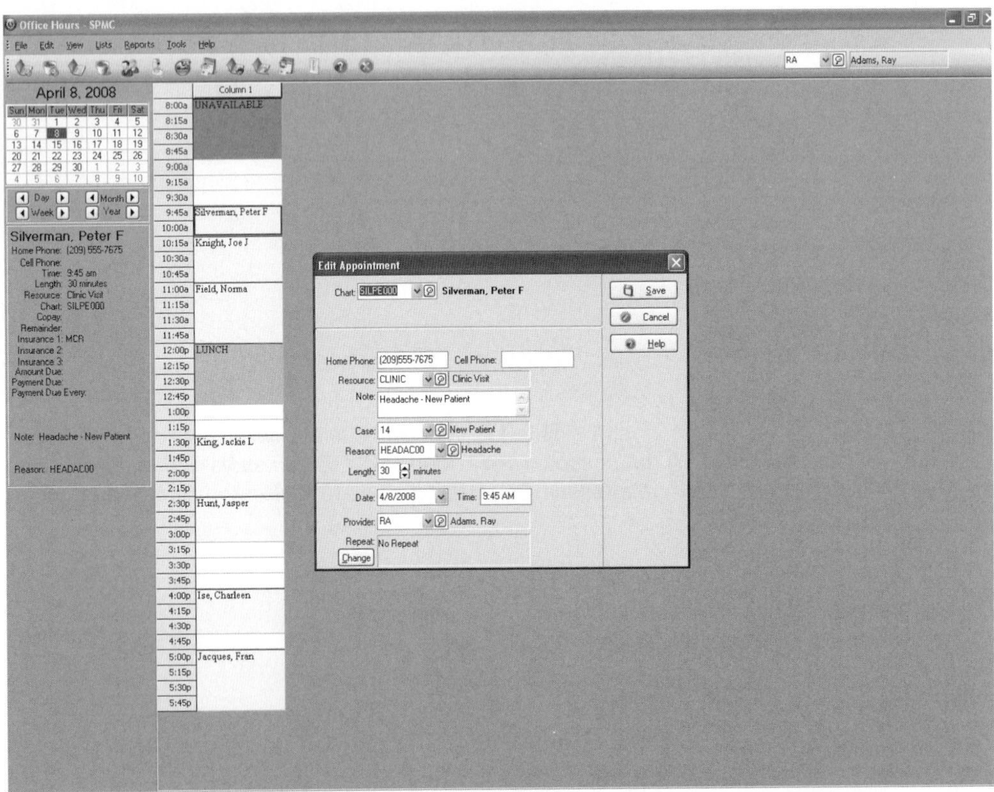

Figure **SI 6-19** *Medisoft® is a registered trademark of McKesson Corporation and/or one of its subsidiaries. Medisoft® screen shots and materials used with the permission of McKesson Corporation. © 2010 McKesson Corporation. All rights reserved.*

To delete an existing break or appointment, select the break or appointment and open the scheduling menu. From the scheduling menu select Delete **(Figure SI 6-20)**. A prompt will appear asking, "Delete this appointment?" Clicking on the *Yes* button will delete the break or appointment.

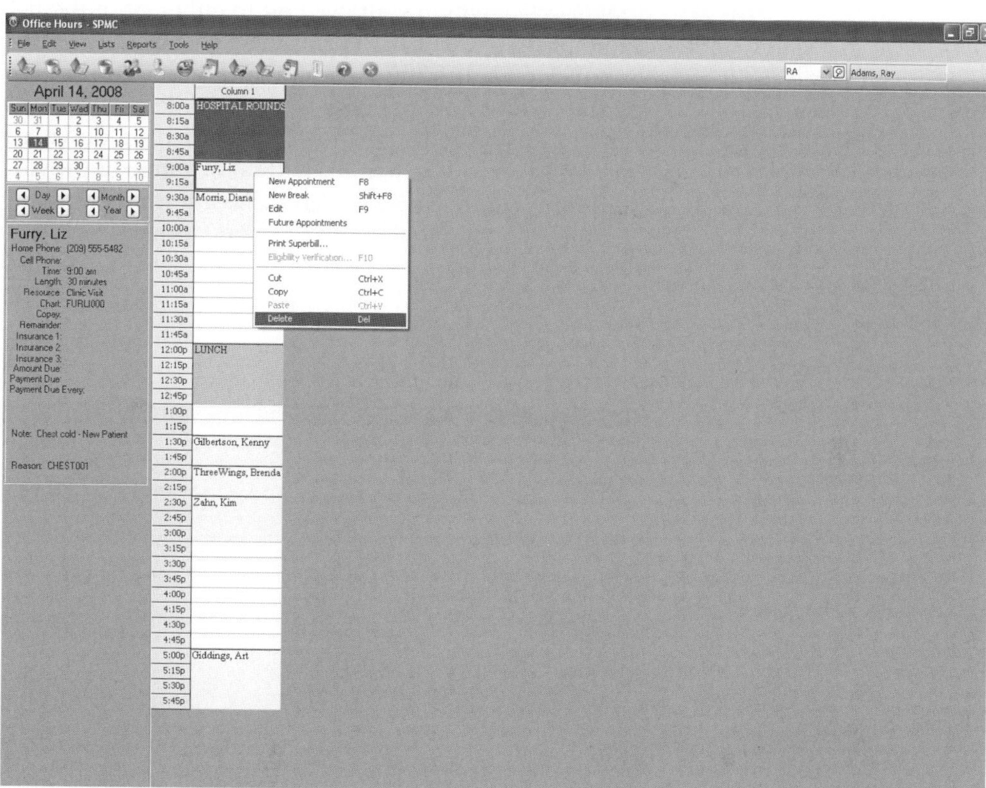

Figure **SI 6-20** *Medisoft® is a registered trademark of McKesson Corporation and/or one of its subsidiaries. Medisoft® screen shots and materials used with the permission of McKesson Corporation. © 2010 McKesson Corporation. All rights reserved.*

MEDISOFT SOFTWARE INSTRUCTIONS

D. Appointment List

An *Appointment List* prints a list, by provider, of all breaks and patients scheduled, each patient's phone number, and the time, length, reason of the visit, and any notes added in the *Appointment Schedule* window for the selected date(s) or provider(s). To print this report, on the Office Hours software program toolbar click on *Reports*. From the drop down menu select *Appointment List* **(Figure SI 6-21)**. The *Report Setup Print Selection* window allows you to either print the list or view it first on screen before printing the list. To print the list, select the radio button for *Print the report on the printer* and click the *Start* button **(Figure SI 6-22)**. In the *Data Selection* window, use the up and down arrows in the date fields to select a date or range of dates for which the list is being generated. Use the drop down arrows or search button in the *Provider* fields to select an individual or range of providers for which the list is being generated **(Figure SI 6-23)**. Verify the information requested is correct and click the *OK* button located in the *Select Data* window.

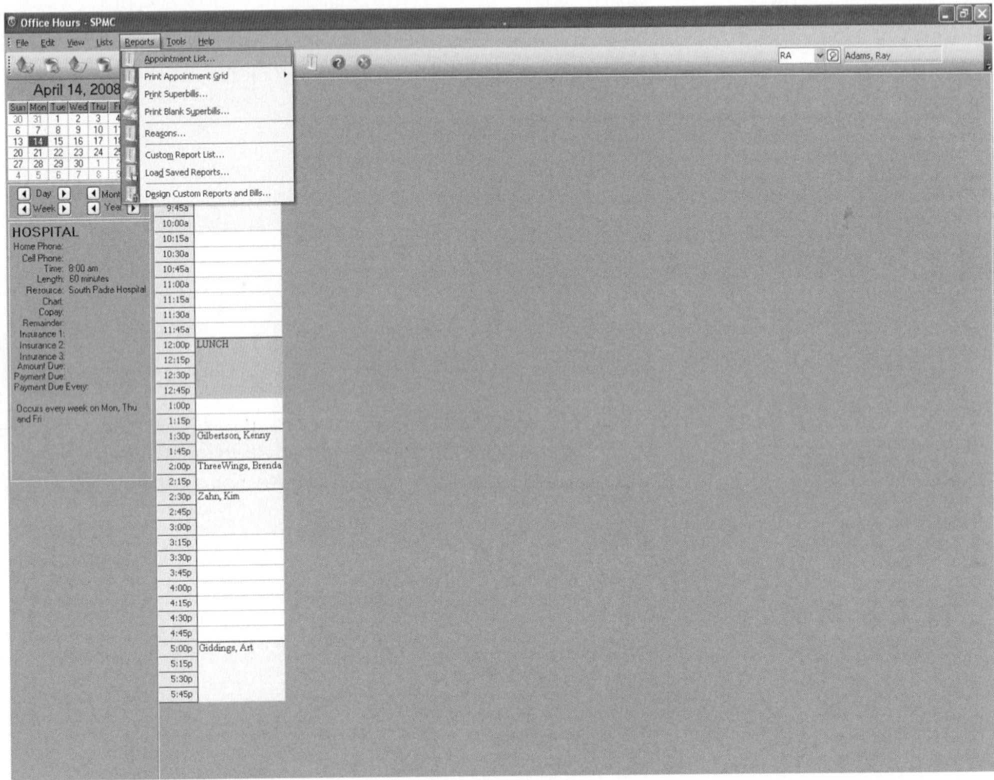

Figure **SI 6-21** *Medisoft® is a registered trademark of McKesson Corporation and/or one of its subsidiaries. Medisoft® screen shots and materials used with the permission of McKesson Corporation. © 2010 McKesson Corporation. All rights reserved.*

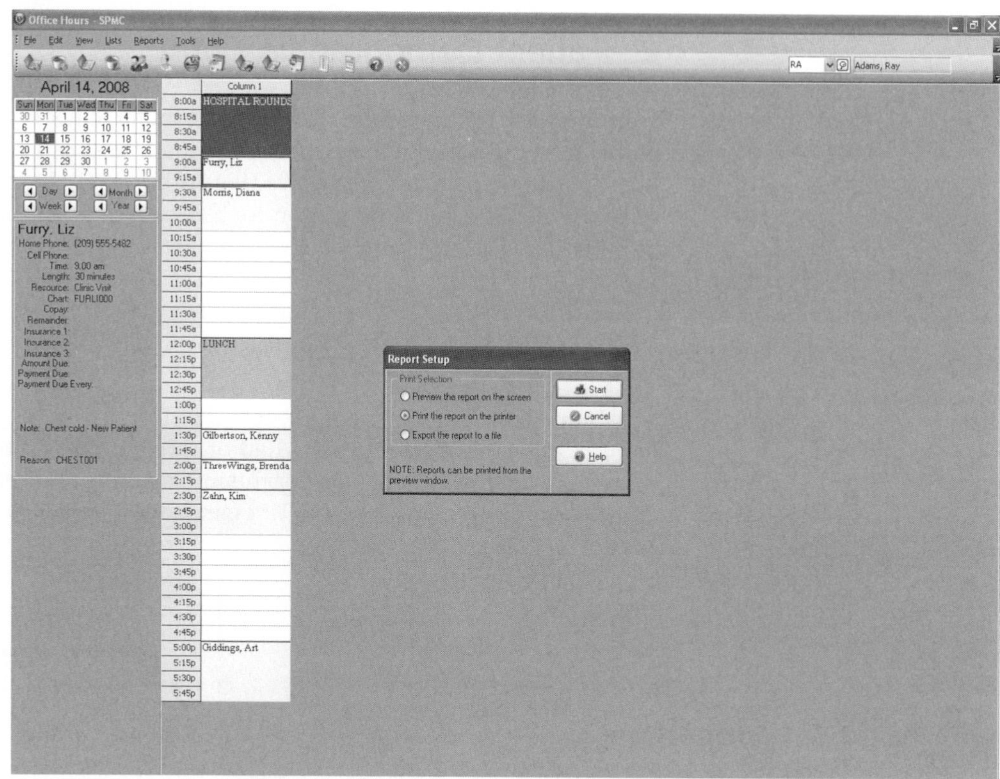

Figure **SI 6-22** *Medisoft® is a registered trademark of McKesson Corporation and/or one of its subsidiaries. Medisoft® screen shots and materials used with the permission of McKesson Corporation. © 2010 McKesson Corporation. All rights reserved.*

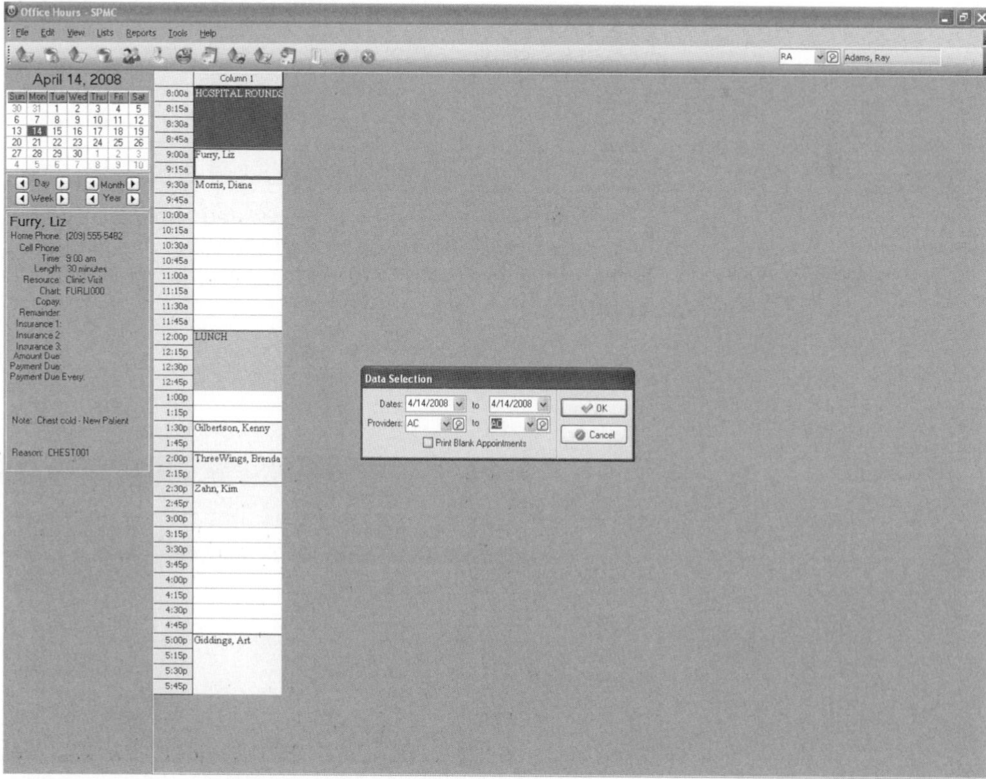

Figure **SI 6-23** *Medisoft® is a registered trademark of McKesson Corporation and/or one of its subsidiaries. Medisoft® screen shots and materials used with the permission of McKesson Corporation. © 2010 McKesson Corporation. All rights reserved.*

E. Patient Demographic Entry

From the Medisoft program main menu toolbar, click on the *Patient List* icon located on the icon toolbar at the top of the screen, or you can click on the *Lists* menu and select *Patients/Guarantors and Cases* **(Figure SI 6-24)**. At the top of the *Patient List* window, click on the radio button for *Patient*. Click on the *New Patient* button **(Figure SI 6-25)**. The *Patient/Guarantor (New)* window is now open.

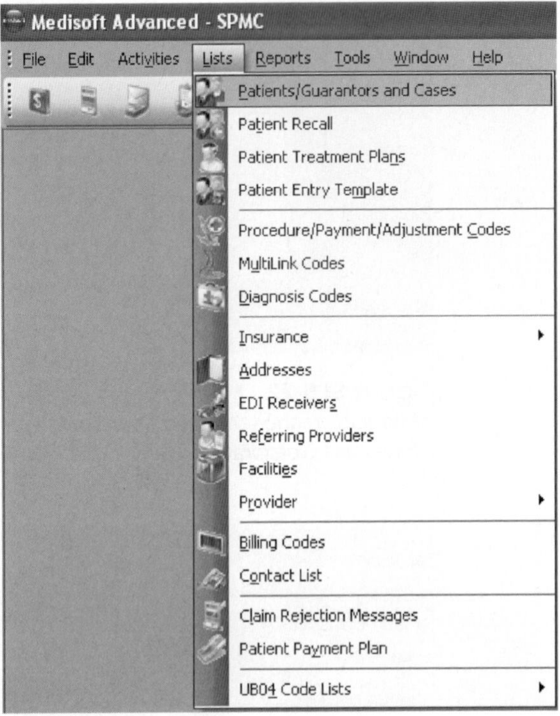

Figure **SI 6-24** *Medisoft® is a registered trademark of McKesson Corporation and/or one of its subsidiaries. Medisoft® screen shots and materials used with the permission of McKesson Corporation. © 2010 McKesson Corporation. All rights reserved.*

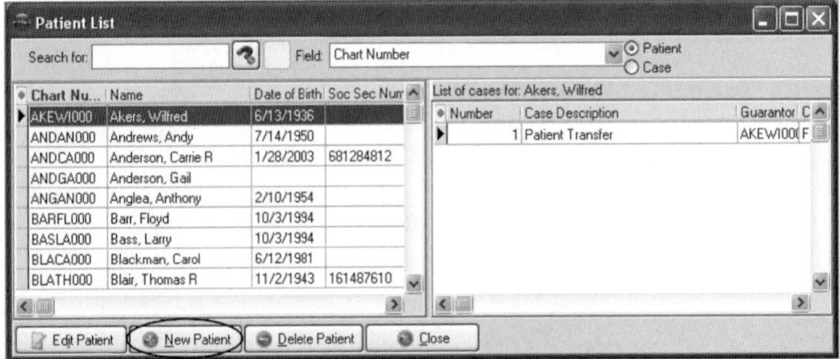

Figure **SI 6-25** *Medisoft® is a registered trademark of McKesson Corporation and/or one of its subsidiaries. Medisoft® screen shots and materials used with the permission of McKesson Corporation. © 2010 McKesson Corporation. All rights reserved.*

Beginning on the *Name, Address* tab, *Last Name* field, enter the patient's demographic information **(Figure SI 6-26)**. On the *Other Information* tab, use the drop down arrow in the *Type* field to indicate if this record is for a patient or guarantor **(Figure SI 6-27)**. For a patient record, use the drop down arrow in the *Assigned Provider* field to indicate the patient's provider and complete the *Emergency Contact* fields. The search buttons located to the right of the *Employer* fields may be used to find the information needed to populate these fields. If this information is not available, leave these fields blank, as they will be reviewed by Kerri Marshall, insurance specialist, before a claim is submitted. When entering a Guarantor's record, this information does not need to be completed.

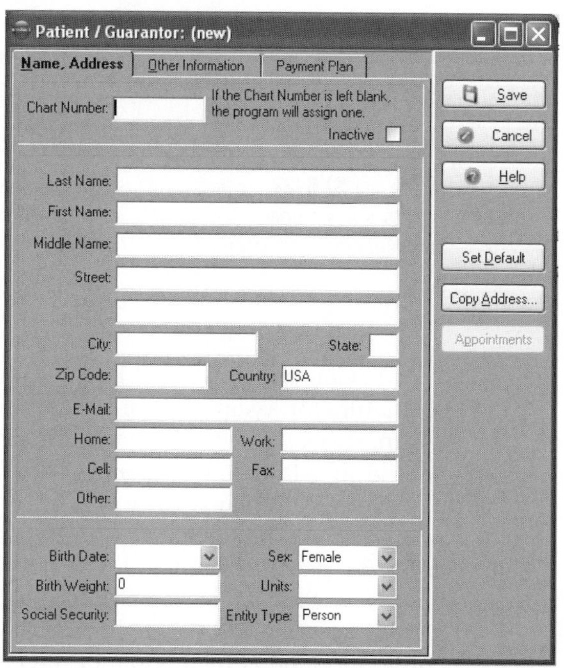

Figure **SI 6-26** *Medisoft® is a registered trademark of McKesson Corporation and/or one of its subsidiaries. Medisoft® screen shots and materials used with the permission of McKesson Corporation. © 2010 McKesson Corporation. All rights reserved.*

MEDISOFT SOFTWARE INSTRUCTIONS

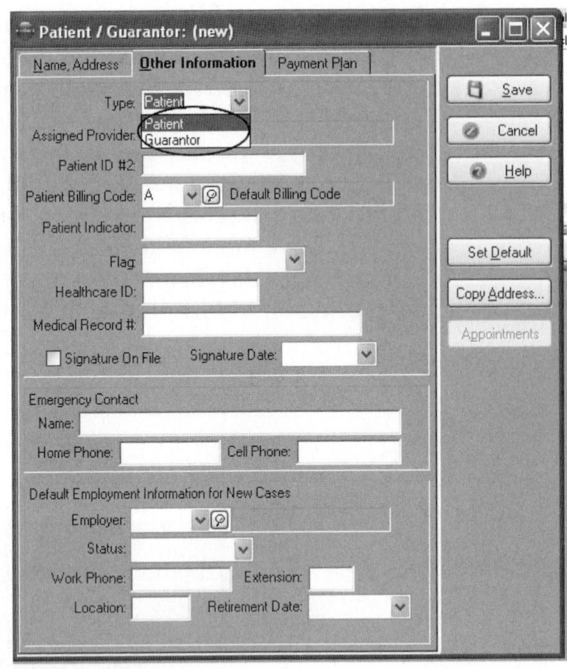

Figure **SI 6-27** *Medisoft® is a registered trademark of McKesson Corporation and/or one of its subsidiaries. Medisoft® screen shots and materials used with the permission of McKesson Corporation. © 2010 McKesson Corporation. All rights reserved.*

Review the completed Patient Information form for the patient's or guarantor's signature for assignment of benefits and release of information. If completed on this form, check the *Signature on File* box on the *Other Information* tab and enter the date of the signature. The remaining fields and tab have been populated by default or should remain blank. Once you have verified that the information entered is correct, click the *Save* button located on the right side of the *Patient/Guarantor* window to save the patient record and return to the *Patient List* window.

Now click on the radio button for *Case*, located at the top of the *Patient List* window. Select and highlight the patient being added and click on the *New Case* button located at the bottom of the *Patient List* window **(Figure SI 6-28)**. In the *Case entry* window, *Personal* tab, *Description* field, enter **New Patient (Figure SI 6-29)**. Using the drop down arrows located in the *Marital* and *Student* fields, complete each of these fields. With the information available from the Patient Information forms or additional source documents complete the *Employment* fields.

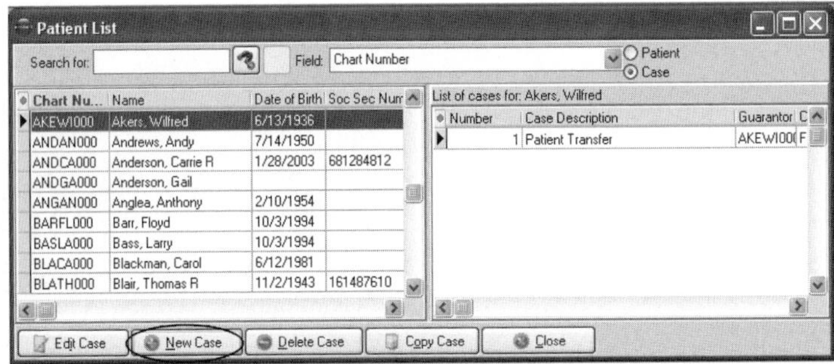

Figure **SI 6-28** *Medisoft® is a registered trademark of McKesson Corporation and/or one of its subsidiaries. Medisoft® screen shots and materials used with the permission of McKesson Corporation. © 2010 McKesson Corporation. All rights reserved.*

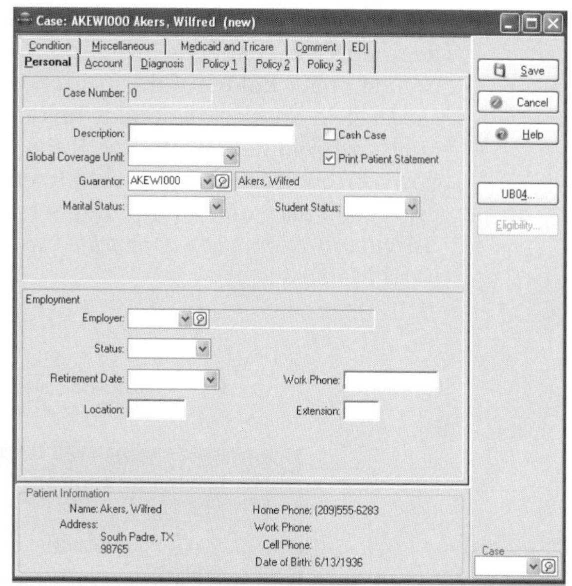

Figure **SI 6-29** *Medisoft® is a registered trademark of McKesson Corporation and/or one of its subsidiaries. Medisoft® screen shots and materials used with the permission of McKesson Corporation. © 2010 McKesson Corporation. All rights reserved.*

On the *Account* tab, using the drop down arrows located in each field and the source document information available, complete the *Assigned*, *Referring*, and *Operating Provider* fields **(Figure SI 6-30)**. Leave the remaining fields blank; these will be completed by Kerri Marshall at a later date.

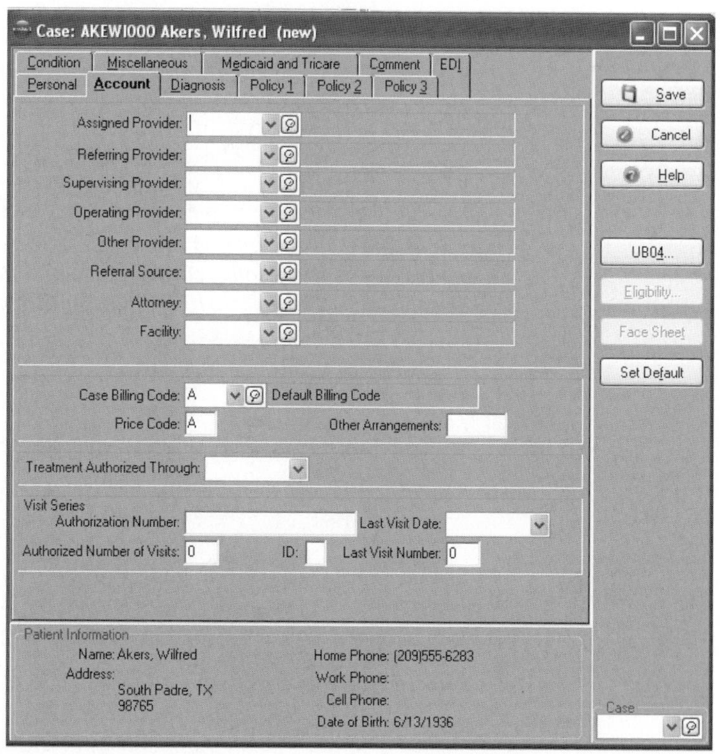

Figure **SI 6-30** *Medisoft® is a registered trademark of McKesson Corporation and/or one of its subsidiaries. Medisoft® screen shots and materials used with the permission of McKesson Corporation. © 2010 McKesson Corporation. All rights reserved.*

Next, click on the *Policy 1* tab. Using the drop down arrow in the *Insurance 1* field, select the patient's primary insurance. If the patient is a minor or the patient is not the policy holder of the insurance, use the drop down arrow located in the *Policy Holder* field to select the policy holder from the *Patient/Guarantor* list. The *Relationship to Insured* field defaults to *Self*. If the patient is not the policy holder, use the drop arrow located in this field to enter the correct relationship **(Figure SI 6-31)**. Enter the Policy and Group numbers in each of these fields and check the *Accept Assignment/Assignment of Benefits* box. The remaining fields will be completed by Kerri Marshall.

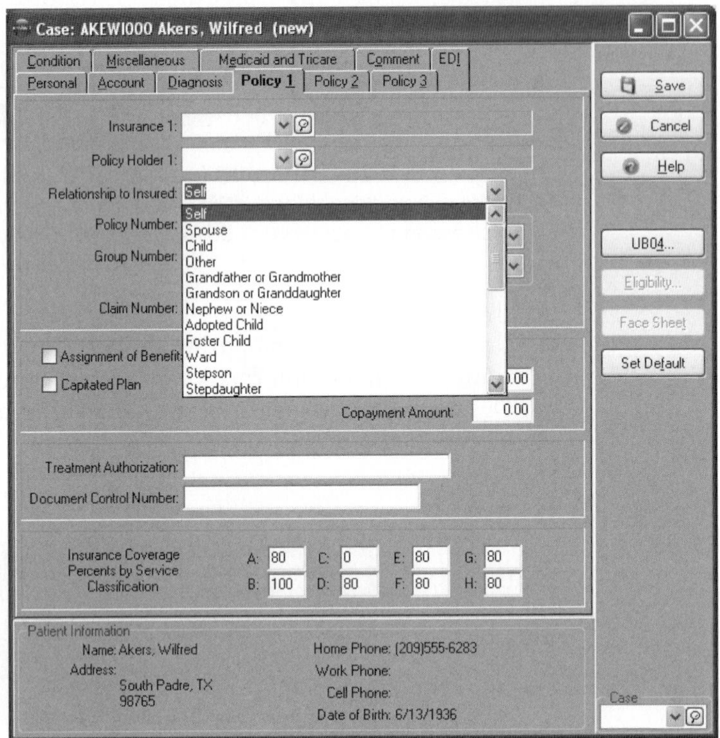

Figure **SI 6-31** *Medisoft® is a registered trademark of McKesson Corporation and/or one of its subsidiaries. Medisoft® screen shots and materials used with the permission of McKesson Corporation. © 2010 McKesson Corporation. All rights reserved.*

F. Printing Patient Face Sheets

From the main menu, click on *Reports*, located on the toolbar at the top of the screen. On the *Reports* menu, select *Custom Reports List* **(Figure SI 6-32)**. In the *Open Report* menu, scroll to and select *Patient Face Sheet*. Click the *OK* button located in the *Open Reports* menu. In the *Print Reports Where* window, click on the radio button for *Print the report on the printer* and select *Start*. In the *Patient Face Sheet: Data Selection Questions* window **(Figure SI 6-33)**, use the search button located in the *Chart Number Range* field to open the *Patient Search* window. Enter the patient's last name in the *Search for* field. Select and highlight the patient from the list and click the *OK* button located at the bottom of the *Patient Search* window. You will need to complete this step for both *Chart Number Range* fields. Click the *OK* button located in the *Patient Face Sheet: Data Selection Questions* window.

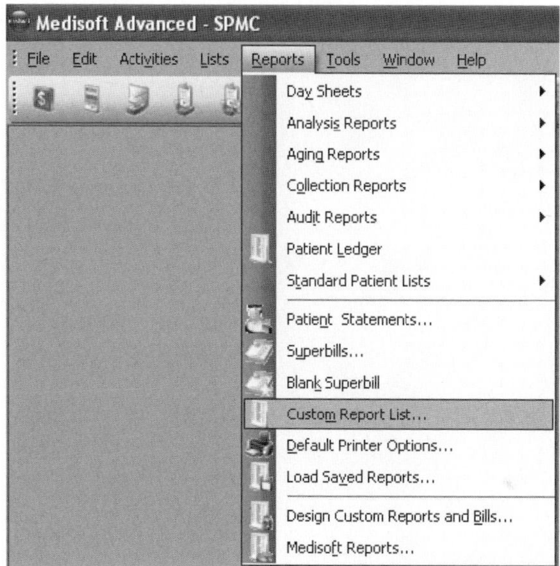

Figure **SI 6-32** *Medisoft® is a registered trademark of McKesson Corporation and/or one of its subsidiaries. Medisoft® screen shots and materials used with the permission of McKesson Corporation. © 2010 McKesson Corporation. All rights reserved.*

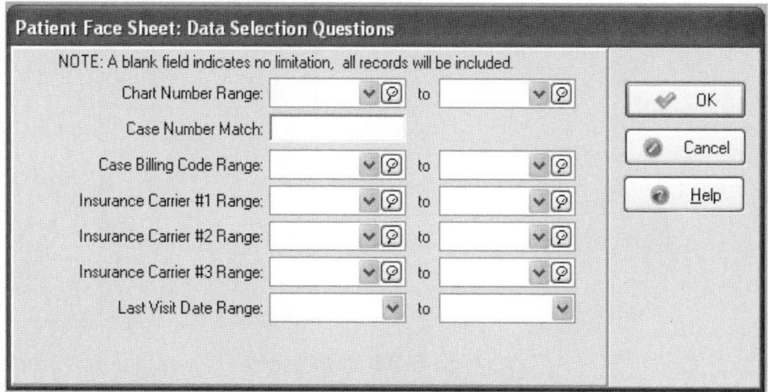

Figure **SI 6-33** *Medisoft® is a registered trademark of McKesson Corporation and/or one of its subsidiaries. Medisoft® screen shots and materials used with the permission of McKesson Corporation. © 2010 McKesson Corporation. All rights reserved.*

G. Charge Entry

From the main menu, click on *Activities*, located on the toolbar at the top of the main menu Medisoft program. From the drop down menu, select *Enter Transactions* **(Figure SI 6-34)**. The *Transaction Entry* window is now available **(Figure SI 6-35)**. Using the search button (magnifying glass) located in the *Chart* field, open the *Patient Search* window and select the patient for which you are entering charges. You will be returned to the *Transaction Entry* window. Use the dropdown arrow in the *Case* field to select the case for this patient. The software program will populate the *Chart* field with the ID number of the patient. Clicking in each field of the *Charges* portion of the *Transaction Entry* window will activate a drop down list for each field. Enter the date of the service(s) in the *Date* field. For example, clicking on the drop down arrow in the *Date* field will open a calendar on which you may indicate the date of service for the transaction being entered **(Figure SI 6-36)**. Using the drop down arrows in each field, enter the *Procedure* and *Diagnosis* fields from the patient's superbill. Repeat these steps until all services and diagnoses have been entered. Tab or enter past the remaining charge entry fields; Kerri Marshall will review and, if needed, complete these fields.

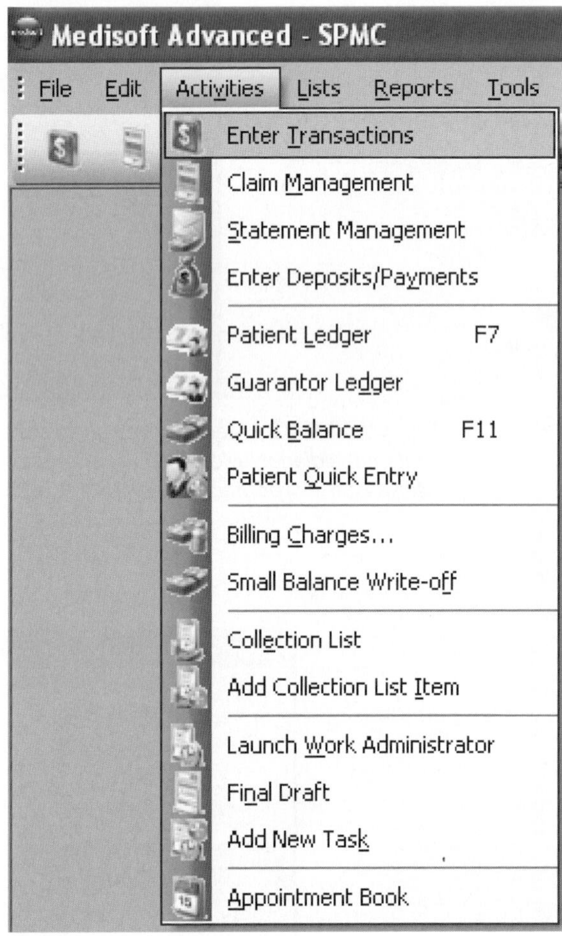

Figure **SI 6-34** *Medisoft® is a registered trademark of McKesson Corporation and/or one of its subsidiaries. Medisoft® screen shots and materials used with the permission of McKesson Corporation. © 2010 McKesson Corporation. All rights reserved.*

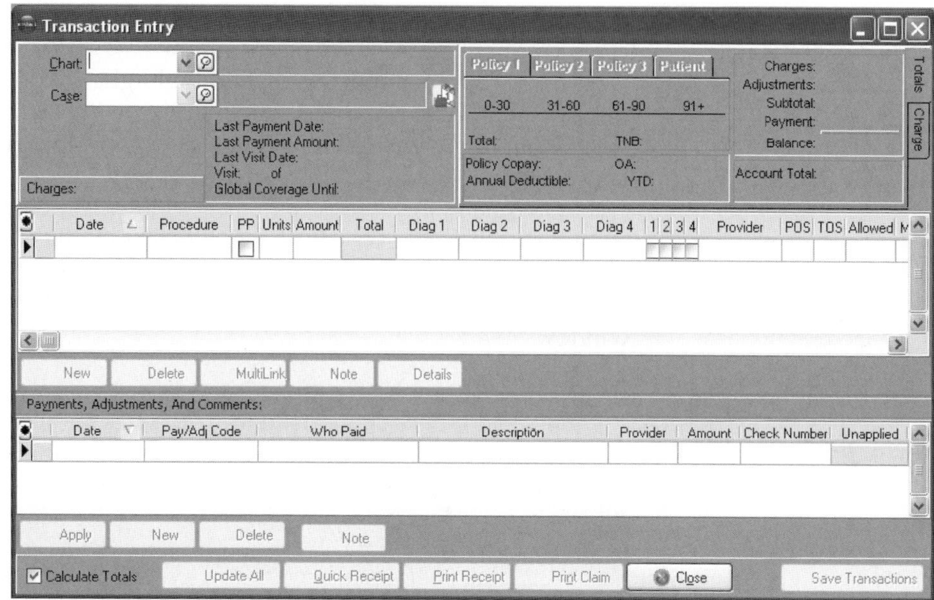

Figure **SI 6-35** *Medisoft® is a registered trademark of McKesson Corporation and/or one of its subsidiaries. Medisoft® screen shots and materials used with the permission of McKesson Corporation. © 2010 McKesson Corporation. All rights reserved.*

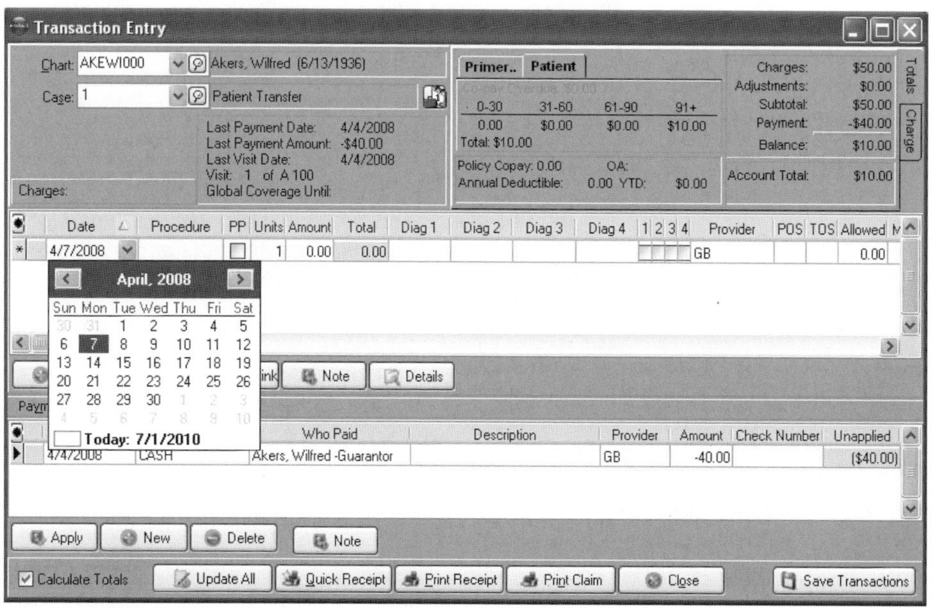

Figure **SI 6-36** *Medisoft® is a registered trademark of McKesson Corporation and/or one of its subsidiaries. Medisoft® screen shots and materials used with the permission of McKesson Corporation. © 2010 McKesson Corporation. All rights reserved.*

Verify that the *Date*, *Procedure*, and *Diagnosis* fields have been completed correctly. If any errors have occurred, the charge line may be deleted while in the *Transaction Entry* window. Select and highlight the date of service for the charge line to be deleted. With the charge line highlighted click on the *Delete* button located at the bottom of the *Transaction Entry, Charges* window **(Figure SI 6-37)**. If all charges are correct as entered, payments received and included on the superbill may also be entered while in the *Transaction Entry* window. To enter payments, see the following section on payment entry. If no payments are to be entered at this time, click on the *Update All* button located at the bottom of the *Charge Entry* window. Next, close the *Transaction Entry* window by clicking on the *Close* button located at the bottom of this window.

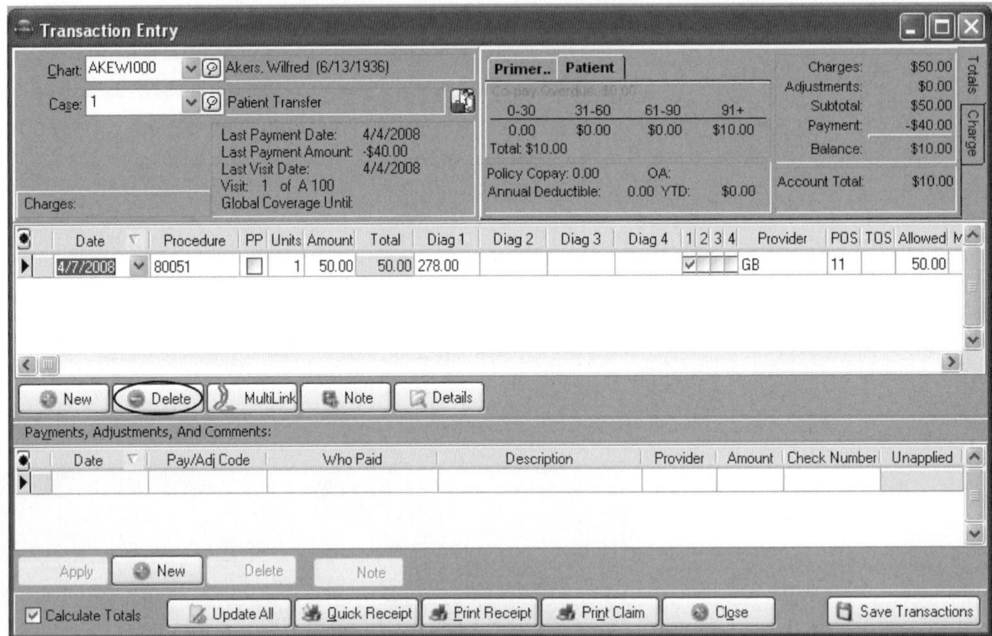

Figure **SI 6-37** *Medisoft® is a registered trademark of McKesson Corporation and/or one of its subsidiaries. Medisoft® screen shots and materials used with the permission of McKesson Corporation. © 2010 McKesson Corporation. All rights reserved.*

H. Payment Entry

From the main menu click on *Activities* located on the toolbar at the top of the main menu of the Medisoft program. From the drop down menu, select *Enter Transactions* **(Figure SI 6-34)**. The *Transaction Entry* window is now available **(Figure SI 6-35)**. Using the search button located in the *Chart* field, open the *Patient Search* window and select the patient for which you are entering charges. Use the drop down arrow in the *Case* field to select the case for this patient. The software program will populate the *Chart* field with the ID number of the patient. Clicking in each field of the *Payments, Adjustments, and Comments* portion of the *Transaction Entry* window will activate a drop down list for each field **(Figure SI 6-36)**. Enter the date the payment was received in the *Date* field. Using the drop down arrows in the *Pay/Adj Code* and *Who Paid* fields, complete these fields with the information from each source document (superbill, EOB, etc.). Enter the amount received in the *Amount* field.

Verify that all information entered is correct. Next, the payment will need to be applied to the patient's account. Click on the *Apply* button, located at the bottom of the *Payments, Adjustments, and Comments* portion of the *Transaction Entry* window. In the *Apply Payments to Charges* window **(Figure SI 6-37)**, click *This Payment* field to enter the amount to be applied to each charge. Verify that all funds have been applied by reviewing the *Unapplied* field located at the top of the *Apply Payments to Charges* window **(Figure SI 6-38)**. If all funds have been applied, the *Unapplied* field should be 0.00. Once all information has been verified as correct, click the *Close* button located at the bottom of the *Apply Payments to Charges* window. In the *Transaction Entry* window, click the *Update All* and then *Close* button located at the bottom of the window.

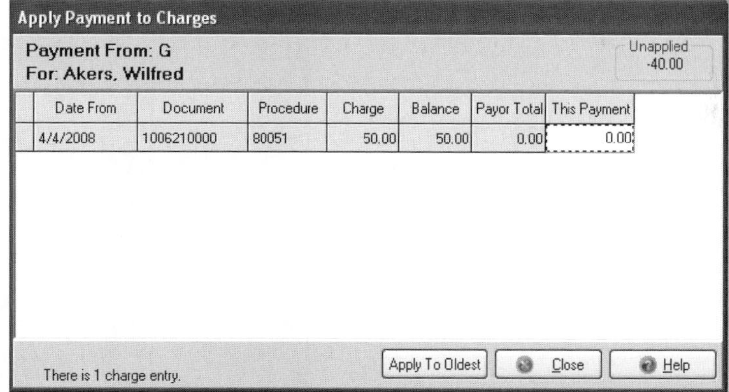

Figure **SI 6-38** *Medisoft® is a registered trademark of McKesson Corporation and/or one of its subsidiaries. Medisoft® screen shots and materials used with the permission of McKesson Corporation. © 2010 McKesson Corporation. All rights reserved.*

DELETING OR EDITING CHARGES/PAYMENTS

Once applied, charges and/or payments may be deleted from the patient's account. From the main menu click on *Activities*, located on the toolbar at the top of the main menu. From the drop down menu, select *Patient Ledger* **(Figure SI 6-39)**. The *Quick Ledger* window is now available **(Figure SI 6-40)**. Use the search button in the *Chart* field to locate and select the patient. Select and highlight the transaction line to be deleted and right click to open the *Quick Ledger* menu. Selecting *Edit* from this menu will return you to the *Transaction Entry* window for the charge/payment **(See Charge/Payment Entry)**. To delete the charge/payment, select *Delete Transaction* from the *Quick Ledger* menu **(Figure SI 6-41)**. A confirmation window will open. Confirm the deletion by clicking the *Yes* button in this window. Once all transactions have been deleted, click the *Update All* button to save your changes.

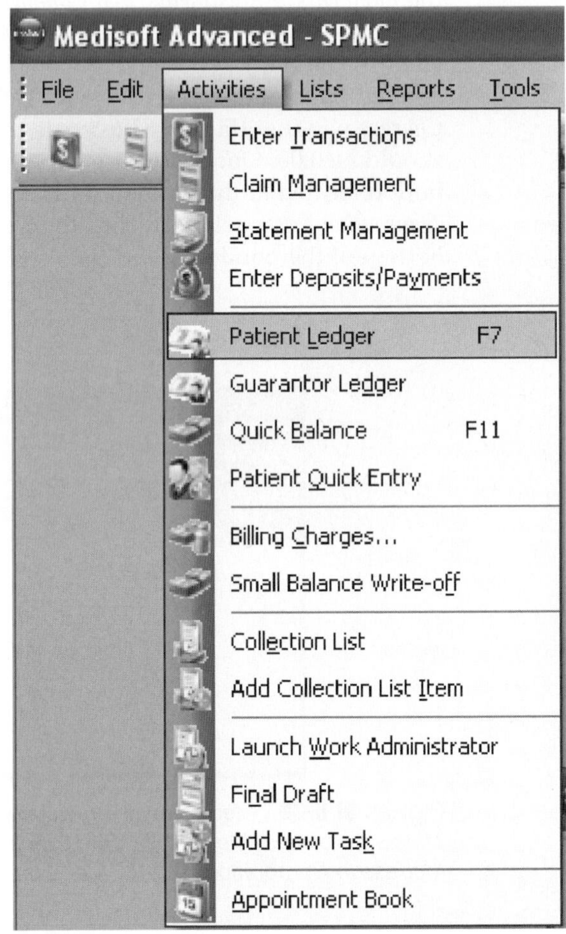

Figure **SI 6-39** *Medisoft® is a registered trademark of McKesson Corporation and/or one of its subsidiaries. Medisoft® screen shots and materials used with the permission of McKesson Corporation. © 2010 McKesson Corporation. All rights reserved.*

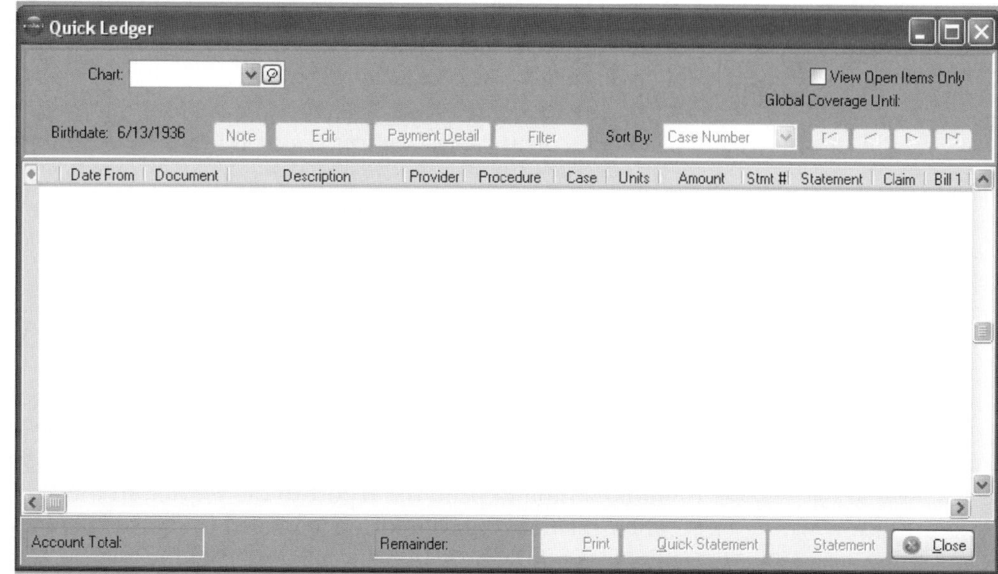

Figure **SI 6-40** *Medisoft® is a registered trademark of McKesson Corporation and/or one of its subsidiaries. Medisoft® screen shots and materials used with the permission of McKesson Corporation. © 2010 McKesson Corporation. All rights reserved.*

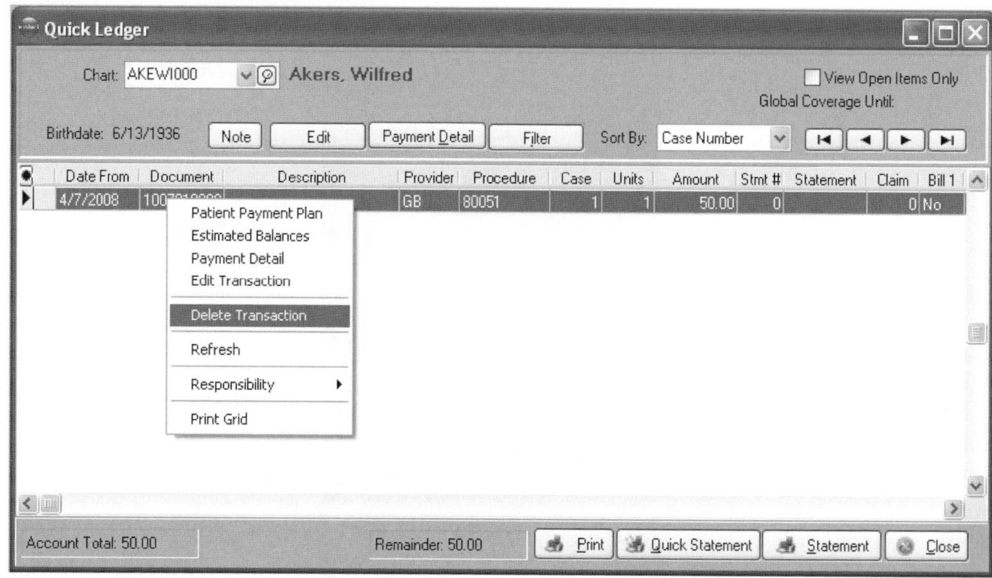

Figure **SI 6-41** *Medisoft® is a registered trademark of McKesson Corporation and/or one of its subsidiaries. Medisoft® screen shots and materials used with the permission of McKesson Corporation. © 2010 McKesson Corporation. All rights reserved.*

I. Patient Ledger

To print a patient ledger, select *Activities* from the main menu toolbar. From the *Activities* menu, select *Patient Ledger* **(Figure SI 6-39)**. In the *Quick Ledger* window, use the *Search* button in the *Chart* field to locate and select the patient. Click on the *Print* button located at the bottom of the *Quick Ledger* window. Verify the ledger is correct and click the *Print* button located at the top of the *Preview Report* window.

J. Day Sheet with Transaction Detail

From the main menu, click on *Reports* located on the toolbar at the top of the screen. Click on *Day Sheets* in the drop down menu, then *Patient Day Sheet* from the next drop down menu **(Figure SI 6-42)**. In the *Print Report Where?* window, click on the radio button to print the report to the printer. In the *Print Report Where?* window, enter the date the charges were posted in the *and the Date Created is between* fields. Enter the date the charges were posted in the *and the Date From is between* fields **(Figure SI 6-43)**. Once you have verified the information requested is correct, click the *OK* button located at the bottom of the *Search* window.

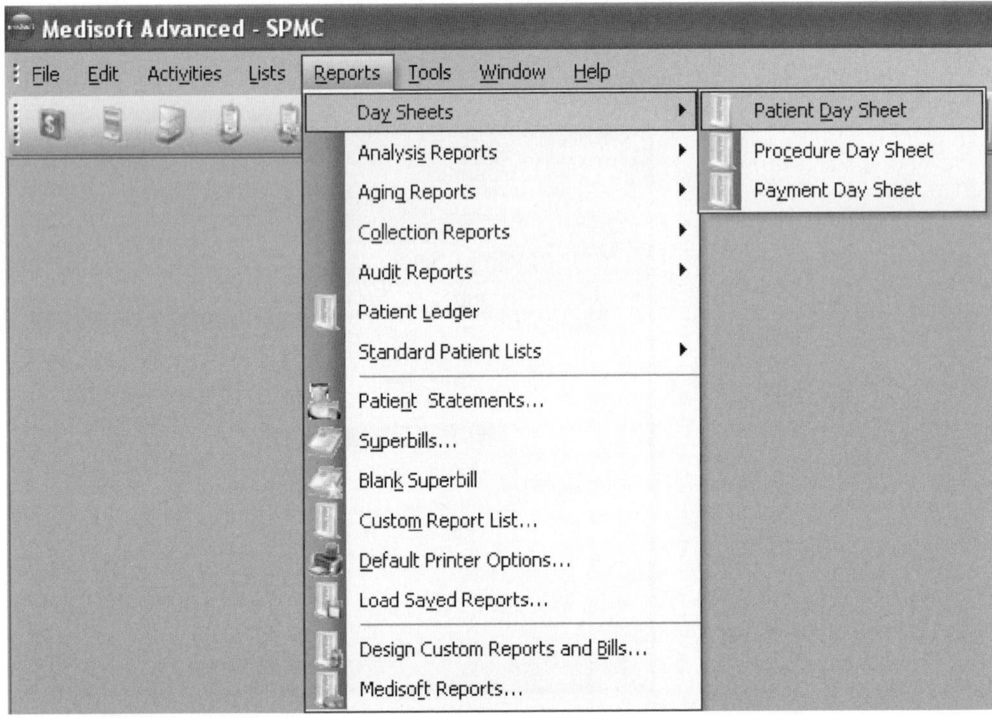

Figure **SI 6-42** *Medisoft® is a registered trademark of McKesson Corporation and/or one of its subsidiaries. Medisoft® screen shots and materials used with the permission of McKesson Corporation. © 2010 McKesson Corporation. All rights reserved.*

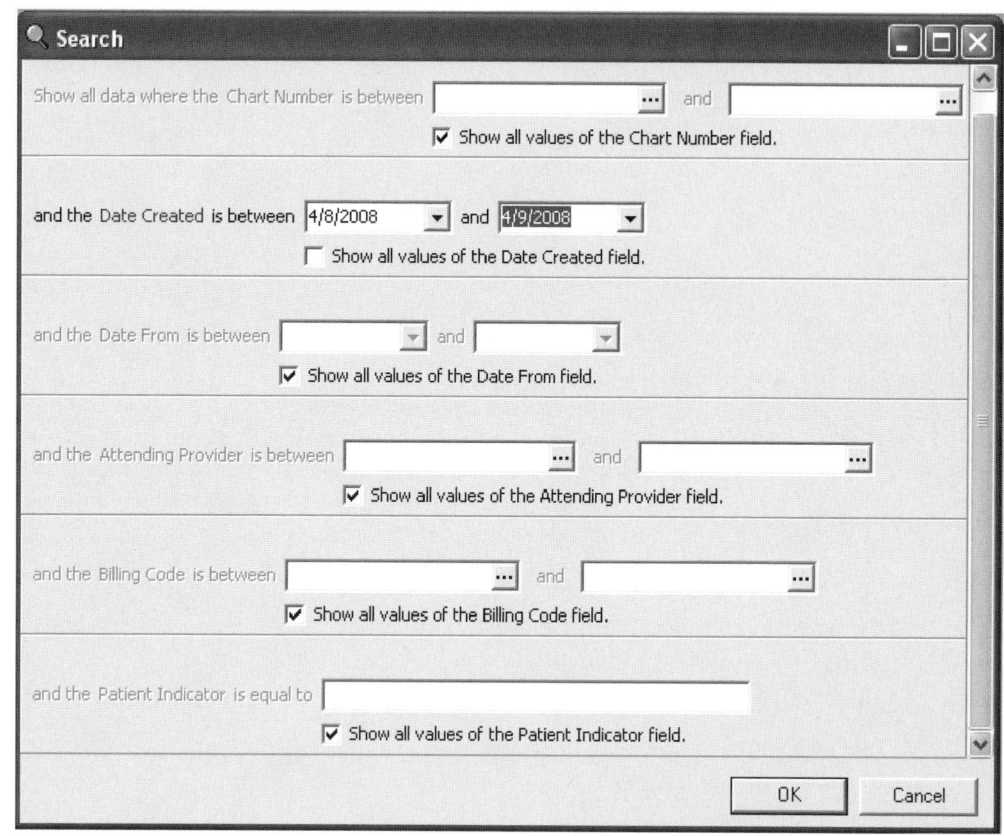

Figure **SI 6-43** *Medisoft® is a registered trademark of McKesson Corporation and/or one of its subsidiaries. Medisoft® screen shots and materials used with the permission of McKesson Corporation. © 2010 McKesson Corporation. All rights reserved.*

MEDISOFT SOFTWARE INSTRUCTIONS

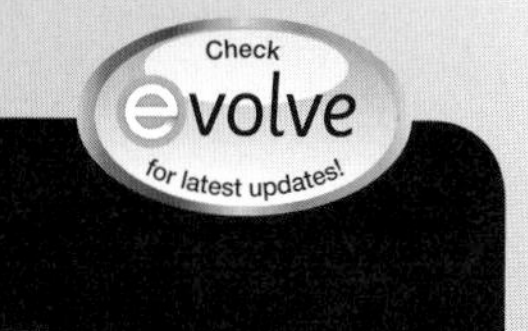
Check
evolve
for latest updates!

STUDENT MANUAL

Supplies from the Supplies section (p. 221) are also located in the forms library on the Evolve site at http://evolve.elsevier.com/Buck/practicekit/.

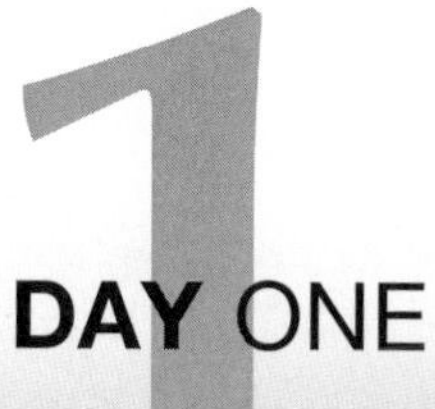

DAY ONE

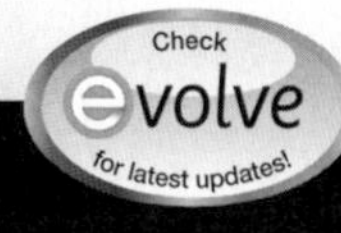

Monday, April 7, 2008

TASK **1.1**

Risk Management

Today, before you begin your internship, Gladys, medical office assistant, tells you that she would like to share a very important part of her job with you—risk management. She explains that risk management procedures are used in the Center and are the responsibility of all staff members. *Risk* is defined as any occurrence that may result in a patient, staff member, or visitor being injured or any liability that could result in financial loss to the Center. A major risk factor to any health care facility is management of patient information, and it is an important aspect of every health care facility member's job. Gladys has been designated the privacy officer for the Center and as such is responsible for ensuring that policies and procedures are in place and that all staff are trained in patient rights and the Health Insurance Portability and Accountability Act of 1996 (HIPAA). The primary function of HIPAA is to provide continuous insurance coverage for employees and their dependents when they change jobs or lose their jobs. Another function of HIPAA is to reduce the costs of managing the exchange of patient data. One part of the management of patient data is standardization of electronic transactions, and another part is the implementation of security and privacy procedures that ensure confidentiality of patient information. Further, the Act ensures that the patients have the legal right to restrict access to their health records and know who accesses their records. All staff members are responsible for complying with HIPAA and safeguarding all patient information.

Another important component of risk management reduction in the health care setting is for each employee to report any situation that may place patients, employees, or the facility at risk. For example, if you witness any behavior that would be considered risky, such as the odor of alcohol on a fellow employee, you should immediately report the behavior to your supervisor. Also, your attention to details that may present a risk in the Center, such as a rug with a turned-up corner or a chair that is placed too far into a traffic path in the waiting room, is essential. You are to be alert to every possible detail in the office to ensure that the office space is as safe as we can make it. Each member of the health care team must assume the responsibility for safety in the Center.

You also will find a confidentiality statement in the Supplies section (p. 225). You are to now read the statement, sign it, and place it in the General file.

TASK **1.2**

Preparing the Schedules

Gladys has asked you to prepare the schedule for November 10 to November 21 for appointments by blocking off the times when the physicians will not be available. Gladys previously prepared the schedules through November 9. If you are completing the scheduling activities using the paper appointment sheets, please enter all information onto the schedule in pencil and print clearly. For all other handwritten documents you will use a pen.

SUPPLIES NEEDED

- 10 appointment sheets dated Monday, November 10, to Friday, November 21
- 1 file folder and 1 file folder label

November 2008						
S	M	T	W	T	F	S
						1
2	3	4	5	6	7	8
9	10	11	12	13	14	15
16	17	18	19	20	21	22
23	24	25	26	27	28	29
30						

1. **Write the physicians' names on the appointment sheets.**
   - Note that on the Monday, November 10, appointment sheet, not only has the date been entered, but also the last names of each of the Center's four physicians. Using Monday's appointment sheet as a model, write the physicians' names at the top of each column on the schedule's remaining 9 days of the appointment sheets.

2. **Read about establishing an appointment sheet matrix.**
   - Matrixing means you mark off the times when a physician is not available for appointments. Referring to Appendix 2, Policies and Procedures (p. 163), in this text, locate Items I through M. These items contain the scheduling preferences of each physician.
   - *Caution:* Be sure to read all information regarding schedules contained in Items I through M **before** you begin to matrix the appointment schedules. Use a pencil for all entries on the schedule.
   - You will begin by marking off the times when Dr. Bond is unavailable for appointments for the weeks of November 10-21. According to Item I, Dr. Bond is unavailable before 10 AM on Mondays. You will note that on the Monday, November 10, appointment sheet, under Dr. Bond's name, the hours from 8 AM to 10 AM have been marked off by placing an X over the time period and writing "Unavailable" in the space. By marking off the

times when the physician is unavailable for appointments, you can be certain that all office employees know not to schedule appointments for Dr. Bond before 10 AM on Monday.

3. **Read about and mark off lunch breaks on Dr. Bond's schedule.**
   - The directions in Item J, Physicians' Lunch Hours, indicate that when a physician begins his/her appointments at 10 AM, the lunch break is to be scheduled from 1 PM to 2 PM. Note that Dr. Bond's lunch has been previously marked off on the Monday, November 10, appointment schedule from 1 PM to 2 PM in accordance with his stated preference. Referring to Dr. Bond's office hours in Item I and his lunch hour preferences in Item J, mark off Dr. Bond's lunch hours for the remainder of the week, Tuesday, November 11, through Friday, November 14.

4. **Mark off Dr. Bond's hospital rounds.**
   - According to Item M, Other Physician Scheduling Preferences, Dr. Bond has a board meeting scheduled from 7:30 AM to 8:45 AM on Thursday, and he has requested that you allow an additional 15 minutes after his meeting to allow him time to return to the Center. Mark off from 8 AM to 9 AM on Dr. Bond's Thursday appointment schedule and write "Board Meeting" on the schedule, as illustrated in **Figure 1-1.** This will ensure that all employees referencing Dr. Bond's schedule for that day will know that he is at a board meeting during that time period. The office staff does not schedule appointments in the times the physician has indicated he does not want to be scheduled. The office staff is not responsible for scheduling Dr. Bond's or any of the physicians' time before 8 AM or after 6 PM, unless specifically requested to do so.
   - On Tuesday and Wednesday, Dr. Bond has hospital rounds from 6 AM until 8:45 AM, plus the additional 15 minutes after his rounds to allow for time to return to the clinic. Mark off his schedule on Tuesday and Wednesday from 8 AM to 9 AM and write "Rounds" on the schedule.

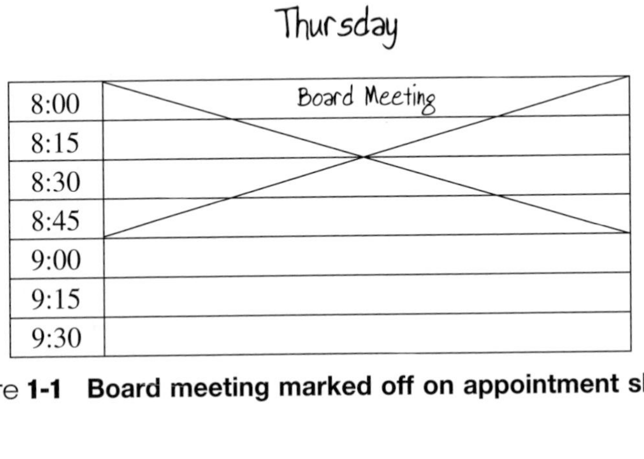

Thursday

8:00	Board Meeting
8:15	
8:30	
8:45	
9:00	
9:15	
9:30	

Figure **1-1** **Board meeting marked off on appointment sheet.**

5. **Mark off Dr. Bond's surgery schedule.**
   - According to Item M, Other Physician Scheduling Preferences, Dr. Bond has requested his surgical procedures be scheduled beginning at 1 PM, with the last procedure scheduled with a starting time of no later than 4 PM on Wednesday and Thursday.
   - Mark off the 1 PM up to the 4:15 PM time period on Dr. Bond's schedule by placing a heavy line around the times reserved for scheduling surgeries.

- **Figure 1-2** illustrates the placement of surgery hours on a physician's schedule. Note that in order to schedule a 4 PM surgery, you must leave the 4 PM to 4:15 PM line in the surgery block open to allow a patient's name to be placed on the 4 PM line.
- Dr. Bond also has requested that the hour before his surgery schedule be marked off to allow him desk time and lunch and to ensure he will be on time for his first surgery. Mark off 12 to 1 PM on Wednesday and Thursday by placing an X though the time as illustrated in **Figure 1-2.**
- The time from 4:15 PM to 6 PM on Dr. Bond's surgery days is to be marked off to allow for time to complete the surgical procedures begun between 1 PM and 4:00 PM. Mark off 4:15 PM to 6 PM on Dr. Bond's schedule on Wednesday and Thursday as "Unavailable," as illustrated in **Figure 1-3.**

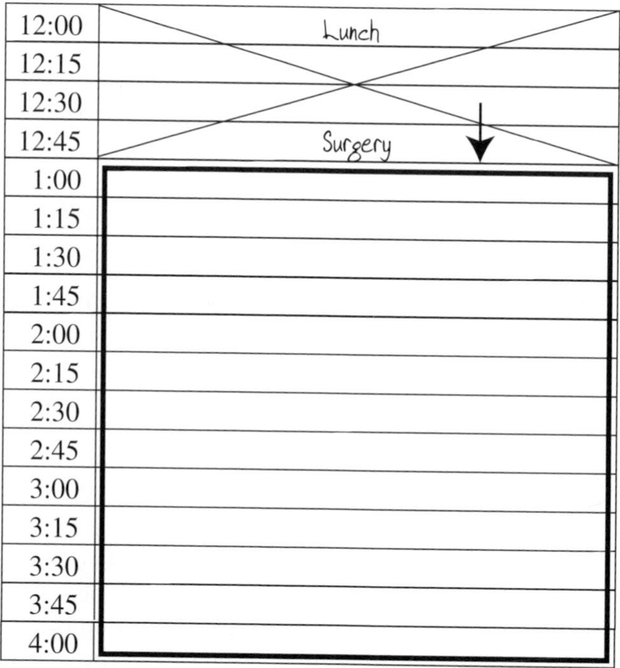

Figure **1-2 Surgery hours marked off on appointment sheet.**

DAY ONE TASK 1.2

Time	
1:00	
1:15	
1:30	
1:45	
2:00	
2:15	
2:30	
2:45	
3:00	
3:15	
3:30	
3:45	
4:00	
4:15	Unavailable
4:30	
4:45	
5:00	
5:15	
5:30	
5:45	

Figure **1-3** **Unavailable time periods marked off on appointment sheet.**

6. **Mark off the end-of-day time blocks.**
   - On Tuesday and Friday Dr. Bond works until 5 PM. The time from 5 PM to 6 PM needs to be marked off so no one will inadvertently schedule an appointment that will begin at or continue past 5 PM. According to Item L, you are to do this by placing an X over the four time slots from 5 PM to 6 PM. Refer to **Figure 1-4** for an example of how this time is marked off. Mark off the time at the end of the day and label the time from 5 PM to 6 PM as "Unavailable."

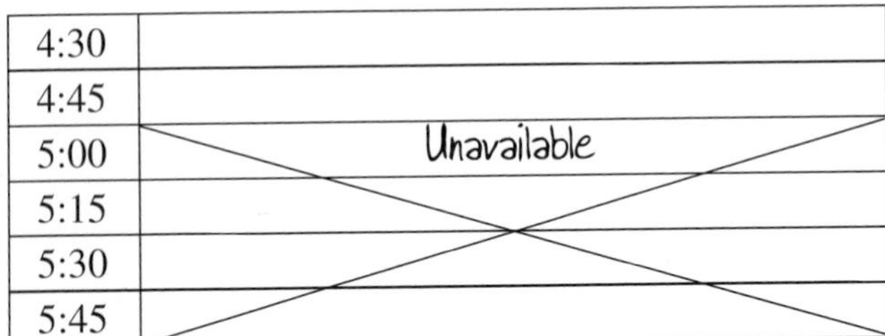

4:30
4:45
5:00
5:15
5:30
5:45
Unavailable

Figure **1-4** **End-of-day time marked off on appointment sheet.**

7. **Review Dr. Bond's schedule.**
   - Dr. Bond's first weekly schedule is now completely matrixed and ready for scheduling appointments. Review Dr. Bond's Monday through Friday schedule again and ensure that you have written down the reason for each block of time marked off. All time marked off on the physician's schedule should be accounted for. If you do not know the reason, write "Unavailable" over the marked-off time. If you followed the preceding directions correctly, the five days of schedules for Dr. Bond should look similar to those illustrated in **Figure 1-5.**

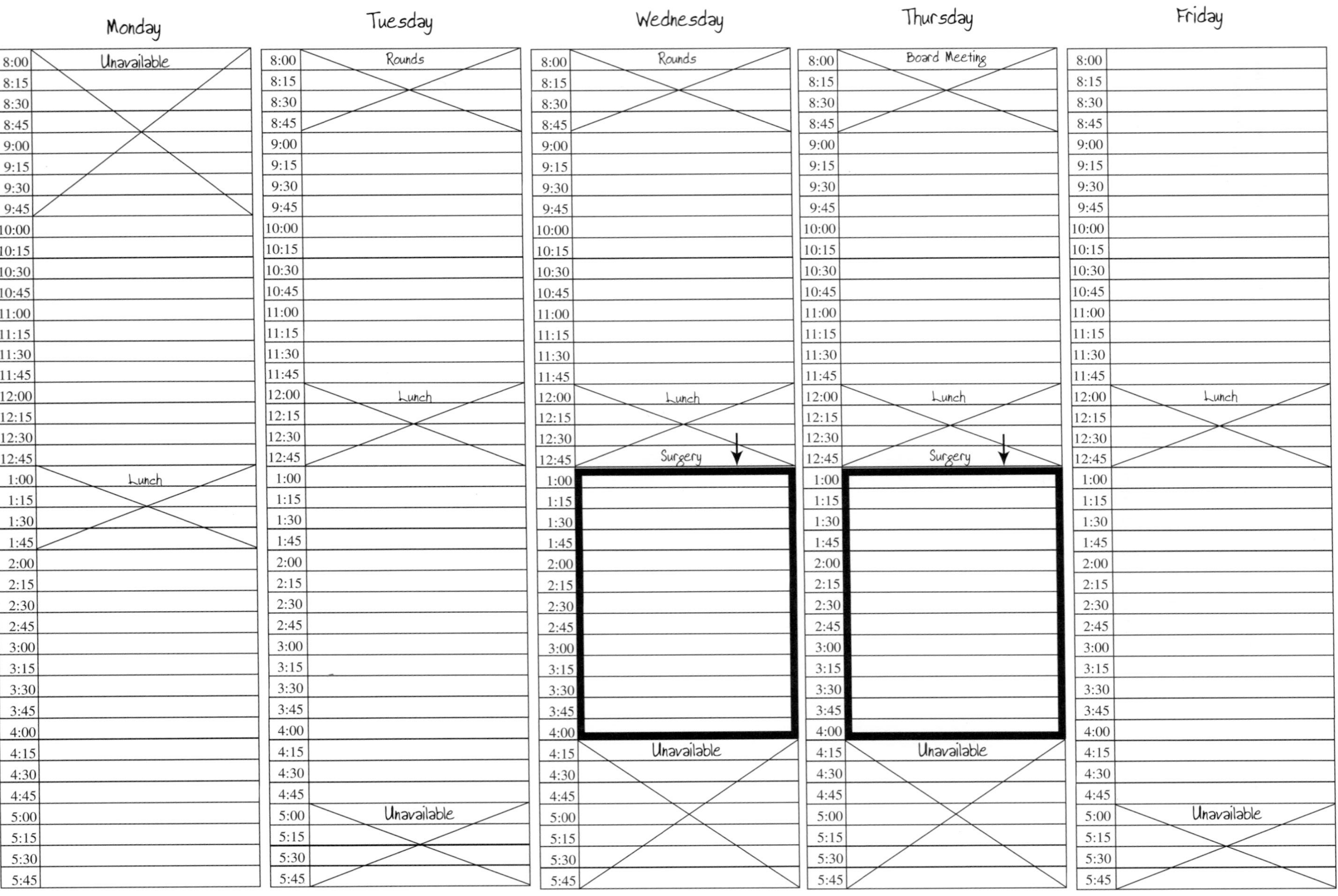

Figure **1-5 Dr. Bond's matrixed schedule for the week of November 10 to November 14.**

8. **Matrix the remaining schedules for the week of Monday, November 10, to Friday, November 14.**
   - Mark off the remaining physicians' schedules using the information about their individual preferences provided to you in Items I through M.
   - Remember to mark off the entire day when Dr. Harkness and Dr. Clark are not in the office and indicate "Unavailable."

9. **Matrix the four physicians' schedules for the week of November 17-21 using the same directions you used for the week of November 10-14.**

10. **Write "COMPLETED WORK" on the file folder label and place the label on the file folder. Place the completed matrixed schedules for November 10-21 in the Completed Work folder.**

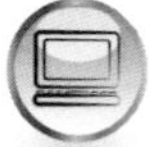

If your instructor has directed the use of the medical practice software, follow these directions: Gladys has asked that you also prepare the schedule for each physician from November 10 to November 21 using the new software scheduling program. She has provided step-by-step instructions for blocking and labeling the time slots. These instructions are located in Software Instructions, Item A (p. SI-29). Following the physician scheduling preferences located in Appendix 2, Items I through M (pp. 170–172), matrix the schedules for each physician. Place the printed schedules in the following order:

- Dr. Bond
- Dr. Adams
- Dr. Harkness
- Dr. Clark

All of Dr. Bond's schedules will be in date order (lowest to highest) and placed first in the folder, followed by all Dr. Adams' schedules in date order, and so on.

TASK **1.3**

Scheduling Telephone Appointments and Inpatient Consultations

SUPPLIES NEEDED **(p. 227)****:**

- Appointment sheets for Monday, April 7, to Friday, April 18
- Access Evolve site containing telephone messages from Saturday, April 5, and Sunday, April 6
- 8 blank Telephone Records (as illustrated in **Figure 1-6**) (located in the Supplies section)
- 3 blank Request for Inpatient Consultation forms (as illustrated in **Figure 1-7**) (located in the Supplies section)

1. Locate the "Telephone Messages" area on the Evolve site (Task 1.3).
   - Requests for appointments came into the office over the weekend (April 5 and 6). Gladys has asked you to listen to the voice mail of the calls and complete a Telephone Record for each call.

PRIORITY ☐

Telephone Record

Patient	Age	Message	
Caller			
Telephone			
Referred to		Temp	Allergies
Chart #		Response	
Chart Attached ☐ YES ☐ NO			
Date / /	Time / Rec'd By	PHY/RN Initials	Date / / / Time / Handled By

Figure **1-6** **Telephone Record form.**

- Schedule the Appointments: If the patient requests a specific time for an appointment and the time the patient requested is not available, schedule the patient as close as you can to the requested time. Refer to Appendix 2, Policies and Procedures, Item N, for directions on scheduling appointments.
- Indicate on the Telephone Record the date and time of the tentative appointment in the "Response" block. Gladys will then review the appointments you made and call each of the patients to confirm the tentative appointment you made for them.
- The voice mail messages may contain calls from other physicians who are requesting that a Center physician do a consultation for a hospital inpatient. For these calls, you are to complete a Request for Inpatient Consultation form. Gladys will review these requests for consultations and deliver them to the appropriate physician. You do not need to complete a Telephone Record

for consultation requests for inpatients because all of the necessary information is located on the Request for Inpatient Consultation form. When a physician requests that one of the Center physicians provide a consultation at the hospital, place the consultation on the appointment schedule. For example, Dr. Thompson requests an inpatient consultation Monday afternoon by Dr. Bond. You would identify adequate time on the schedule, at either the requested time or a convenient time for the Center physician, and enter the information about the patient (e.g., name, room number, reason for consultation, requesting physician, and if the patient is a new or established patient) onto the schedule. The necessary information will be provided. Remember to schedule 15 minutes of travel time before the consultation.

REQUEST FOR INPATIENT CONSULTATION

To: ❑ Gerald Bond, MD
❑ Ray Adams, MD
❑ Joyce Harkness, MD
❑ Anthony Clark, MD

ATTENDING: ____________________
TELEPHONE: ____________________
Request Date and Time: ____________________

PATIENT: ____________________ ADMIT DATE: ____________________

FACILITY: ____________________ FLOOR: __________ ROOM: __________

REASON FOR CONSULTATION: ____________________

PLEASE COMPLETE BY: ____________________ (DATE) RECEIVED BY: ____________________

Figure **1-7** **Request for Inpatient Consultation form.**

- Refer to Appendix 2, Policies and Procedures, Item F, for the step-by-step directions on how to complete the Telephone Record and the Request for Inpatient Consultation forms.

2. Gladys has spoken with Dr. Bond about Dr. Thomas Thompson's request for a consultation on Charlie Burke at the SPH. Dr. Bond has indicated that he would like to go over to the hospital after lunch today and do the consultation. Gladys wants you to write the consultation information on Dr. Bond's schedule to ensure that no one books an appointment for him from 2 PM to 3 PM today, April 7. In addition, she requests you mark off the remainder of the day because Dr. Bond has decided not to return to the office after the hospital consultation.

3. Gladys informs you that Dr. Harkness wants Marion Wilbert seen in consultation after Harriet Muir on Wednesday, April 9. Gladys directs you to schedule the travel from 5:00 PM to 5:15 PM, followed by the consultation, even though only 30 minutes remain on the schedule. Gladys indicates that Bridget Larson should be scheduled for a 30-minute preoperative visit as per directions in Appendix 2,

Item N (p. 173). Place the completed telephone messages, Request for Inpatient Consultation forms, and appointment sheets into the Completed Work folder behind the completed schedules from Task 1.2.

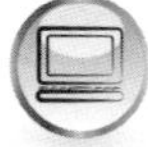

1. Using the completed Telephone Records, Request for Inpatient Consultation forms, and completed appointment sheets from Task 1.3, transfer the new appointments to the office software scheduling program. Gladys has provided step-by-step instructions for scheduling new, established, surgery, emergent, and nursing home appointments in Software Instructions, Item B.
   - Once you have completed scheduling the appointments, Gladys has asked that you print an Appointment List for Monday, April 7, and Wednesday, April 9, for physicians' schedules that changed. This report will allow her to compare the current paper schedule to the new software schedule. Instructions for printing this list are provided in Software Instructions, Item D.

2. Place the Appointment List in the Completed Work folder behind the completed schedules from Task 1.2.

TASK **1.4**

Written Communications

SUPPLIES NEEDED (p. 237):

- Handwritten History and Physical Examination form by Dr. Adams for Gloria Hydorn (2 pages) (located in the Supplies section)
- Blank History and Physical Examination form (as illustrated in **Figure 1-8**) (located in the Supplies section and the Forms Library on the companion Evolve site)
- Handwritten Continuation note by Dr. Adams for Gloria Hydorn (located in the Supplies section)
- Blank Continuation form (as illustrated in **Figure 1-9**) (located in the Supplies section)

1. **History and physical examination.**
   - Last Thursday, April 3, 2008, Dr. Ray Adams saw a new patient, Gloria Hydorn, who recently moved to the area and wanted to establish a family practitioner. Dr. Adams performed a complete history and physical and completed handwritten notes that you will now key onto a History and Physical Examination (H&P) form.

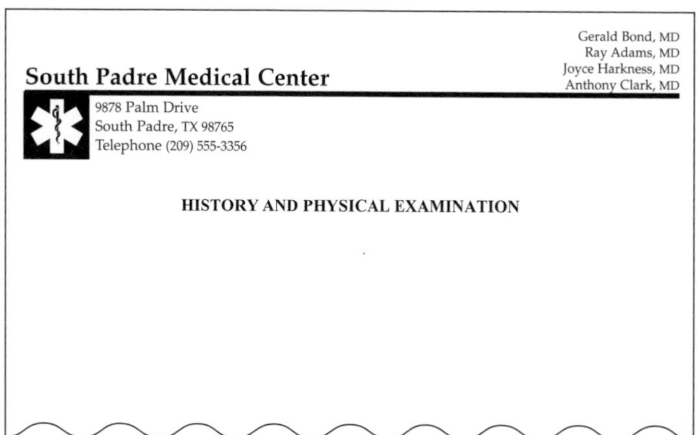
Gerald Bond, MD
Ray Adams, MD
Joyce Harkness, MD
Anthony Clark, MD

South Padre Medical Center

9878 Palm Drive
South Padre, TX 98765
Telephone (209) 555-3356

HISTORY AND PHYSICAL EXAMINATION

Figure **1-8** **History and Physical Examination form.**

2. **Key Dr. Adams's handwritten notes onto the H&P form.**
   - After you have completed the H&P for Gloria Hydorn, set it aside until after the completion of all tasks on Day One because you will be creating a medical record for Gloria Hydorn in Task 1.5 and then you will place both the H&P and Continuation form into the record.

3. **Key Dr. Adams's handwritten continuation notes (word for word) onto the Continuation form.**
   - Dr. Adams noted a left breast lump during Gloria's examination on Thursday and has requested that diagnostic mammography be performed on Friday, April 4. The radiologist performed the mammography and notified Dr. Adams of the findings. After completing the Continuation form, set it aside until after the completion of the medical record for this patient in Task 1.5.

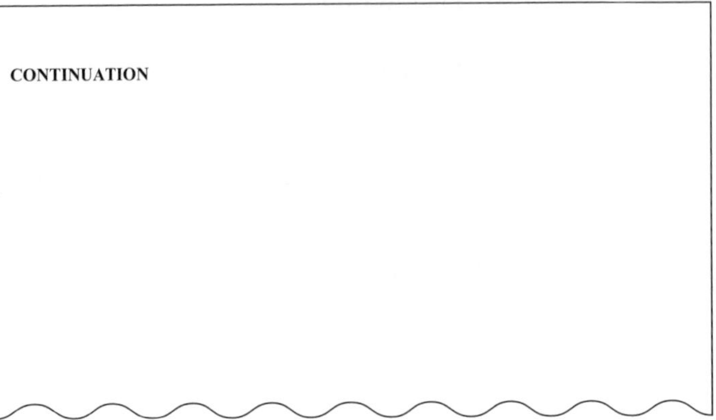
CONTINUATION

Figure **1-9 Continuation form.**

Records Management and Patient List

SUPPLIES NEEDED (p. 247):

- 1 completed Patient Information form for Gloria Hydorn (as illustrated in **Figure 1-10**)
- 11 completed Patient Information sheets
- 11 completed Subsequent Findings sheets
- 12 file folder labels
- 12 file folders
- 2 blank pieces of paper for patient lists
- 1 Filing document

1. Using the completed work from Task 1.3, you will now establish a medical record for Gloria Hydorn.
   - Locate a file folder and a file label in the packet. The patient's name is in capital letters on a label with last name first, then the first name, and then the middle initial (as illustrated in **Figure 1-11**). Secure the label to the file folder.

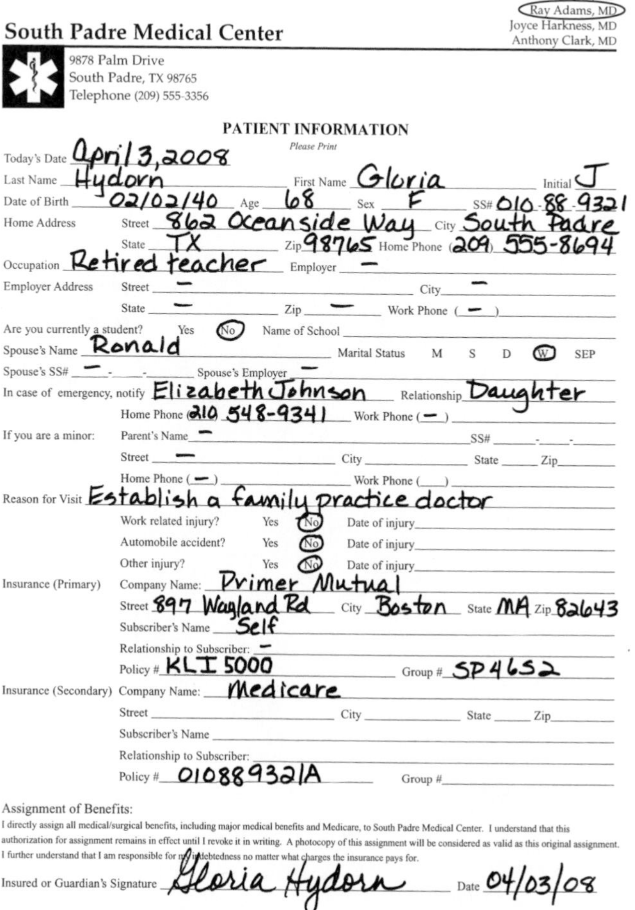

South Padre Medical Center

Gerald Bond, MD
Ray Adams, MD (circled)
Joyce Harkness, MD
Anthony Clark, MD

9878 Palm Drive
South Padre, TX 98765
Telephone (209) 555-3356

PATIENT INFORMATION
Please Print

Today's Date: April 3, 2008
Last Name: Hydorn First Name: Gloria Initial: J
Date of Birth: 02/02/40 Age: 68 Sex: F SS#: 010-88-9321
Home Address: Street: 862 Oceanside Way City: South Padre
State: TX Zip: 98765 Home Phone: (209) 555-8694
Occupation: Retired teacher Employer: —
Employer Address: Street: — City: —
State: — Zip: — Work Phone: (—)
Are you currently a student? Yes No (circled) Name of School:
Spouse's Name: Ronald Marital Status: M S D W (circled) SEP
Spouse's SS#: — Spouse's Employer: —
In case of emergency, notify: Elizabeth Johnson Relationship: Daughter
Home Phone: (210) 548-9341 Work Phone: (—)
If you are a minor: Parent's Name: — SS#:
Street: — City: State: Zip:
Home Phone: (—) Work Phone: ( )
Reason for Visit: Establish a family practice doctor
Work related injury? Yes No (circled) Date of injury:
Automobile accident? Yes No (circled) Date of injury:
Other injury? Yes No (circled) Date of injury:
Insurance (Primary) Company Name: Primer Mutual
Street: 897 Wayland Rd City: Boston State: MA Zip: 82643
Subscriber's Name: Self
Relationship to Subscriber: —
Policy #: KLI 5000 Group #: SP4652
Insurance (Secondary) Company Name: Medicare
Street: City: State: Zip:
Subscriber's Name:
Relationship to Subscriber:
Policy #: 010889321A Group #:

Assignment of Benefits:
I directly assign all medical/surgical benefits, including major medical benefits and Medicare, to South Padre Medical Center. I understand that this authorization for assignment remains in effect until I revoke it in writing. A photocopy of this assignment will be considered as valid as this original assignment. I further understand that I am responsible for my indebtedness no matter what charges the insurance pays for.

Insured or Guardian's Signature: Gloria Hydorn Date: 04/03/08

Figure **1-10** **Patient Information sheet for Gloria Hydorn.**

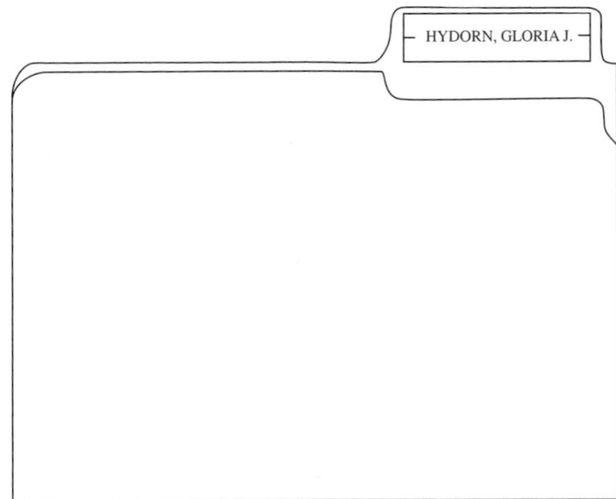

Figure **1-11** **Gloria Hydorn's patient medical record file folder.**

2. Assemble the patient's medical record.
   - In the Supplies section you will find a completed Patient Information form for Gloria Hydorn. Place the information form first in the file with the top of the form to the left edge of the file. This way, when you place the file on the desk in front of you and open it, the information sheet will be the first document and the heading will be at the top of the file (as shown in **Figure 1-12**).

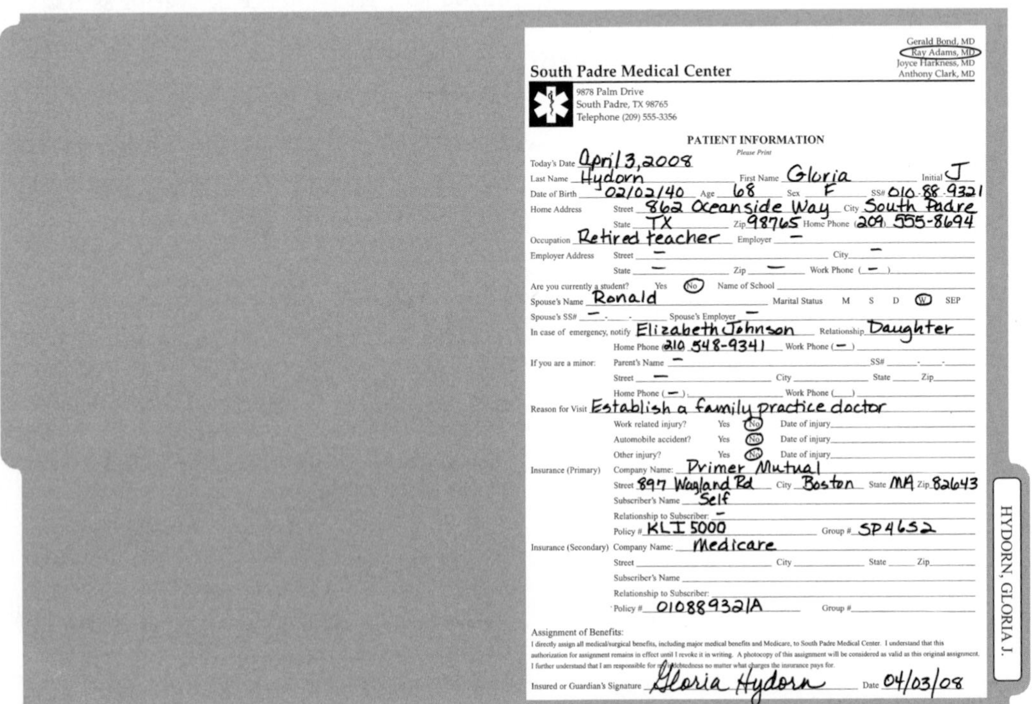

South Padre Medical Center

Gerald Bond, MD
Ray Adams, MD
Joyce Harkness, MD
Anthony Clark, MD

9878 Palm Drive
South Padre, TX 98765
Telephone (209) 555-3356

PATIENT INFORMATION

Please Print

Today's Date April 3, 2008
Last Name Hydorn First Name Gloria Initial J
Date of Birth 02/02/40 Age 68 Sex F SS# 010-88-9321
Home Address Street 862 Oceanside Way City South Padre
State TX Zip 98765 Home Phone (209) 555-8694
Occupation Retired teacher Employer —
Employer Address Street — City —
State — Zip — Work Phone (—)
Are you currently a student? Yes (No) Name of School
Spouse's Name Ronald Marital Status M S D (W) SEP
Spouse's SS# —-- Spouse's Employer —
In case of emergency, notify Elizabeth Johnson Relationship Daughter
Home Phone (210) 548-9341 Work Phone (—)
If you are a minor: Parent's Name — SS# --
Street — City State Zip
Home Phone (—) Work Phone ( )
Reason for Visit Establish a family practice doctor
Work related injury? Yes (No) Date of injury
Automobile accident? Yes (No) Date of injury
Other injury? Yes (No) Date of injury
Insurance (Primary) Company Name: Primer Mutual
Street 897 Wagland Rd City Boston State MA Zip 82643
Subscriber's Name Self
Relationship to Subscriber: —
Policy # KLI 5000 Group # SP4652
Insurance (Secondary) Company Name: Medicare
Street City State Zip
Subscriber's Name
Relationship to Subscriber:
Policy # 010889321A Group #

Assignment of Benefits:
I directly assign all medical/surgical benefits, including major medical benefits and Medicare, to South Padre Medical Center. I understand that this authorization for assignment remains in effect until I revoke it in writing. A photocopy of this assignment will be considered as valid as this original assignment. I further understand that I am responsible for my indebtedness no matter what charges the insurance pays for.

Insured or Guardian's Signature Gloria Hydorn Date 04/03/08

Figure **1-12** **Placement of Patient Information sheet in medical record file folder.**

- The second and third items in the file should be the History and Physical Examination form and the Continuation page you completed in Task 1.4. Place the papers in reverse chronological order. The order of the medical record for Gloria Hydorn from the first page to the last will be:
- Completed Patient Information sheet (first)
- Continuation page (second)
- History and Physical Examination form (pages 1 and 2) (last)

3. Assemble the established patient's medical records.
    - Using the supplies located in this packet, you will now assemble the established patients' medical records for Monday, April 7, 2008.
    - Prepare a file folder for each of the established patients scheduled with Dr. Bond and Dr. Adams on Monday, April 7, 2008. Note that the patient's name is on the label in capital letters—last name, first name, middle initial.
    - Place the Patient Information form and the Subsequent Findings form into the file folder with the Patient Information form first.
    - After completing the files, place all files in *alphabetic* order.

4. Using the information regarding a color-coded filing system in Appendix 2, Policies and Procedures, Item Q, of this Student Manual, indicate on the form in the Supplies section for this task the first two colors used on these patients' charts. For example, Carrie Anderson would be filed "Anderson, Carrie" and the color for the letter "A" is gray and the color for the letter "N" is green.

5. On the same form (from the Supplies section for this task), place in numeric order the 10 patient numbers previously taken from an accession ledger by Monday. Indicate the first two colors used in the color coding of these patient numbers. For example, 5678 (Kathy Sue Thompson) would be represented by 005678 and would be the first number in the list of 10. The color for the number "0" is gray, and the first two colors for 005678 would be gray and gray.

6. Prepare a Patient List for Dr. Bond and Dr. Adams for Monday, April 7, 2008. An example of the format used for the Patient List is illustrated in **Figure 1-13**. Refer to Appendix 2, Item O, for directions on Patient Lists.

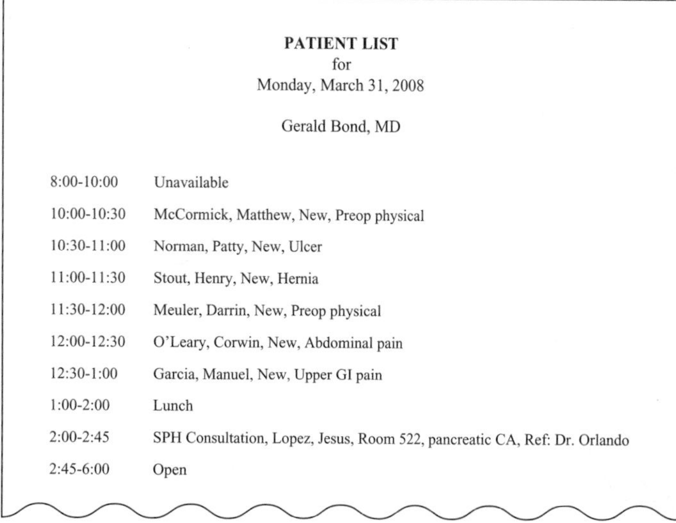

PATIENT LIST
for
Monday, March 31, 2008

Gerald Bond, MD

8:00-10:00	Unavailable
10:00-10:30	McCormick, Matthew, New, Preop physical
10:30-11:00	Norman, Patty, New, Ulcer
11:00-11:30	Stout, Henry, New, Hernia
11:30-12:00	Meuler, Darrin, New, Preop physical
12:00-12:30	O'Leary, Corwin, New, Abdominal pain
12:30-1:00	Garcia, Manuel, New, Upper GI pain
1:00-2:00	Lunch
2:00-2:45	SPH Consultation, Lopez, Jesus, Room 522, pancreatic CA, Ref: Dr. Orlando
2:45-6:00	Open

Figure **1-13** **Sample Patient List.**

7. Place the filing form, all file folders, and the Patient Lists into the Competed Work folder behind the work from Task 1.3.

Always place your completed work from one task behind the work from the previous task. So, the completed work from Task 1.2 is placed behind the work from Task 1.1. In this way, the completed work from Task 1.1 is always first in the Completed Work folder. If, as in this task, the completed work is folders, always place the work in alphabetic order. Anderson is in the first position, Burthold in the second, Carlisle in the third, and so on. Once alphabetized, place the work in the completed work folder.

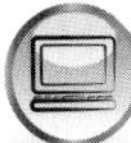

1. Enter Gloria Hydorn's patient information into the new software system using the completed Patient Information form. The step-by-step instructions for entering patient information are located in Software Instructions, Item E. Once all the demographic information has been entered, print a Patient Face Sheet to review the information for errors. The instructions for printing the Patient Face Sheet are located in Software Instructions, Item F.

2. Place the printed Patient Face Sheet in the Completed Work folder behind the work from Task 1.3.

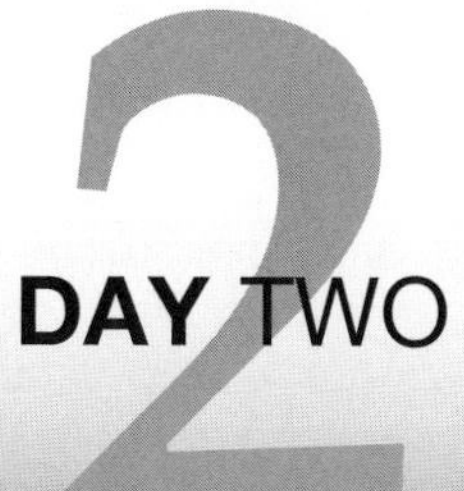

DAY TWO

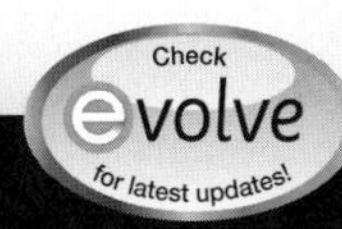
Check
evolve
for latest updates!

Tuesday, April 8, 2008

TASK **2.1**

Patient List

SUPPLIES NEEDED:

- Appointment schedule for Tuesday, April 8, from Completed Work file
- 2 sheets of plain white paper

1. Prepare today's Patient Lists for Dr. Bond and Dr. Adams using the same format that you used in Task 1.5.

2. Place the completed Patient Lists in the Completed Work file.

1. Print today's Appointment List for Dr. Bond and Dr. Adams following the instructions listed in Software Instructions, Item D.

2. Place the Schedule Reports in the Completed Work file.

TASK **2.2**

Patient Reception

SUPPLIES NEEDED (p. 297):

- Appointment schedule for Tuesday, April 8, 2008, from Completed Work file
- 6 file folders
- 6 completed file labels
- 6 completed Patient Information forms **(Figure 2-1)**
- 6 completed Patient Face Sheets from Medisoft **(Figure 2-2)**
- 6 blank Subsequent Findings forms **(Figure 2-3)**

1. This morning you will be working at the reception desk, greeting the patients as they arrive. You will first need to read the Patient Reception directions in Appendix 2, Policies and Procedures, Item P.

2. Assemble the patient's medical record.
   - Locate the 6 file folders and 6 completed labels.
   - Secure the completed label to each file folder.

3. In the Supplies section you will find 6 completed Patient Information forms **(Figure 2-1)** and 6 completed Patient Face Sheets from the new office management software **(Figure 2-2)** for Task 2.2. Using the Patient Information forms, locate and circle any errors on the 6 Patient Face Sheets. Assume the patient is the stated age and that the policy number is correct. Place the Patient Information form in the file with the top of the form to the left edge of the file (see Figure 1-12).

Gerald Bond, MD
Ray Adams, MD
Joyce Harkness, MD
Anthony Clark, MD

South Padre Medical Center

9878 Palm Drive
South Padre, TX 98765
Telephone (209) 555-3356

PATIENT INFORMATION

Please Print

Today's Date ________________

Last Name ______________________________ First Name ________________________ Initial ______

Date of Birth ____________________ Age __________ Sex __________ SS# _____-____-_____

Home Address Street ______________________________________ City ________________
State ________________ Zip_________ Home Phone (_____)________________

Occupation ______________________________ Employer ______________________________

Employer Address Street ____________________________________ City________________
State ________________ Zip __________ Work Phone (_____)______________

Are you currently a student? Yes No Name of School ______________________________

Spouse's Name ____________________________ Marital Status M S D W SEP

Spouse's SS# _____-____-_______ Spouse's Employer ______________________________

In case of emergency, notify ______________________________ Relationship______________

Home Phone (___) ________________ Work Phone (___) ________________

If you are a minor: Parent's Name ______________________________________SS# _____-____-_____
Street ______________________ City ______________ State _____ Zip________
Home Phone (___) ________________ Work Phone (___) ________________

Reason for Visit ____

Work related injury? Yes No Date of injury______________________
Automobile accident? Yes No Date of injury______________________
Other injury? Yes No Date of injury______________________

Insurance (Primary) Company Name: ____
Street ______________________ City ______________ State _____ Zip________
Subscriber's Name ____
Relationship to Subscriber: ____________________________________
Policy #______________________________ Group #____________________

Insurance (Secondary) Company Name: ____
Street ______________________ City ______________ State _____ Zip________
Subscriber's Name ____
Relationship to Subscriber: ____________________________________
Policy #______________________________ Group #____________________

Assignment of Benefits:
I directly assign all medical/surgical benefits, including major medical benefits and Medicare, to South Padre Medical Center. I understand that this authorization for assignment remains in effect until I revoke it in writing. A photocopy of this assignment will be considered as valid as this original assignment. I further understand that I am responsible for my indebtedness no matter what charges the insurance pays for.

Insured or Guardian's Signature ______________________________ Date ______________

Figure **2-1** **Patient Information form.**

South Padre Medical Center

Patient Face Sheet

4/8/2008

Patient Chart #:
Patient Name:
Street 1:
Street 2:
City:
Phone:

D.O.B:
Sex:
SSN:
Mar Status:
S.O.F:
Assigned Provider:

Age:

Employer Name:
Street 1:
City:
Phone:

Case Information

Case Desc:
Last Visit:
Referral:
Guarantor Name:
Street 1:
City:
Phone:
SSN:

Diagnosis 1:
Diagnosis 2:
Diagnosis 3:
Diagnosis 4:

Ins Co #:
Insurance 1:
Street 1:
Street 2:
City:
Phone:
Ins-Start:
End:

Insured 1 Name:
Street 1:
Street 2:
Phone:
D.O.B.:
Policy Number:
Group Number:

Sex:Male

Ins Co #:
Insurance 2:
Street 1:
Street 2:
City:
Phone:
Ins-Start:
End:

Insured 2 Name:
Street 1:
Street 2:
City:
Phone:
D.O.B.:
Policy Number:
Group Number:

Sex:

Ins Co #:
Insurance 3:
Street 1:
Street 2:
City:
Phone:
Ins-Start:
End:

Insured 3 Name:
Street 1:
Street 2:
City:
Phone:
D.O.B.:
Policy Number:
Group Number:

Sex:

Figure **2-2** **Patient Face Sheet.**

DAY TWO TASK 2.2

South Padre Medical Center

Patient's Name ______ Age ____ Sex ____ Marital Status S M W D

Address ______ Insurance ______

Telephone ______ Referred ______

Date	Subsequent Findings

Figure **2-3** **Subsequent Findings form.**

4. The second item in the file should be the Subsequent Findings form, so the order of the medical record will be:
    1. Patient Information form
    2. Subsequent Findings form

Once you have completed this task, place the completed files and Patient Face Sheets in your Completed Work folder directly behind Task 2.1.

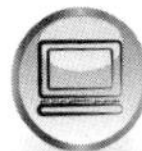

1. Gladys has requested that you correct the demographic errors found on the Patient Face Sheets. Using the instructions from Software Instructions, Item E, correct the patient demographics within the software system.

2. Print a new Patient Face Sheet for each patient and place it in the Completed Work file behind the rest of the work for Task 2.2.

TASK 2.3

Scheduling Appointments

SUPPLIES NEEDED:

- Appointment schedules from your Completed Work file

1. Schedule patients for follow-up appointments
   - Using the patient information from Task 2.2, this morning you will be scheduling three patients for follow-up visits with Dr. Bond for April 16 and 17:
     - Lewis Rock will need a recheck appointment on April 17 at 9 AM for 30 minutes.
     - Ed Goldman will need a recheck appointment on April 17 at 10 AM for 30 minutes. Note the patient's age and the mother's name on the appointment sheet.
     - Thomas Blair will need a recheck appointment on April 16 at 9 AM for 30 minutes for a varicocele recheck.
2. Once you have completed this task, place your work in your Completed Work folder directly behind Task 2.2.

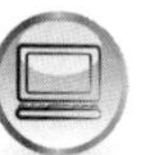

1. Using the step-by-step instructions provided in Software Instructions, Items B and C, reschedule the appointments from Task 2.3 in the software scheduling program.
2. Once all appointments have been scheduled, print an Appointment List for Dr. Bond for April 16 and 17.
3. Place the Appointment List in your Completed Work folder behind Task 2.2.

TASK **2.4**

Medical Transcription

SUPPLIES NEEDED (p. 333):

- Companion Evolve site containing medical dictation for Monday, April 7 (Task 2.4)
- 6 Subsequent Findings forms (located in the Supplies section)

1. Locate the "Transcription" area on the companion Evolve site (Task 2.4).
   - This afternoon Gladys is going to cover the receptionist desk and you are to key in the medical transcription that was dictated Monday, April 7.
   - You will key in dictation for six office visits.
   - Subsequent Findings forms are to be completed by hand and then attached to the transcription. To do this, write the patient's known demographic information at the top of the Subsequent Findings form on the lines provided. In the left-hand column of the form under the "Date" heading, write today's date (April 8) of the visit. In the right-hand column under the "Subsequent Findings" heading, write "See Dr. (physician's name here) dictation dated (April 8)." See **Figure 2-4,** ***A,*** for an example of the format. Then, open a blank document, and start your electronic transcription in the upper left-hand corner with the patient's name (last name, first name, middle initial) on the first line and the date on the second line. Leave two blank spaces and begin to key the physician's dictation. When you have finished keying in the dictation, create a signature line approximately 1½ inches wide double spaced below the last line of the dictation. See **Figure 2-4,** ***B,*** for an illustration of the placement of this line. After the line, key "MD." This is the line that the physician will use to sign the report after he/she has reviewed it. Next, place the physician's initials in capital letters a double space below the physician signature line, followed by a slash and your initials in lower case (refer to Figure 2-4, *B*). Enter another double space and key "DD" for date of dictation in capital letters followed by a colon and two blank spaces. On this line key the date the physician dictated the report. On the next line, key "DT" for date of transcription in capital letters followed by a colon and two blank spaces. On this line key the date you are transcribing the report.
2. Once you have completed this task, place all forms in your Completed Work file.

A

South Padre Medical Center

Patient's Name Adam G. Hoverson Age 14 Sex M Marital Status (S) M W D

Address ______ Insurance ______

Telephone ______ Referred ______

Date	Subsequent Findings
04/08/08	See Dr. Adams' dictation dated 04/07/08.

B

Hoverson, Adam G.
04/07/08

PROBLEM: Clogged ears.

SUBJECTIVE: Adam returns to the clinic. He has had some clogged ears for the last couple of weeks. He denies any specific pain. He tried to clean his ears out and did not really get anything. He did have PE tubes about a year ago and he had apparently flat tympanograms at that time. He denies any runny nose, fever, or chills.

PAST MEDICAL HISTORY: He is on no meds and has no allergies.

PHYSICAL EXAMINATION reveals a well-developed, well-nourished young male in no obvious distress. Temperature is 96.6. Pulse is 72 and regular. Respirations 14 and unlabored. TMs are both slightly dull and red. They have tympanosclerosis. I cannot detect an obvious effusion but the TMs appear retracted.

ASSESSMENT:
1. Otitis media.
2. Tympanosclerosis.

PLAN: I have given him Bactrim DS b.i.d. for two weeks and Claritin-D one p.o. b.i.d., for two weeks. If he is not symptom free in two weeks he will let us know and we will have to do another tympanogram.

______________, MD

RA/si

DD: 04/07/08

DT: 04/08/08

Figure **2-4** **A, Subsequent Findings form and B, transcription format.**

TASK **2.5**

Scheduling Emergency or Urgent Appointments

SUPPLIES NEEDED:

- Appointment schedule for Tuesday, April 8, 2008

1. Work the reception desk to schedule appointments.
    - The rest of the afternoon you will be working the reception desk. During the time you are at the reception desk, three patients will present in need of emergency or urgent appointments.
    - Upon checking the appointment schedule, you will see that both Dr. Bond and Dr. Adams are available.
2. Schedule patients for emergency appointments.
    - Note that if there is not an exact time frame open when the patient arrives, you are to schedule with the physician who has the next available appointment time slot open. You would immediately notify the physician's nurse when an emergency patient arrives.
    - The patients will be arriving between 1 PM and 5 PM. All patients are established patients.
        - David Oakland (Est) arrives at 12:45 PM with a dog bite to the left hand. Schedule the patient with the physician who has an appointment time available. Block off 30 minutes for the appointment.
        - Larry Smith arrives at 3 PM with severe RLQ pain. Schedule this patient with the physician who has an appointment time open. Block off 45 minutes for the appointment.
        - Anne Meires (Est) arrives at 4:15 PM with a severe headache and some dizziness. Schedule this patient with the physician who has an appointment time open. Block off 30 minutes.
3. Once you have completed this task, place the appointment schedule into your Completed Work file. Make sure that your work is placed in order of day and task.

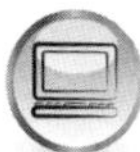

1. Using the step-by-step instructions provided in Software Instructions, Item B, schedule the appointments from Task 2.5 in the software scheduling program.
2. Once all appointments have been scheduled, print an Appointment List for Dr. Bond and Dr. Adams for today's schedule.
3. Place the Appointment List in your Completed Work folder behind Task 2.5.

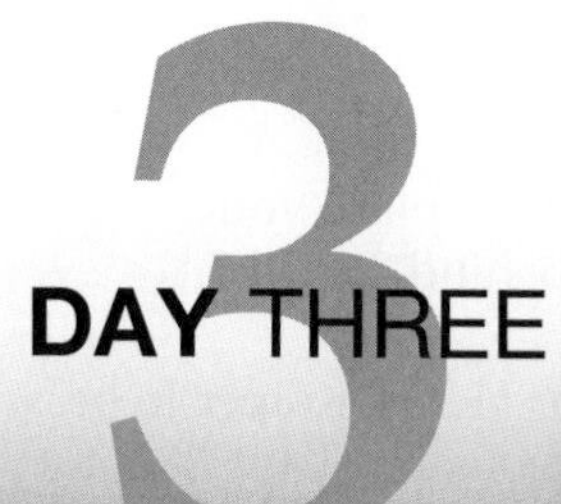

DAY THREE

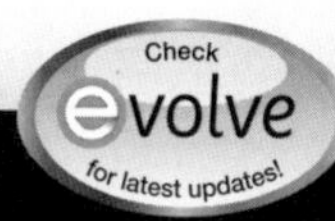
Check
evolve
for latest updates!

Wednesday, April 9, 2008

TASK **3.1**

Patient Reception and Referral

SUPPLIES NEEDED (p. 345):

- Appointment schedule for Wednesday, April 9, from Completed Work folder
- 2 completed Patient Face Sheets for Task 3.1 for Eskew and Kolper (located in the Supplies section)
- 2 blank Patient Information forms (located in the Supplies section)
- 2 blank Subsequent Findings forms (located in the Supplies section, Appendix 4 of the Student Manual, and in the Forms Library on the Evolve site)
- 1 blank referral form (located in the Supplies section)
- 2 file folders (located in the general *Practice Kit* envelope)
- 2 preprinted file labels (located in the general *Practice Kit* envelope)

1. This morning you will be working at the reception desk greeting patients as they arrive. There are two new patients scheduled with Dr. Harkness and Dr. Bond. Gladys has asked you to assemble a medical record for these two new patients scheduled today (Eskew and Kolper).

2. Assemble the patient's medical record.
   - Locate the file folders and preprinted file labels in the envelope. Secure the label to each file folder.
   - In the Supplies section you will find the Patient Face Sheets for Task 3.1 (see Figure 2-2 for the blank form). The information from the Patient Face Sheets and appointment schedule will be used to fill out Patient Information forms for each patient. Although the patients would complete the Patient Information forms themselves, today you will complete the forms to familiarize yourself with the data on the form. Also, there are patients who, due to physical limitations, are unable to complete the forms themselves. Once you have completely filled out each Patient Information form, you will place the Patient Information form first in the file with the top of the form to the left edge of the file. Complete the top portion of the Subsequent Findings form and place it behind the Patient Information form.

3. Once you have completed all file folders for each new patient, place your completed work in your Completed Work folder directly behind Task 2.5.

4. Dr. Harkness has asked Gladys to handle arrangements for Henry Kolper to be referred to Dr. Morton Samson (1256 56th Avenue South, Houston, TX 99881) for his heart murmur. Dr. Morton Samson's office number is 956-934-6120. Gladys has asked you to complete a Referral form (located in the Supplies section, p. 357) and request an appointment as soon as possible (ASAP). Directions for completing Referral forms are in Appendix 2, Policies and Procedures, Item S. Place the form in the Completed Work folder.

TASK **3.2**

Medical Transcription

SUPPLIES NEEDED (p. 359):

- Companion Evolve site for Task 3.2—medical dictation from April 8
- 2 blank Subsequent Findings forms (located in the Supplies section)

Gladys will now take over the reception desk for the rest of the morning. Gladys has asked you to transcribe two of the emergency appointments that were dictated on Tuesday, April 8.

1. Key medical transcription. Locate the "Medical Transcription" area on the companion Evolve site (Task 3.2).

2. Locate the Subsequent Findings forms. If necessary, see specific instructions regarding the format provided in Task 2.4. You are to write the patient's name, age, and sex on the form, but leave the other patient data areas blank (marital status, etc.). Another employee is responsible for obtaining and entering the data.

3. Once you have completed this task, place your completed work in the Completed Work folder directly behind Task 3.1.

TASK **3.3**

Insurance Claim Form

SUPPLIES NEEDED (p. 363):

- 6 blank CMS-1500 health insurance forms (located in the Supplies section)
- 6 Patient Information and 6 Patient Face sheets from the Completed Work file from Task 2.2 for:
  - Lewis Rock
  - Edward Goldman
  - Thomas Blair
  - Jackie King
  - Joe Knight
  - Peter Silverman
- 6 superbills completed for the patients listed above from the Supplies section

1. Completion of CMS-1500 health insurance forms.
   - This afternoon you will be completing CMS-1500 health insurance forms on the six new patients that were seen yesterday, April 8 (Task 2.2). The CMS-1500 form is located in the Supplies section of the Student Manual and in the Forms Library on the companion Evolve site. Appendix 3, Third-Party Payer List and Directions, contains a list of the information entered in each block of the form and the physicians' NPI numbers.
   - To complete each CMS-1500 health insurance claim form (as illustrated in **Figure 3-1**), you will need to use the Patient Information forms from Task 2.2. All patient information for Items 1 through 13 is included on the Patient Face Sheet or the Patient Information sheets completed in Task 2.2. Refer to the superbills to find additional required information.

1500

HEALTH INSURANCE CLAIM FORM

APPROVED BY NATIONAL UNIFORM CLAIM COMMITTEE 08/05

PICA PICA

1. MEDICARE (Medicare #) MEDICAID (Medicaid #) TRICARE CHAMPUS (Sponsor's SSN) CHAMPVA (Member ID#) GROUP HEALTH PLAN (SSN or ID) FECA BLK LUNG (SSN) OTHER (ID) | 1a. INSURED'S I.D. NUMBER (For Program in Item 1)

2. PATIENT'S NAME (Last Name, First Name, Middle Initial) | 3. PATIENT'S BIRTH DATE MM DD YY SEX M F | 4. INSURED'S NAME (Last Name, First Name, Middle Initial)

5. PATIENT'S ADDRESS (No., Street) | 6. PATIENT RELATIONSHIP TO INSURED Self Spouse Child Other | 7. INSURED'S ADDRESS (No., Street)

CITY STATE | 8. PATIENT STATUS Single Married Other | CITY STATE

ZIP CODE TELEPHONE (Include Area Code) ( ) | Employed Full-Time Student Part-Time Student | ZIP CODE TELEPHONE (Include Area Code) ( )

9. OTHER INSURED'S NAME (Last Name, First Name, Middle Initial) | 10. IS PATIENT'S CONDITION RELATED TO: | 11. INSURED'S POLICY GROUP OR FECA NUMBER

a. OTHER INSURED'S POLICY OR GROUP NUMBER | a. EMPLOYMENT? (Current or Previous) YES NO | a. INSURED'S DATE OF BIRTH MM DD YY SEX M F

b. OTHER INSURED'S DATE OF BIRTH MM DD YY SEX M F | b. AUTO ACCIDENT? PLACE (State) YES NO | b. EMPLOYER'S NAME OR SCHOOL NAME

c. EMPLOYER'S NAME OR SCHOOL NAME | c. OTHER ACCIDENT? YES NO | c. INSURANCE PLAN NAME OR PROGRAM NAME

d. INSURANCE PLAN NAME OR PROGRAM NAME | 10d. RESERVED FOR LOCAL USE | d. IS THERE ANOTHER HEALTH BENEFIT PLAN? YES NO *If yes, return to and complete item 9 a-d.*

READ BACK OF FORM BEFORE COMPLETING & SIGNING THIS FORM.

12. PATIENT'S OR AUTHORIZED PERSON'S SIGNATURE I authorize the release of any medical or other information necessary to process this claim. I also request payment of government benefits either to myself or to the party who accepts assignment below.

SIGNED DATE

13. INSURED'S OR AUTHORIZED PERSON'S SIGNATURE I authorize payment of medical benefits to the undersigned physician or supplier for services described below.

SIGNED

14. DATE OF CURRENT: MM DD YY ILLNESS (First symptom) OR INJURY (Accident) OR PREGNANCY(LMP) | 15. IF PATIENT HAS HAD SAME OR SIMILAR ILLNESS. GIVE FIRST DATE MM DD YY | 16. DATES PATIENT UNABLE TO WORK IN CURRENT OCCUPATION FROM MM DD YY TO MM DD YY

17. NAME OF REFERRING PROVIDER OR OTHER SOURCE | 17a. 17b. NPI | 18. HOSPITALIZATION DATES RELATED TO CURRENT SERVICES FROM MM DD YY TO MM DD YY

19. RESERVED FOR LOCAL USE | 20. OUTSIDE LAB? YES NO $ CHARGES

21. DIAGNOSIS OR NATURE OF ILLNESS OR INJURY (Relate Items 1, 2, 3 or 4 to Item 24E by Line) 1. 2. 3. 4. | 22. MEDICAID RESUBMISSION CODE ORIGINAL REF. NO. | 23. PRIOR AUTHORIZATION NUMBER

24. A. DATE(S) OF SERVICE From MM DD YY To MM DD YY	B. PLACE OF SERVICE	C. EMG	D. PROCEDURES, SERVICES, OR SUPPLIES (Explain Unusual Circumstances) CPT/HCPCS MODIFIER	E. DIAGNOSIS POINTER	F. $ CHARGES	G. DAYS OR UNITS	H. EPSDT Family Plan	I. ID. QUAL.	J. RENDERING PROVIDER ID. #
1								NPI	
2								NPI	
3								NPI	
4								NPI	
5								NPI	
6								NPI	

25. FEDERAL TAX I.D. NUMBER SSN EIN | 26. PATIENT'S ACCOUNT NO. | 27. ACCEPT ASSIGNMENT? (For govt. claims, see back) YES NO | 28. TOTAL CHARGE $ | 29. AMOUNT PAID $ | 30. BALANCE DUE $

31. SIGNATURE OF PHYSICIAN OR SUPPLIER INCLUDING DEGREES OR CREDENTIALS (I certify that the statements on the reverse apply to this bill and are made a part thereof.) SIGNED DATE | 32. SERVICE FACILITY LOCATION INFORMATION a. b. | 33. BILLING PROVIDER INFO & PH # ( ) a. b.

NUCC Instruction Manual available at: www.nucc.org PLEASE PRINT OR TYPE APPROVED OMB-0938-0999 FORM CMS-1500 (08-05)

CARRIER — PATIENT AND INSURED INFORMATION — PHYSICIAN OR SUPPLIER INFORMATION

Figure **3-1** **CMS-1500 (08/05) health insurance claim form.**

- Complete Lewis Rock's form and then compare it to the information on the next page. Once you are certain of how to complete the form, complete the remaining 5 forms using the directions that begin on p. 181.
- Using Lewis Rock's form as a guide, complete the CMS-1500 health insurance claim forms for the remaining five patients. The information can be taken from the Patient Information forms used in Task 2.2 and the superbills for April 8, 2008.
- The Center's Federal ID number is 00789200 (p. 181) and is entered in Item 25 of the CMS-1500.

2. Once you have completed the CMS-1500 health insurance claim forms, place all forms in your Completed Work File directly behind Task 3.2. Return the Patient Information sheets to the correct location in the Completed Work folder directly behind Task 2.1.

Item Number	How to Complete the Item
1	Place an X in the Medicare box
1a	201489201A
2	ROCK LEWIS L
3	03 06 1931 Place an X in the "M" box
4	Blank
5	1000 BASS AVENUE SOUTH PADRE TX 97865 (209) 555-2292
6	Place an X in the "Self" box
7	Blank
8	Place an X in the "Married" box
9	Blank
10	Place 3 Xs as follows: Employment, "NO" Auto Accident, "NO" Other Accident, "NO"
11	NONE
12	On "Signed" line place "SOF" (signature on file) Date: 04/09/08
13	On "Signed" line place "SOF"
14	Blank
15	Blank
16	Blank
17	Thomas Thompson MD
17b	1100986210 (see p. 181)
18	Blank
19	Blank
20	Place an X in the "NO" box
21	On line 1, place 171.9
22	Blank
23	Blank
24a	04 08 08
24b	11
24c	Blank
24d	99204
24e	1
24f	105 00

Continued

cont'd

Item Number	How to Complete the Item
24g	Blank
24h	Blank
24i	Blank
24j	4682943911 (see p. 181)
25	00789200, and an X in the "EIN" box (see p. 181)
26	Blank
27	Place an X in the "YES" box
28	105 00
29	Blank
30	105 00
31	Blank
32	SAME
33	(209)555-3356 SOUTH PADRE MEDICAL CENTER 9878 PALM DIRVE SOUTH PADRE TX 98765
33a	Blank
33b	8866905213 (see p. 181)

TASK 3.4

Written Communications

SUPPLIES NEEDED (p. 387):

- 1 blank Subsequent Findings form (located in the Supplies section and in the Forms Library on the companion Evolve site)
- Handwritten progress note by Dr. Bond for Raymond Edwards

1. Progress note.
   - Earlier today Dr. Bond completed a handwritten note on Raymond Edwards, which you will now key onto a Subsequent Findings form (see instructions for completing the form provided in Task 2.4). Dr. Bond saw Mr. Edwards on Friday, April 4, 2008.
2. Once you have completed the progress note, place your completed work in the Completed Work folder directly behind Task 3.3.

Preparing the Superbill

SUPPLIES NEEDED (p. 391):

- 6 blank superbills (illustrated in **Figure 3-2**) (located in the Supplies section)
- April 10, 2008, Appointment Schedule
- 6 completed Patient Face Sheets for Task 3.5 (located in the Supplies section)

1. Preparing superbills for patient services.
   - Gladys has asked you to prepare the superbills for some of the patients scheduled for tomorrow. The shaded areas on the superbill in **Figure 3-2**

South Padre Medical Center

9878 Palm Drive
South Padre, TX 98765
Telephone (209) 555-3356

Gerald Bond, MD
Ray Adams, MD
Joyce Harkness, MD
Anthony Clark, MD

PATIENT'S LAST NAME	FIRST	ACCOUNT #	BIRTHDATE / /	SEX ☐ MALE ☐ FEMALE	TODAY'S DATE / /

INSURANCE COMPANY	SUBSCRIBER	GROUP/PLAN #	SUB. #	TIME

ASSIGNMENT: I hereby assign my insurance benefits to be paid directly to the undersigned physician. I am financially responsible for non-covered services. SIGNED: (Patient, Or parent, if Minor)__________________ DATE: / /	RELEASE: I hereby authorize the physician to release to my insurance carriers any information required to process this claim. SIGNED: (Patient, Or Parent, if Minor) __________________ DATE: / /

✓	DESCRIPTION	CPT	Diag.	FEE
	OFFICE VISIT			
	NEW PATIENT			
	Problem Focused			
	Exp Problem Focused	99202		
	Detailed	99203		
	Comp/ Mod MDM	99204		
	Comp/ High MDM	99205		
	ESTABLISHED PATIENT			
	Minimal/Nurse Visit	99211		
	Problem Focused	99212		
	Exp Problem Focused	99213		
	Detailed	99214		
	Comprehensive	99215		
	CONSULTATION			
	Problem Focused	99241		
	Exp Problem Focused	99242		
	Detailed	99243		
	Comp/ Mod MDM	99244		
	Comp/High MDM	99245		
	Requesting Provider ______________			
	Post-op Exam	99024		0.00
	PREVENTIVE MEDICINE			
	NEW PATIENT			
	Infant – 1 yr	99381		
	1 yr – 4 yr	99382		
	5 yr – 11 yr	99383		
	12 yr – 17 yr	99384		
	18 yr – 39 yr	99385		
	40 yr – 64 yr	99386		
	65 yr and over	99387		
	ESTABLISHED PATIENT			
	Infant – 1 yr	99391		
	1 yr – 4 yr	99392		
	5 yr – 11 yr	99393		
	12 yr – 17 yr	99394		
	18 yr – 39 yr	99395		
	40 yr – 64 yr	99396		
	65 yr and over	99397		
	SUPPLIES			
	Take home burn kit	99070		
	Take home wound kit	99070		
	Miscellaneous			
	MODIFIERS			
	Significant/Sep EM provided with other service	-25		
	Unrelated EM in post op period	-24		
	Repeat procedure, same physician, same day	-76		

✓	DESCRIPTION	CPT	Diag.	FEE
	IMMUNIZATIONS/INJECTIONS			
	Admin of Vaccine 1	90471		
	Admin of Vac 2+	90472		
	TB Tine, skin	86486		
	Pneumococcal	90732		
	Medicare code	G0009		
	Influenza <3	90657	I&D abscess	
	Influenza 3 and >	90658		
	Medicare code	G0008		
	Varicella	90716		
	DPT	90701		
	DT children	90702		
	Td adult	90718		
	DtaP	90700		
	IPV	90713		
	Rubella	90706		
	MMR	90707		
	Hep B Child	90744		
	Hep B Adult	90746		
	IM Administration	96372		
	Compazine	J0780		
	Demerol	J2175		
	Depo-Provera	J1055		
	Dexamethasone	J1100		
	Solumedrol	J1720		
	Antigen admin 1	95115		
	Antigen admin 2+	95117		
	LABORATORY			
	Blood collect Vein	36415		
	Capillary	36416		
	Hemoglobin	85018		
	Glucose, reagent	82948		
	Pregnancy, Serum	84702		
	Pregnancy, Urine	81025		
	Health panel	80050		
	B Met Pan Cal ion	80047		
	B Met Pan Cal tot	80048		
	C Metabolic panel	80053		
	Ob panel	80055		
	Lipid panel	80061		
	UA Auto w/o micro	81003		
	UA dip stck	81000		
	Strep test	87880		
	Hemoccult	82270		
	Lab Handling	99000		

✓	DESCRIPTION	CPT	Diag.	FEE
	PROCEDURES			
	Inhalation treatment	94640		
	Demo/eval treatment	94664		
	Vital Capacity	94150		
	Spirometry	94010		
	EKG w/interpretation	93000		
	10060			
	Remove skin tag <15	11200		
	EXCISION BENIGN LESIONS (inc. margins)			
	Trunk, arms, legs			
	0.5 cm or less	11400		
	0.6 to 1.0 cm	11401		
	1.1 to 2.0 cm	11402		
	2.1 to 3.0 cm	11403		
	Scalp, neck, hand, ft			
	0.5 cm or less	11420		
	0.6 to 1.0 cm	11421		
	1.1 to 2.0 cm	11422		
	2.1 to 3.0 cm	11423		
	Face, ears, eyelids, lip			
	0.5 cm or less	11440		
	0.6 to 1.0 cm	11441		
	1.1 to 2.0 cm	11442		
	2.1 to 3.0 cm	11443		
	EXCISION MALIGNANT LESIONS (inc. margins)			
	Trunk, arms, legs			
	0.5 cm or less	11600		
	0.6 to 1.0 cm	11601		
	1.1 to 2.0 cm	11602		
	2.1 to 3.0 cm	11603		
	Scalp, neck, hand, ft			
	0.5 cm or less	11620		
	0.6 to 1.0 cm	11621		
	1.1 to 2.0 cm	11622		
	2.1 to 3.0 cm	11623		
	Face, ears, eyelids, lip			
	0.5 cm or less	11640		
	0.6 to 1.0 cm	11641		
	1.1 to 2.0 cm	11642		
	2.1 to 3.0 cm	11643		
	Awaiting path report	☐ ***Yes***		☐ ***No***
	Wart destruction < 14	17110		
	Cerumen removal	69210		
	Endometrial biopsy	58100		

30 DAYS	60 DAYS	90 DAYS

DIAGNOSIS:	RETURN APPOINTMENT: (days) (wks) (mos) (PRN)	TODAY'S TOTAL	
1) ______________	NEXT APPOINTMENT: M - T - W - TH - F - S	PREVIOUS BALANCE	
2) ______________			
3) ______________	DATE / / TIME	AMOUNT REC'D TODAY REC'D BY ________	
4) ______________	Provider's Signature:	BALANCE DUE	

Figure **3-2** **Superbill with shading.**

illustrate those areas that you are to complete for this task using information from the appointment schedule and the Patient Face Sheets for Task 3.5.

- You will be completing the aging (length of time the amount has been owed) for each of the superbills you prepare. Complete a superbill for the following patients:

Patient	Previous Balance	30 Days	60 Days	90 Days
a. Mary Bogert	$206.73	$100.73	$106.00	0
b. Elizabeth Fenton	0	0	0	0
c. Amanda Foster	$934.58	0	$900.00	$34.58
d. Jack Masci	$509.00	0	0	$509.00
e. Jean Olson	0	0	0	0
f. Lori Whittaker	0	0	0	0

- In the "Today's Date" (upper right hand corner) space of the superbill, use the date 04/10/2008, as this is the date of service on which the patient will be seen.
- In the "Time" field, enter the time of the patient's appointment located on the Appointment Schedule.
- In the "Subscriber" space, enter "Same" if the patient is also the health insurance subscriber. If not (for instance, when a child is covered by a parent's insurance), enter the name of the subscriber.
- In the "Sub.#" space, enter the subscriber's policy number.
- The "Account #" on the superbill is to be left blank.

2. Once you have completed all 6 superbills, place your completed work in alphabetic order in the Completed Work folder directly behind Task 3.4.

Good job! You have completed Day Three of your internship.

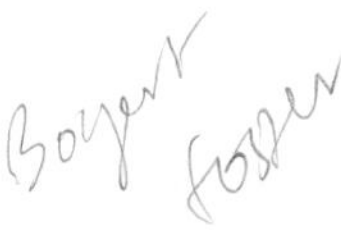

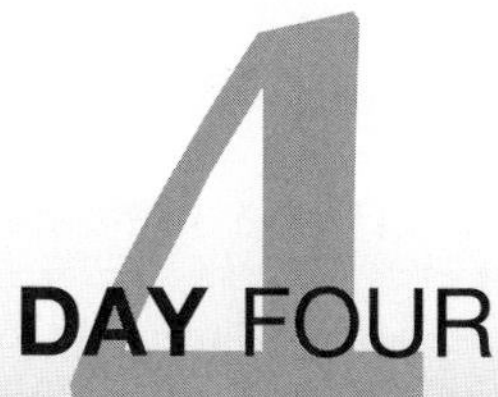

DAY FOUR

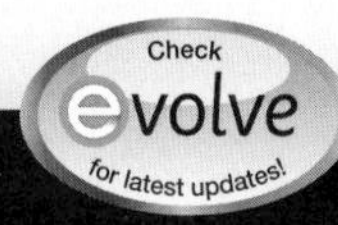
Check
evolve
for latest updates!

Thursday, April 10, 2008

TASK **4.1**

Telephone Messages and Appointment Schedule

SUPPLIES NEEDED (p. 415):

- Appointment sheets for Thursday, April 10, to Friday, April 18, from your Completed Work folder
- Companion Evolve site containing the telephone messages from April 9 (Task 4.1)
- 4 blank Telephone Records (located in the Supplies section)

1. Locate the "Telephone Messages" area on the companion Evolve site (Task 4.1)
   - Telephone messages came into the office during the hours in which the clinic was closed. Gladys has asked you to listen to the voice mail of the calls and complete a Telephone Record for each call.
   - If a patient requests a specific time for an appointment, you are to schedule the appointment as close as possible to the time requested by the patient.
   - Indicate the date and time of the tentative appointment in the "Response" block on the Telephone Record.
   - If a message is left for an employee of the clinic staff, you are to record the message for the appropriate person on the Telephone Record.
2. Once you have completed all messages, place all Telephone Record forms into the Completed Work folder.

1. Using the step-by-step instructions provided in Appendix 2, Item N, schedule the appointments using the Telephone Records from Task 4.1 and the appointment sheets in the software scheduling program.
2. Once all appointments have been scheduled, print an Appointment List for Drs. Bond and Harkness for April 16.
3. Place the Appointment List in alphabetic order in your Completed Work folder behind Task 4.1.

TASK **4.2**

Correspondence and Mail

SUPPLIES NEEDED (p. 417):

- Telephone records from this morning (Task 4.1)
- 2 letterhead forms **(Figure 4-1)** (located in the Supplies section and the Forms Library on the companion Evolve site)
- Incoming Mail form dated April 10 (located in the Supplies section)
- Mail Sorting form **(Figure 4-2)** (located in the Supplies section)

1. **Preparing correspondence and separating of mail.**
   - Per Gladys's instructions, you will be preparing letters for her signature. These letters will be in response to the patients who left telephone messages in Task 4.1, requesting appointments at a later date.
   - The address for Mr. Sven Johnson is 509 Mockingham Road, South Padre, TX 98765, and the address for Mr. George Jones is 79892 Elf Street, South Padre, TX 98765.
   - Prepare responses on letterhead to Sven Johnson and George Jones regarding their requested appointments. Give the date and time you have indicated on the Telephone Record in the "Response" block.
   - On completion of this first part of this task, file the two letters in the Completed Work folder.

Once you have finished the correspondence, you will be sorting mail.

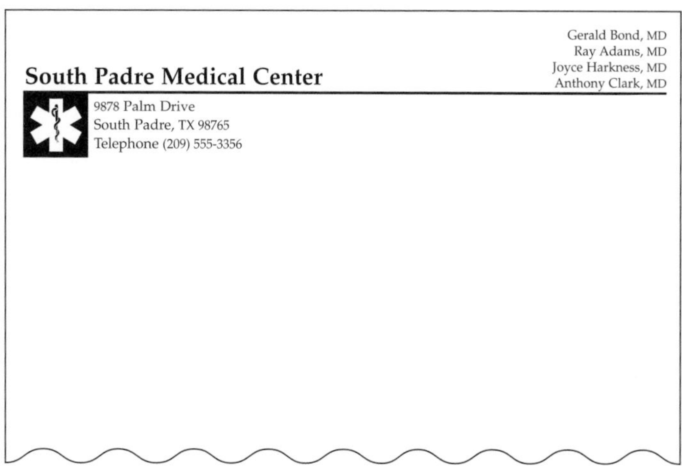
South Padre Medical Center

9878 Palm Drive
South Padre, TX 98765
Telephone (209) 555-3356

Gerald Bond, MD
Ray Adams, MD
Joyce Harkness, MD
Anthony Clark, MD

Figure **4-1** **South Padre Medical Center letterhead.**

1. **Sorting of incoming mail.**
   - Gladys has given the instructions that you are to sort the mail by person and department. You will get all of the mail from the Incoming Mail form. You will sort the mail by doctor, insurance, accounts receivable, human resources, waiting room, and Gladys (refer to Appendix 2, Policies and Procedures, Item G). You will indicate the mail received under the appropriate heading (see **Figure 4-2**).

MAIL SORTING

Dr. Bond
1, 17

Dr. Harkness

Dr. Adams

Dr. Clark

Gladys

Accounts receivable

Insurance

Human Resources

Waiting Room

Figure **4-2 Incoming Mail sorting form for Thursday, April 10.**

2. **Once you have completed this part of Task 4.2, place the form behind the first part of this task and place it in the Completed Work folder directly behind Task 4.1.**

TASK 4.3

Scheduling Appointments

SUPPLIES NEEDED (p. 425):

- Appointment sheets dated Monday, April 7, to Friday, April 18 (located in the general *Practice Kit* box)
- Four previously completed Telephone Records, dated Thursday, April 10 (located in the Supplies section)

1. Work patient reception, answer the telephone, and schedule appointments.
   - The patient information to schedule each appointment is located on the Telephone Record (Task 4.3).
   - You will need to schedule each appointment as requested by the patient on the Telephone Record.
   - Indicate the date, time, and length of appointment on the Telephone Record.

Lilly Rice is known to Dr. Clark, so Gladys directs you to schedule her for 60 minutes rather than the usual 30 minutes. Also, Gladys directs Kristie Olson be scheduled for 30 minutes.

2. Place completed appointment sheets in the Completed Work folder. Place the Telephone Record in the Completed Work folder.

1. Using the step-by-step instructions provided in Appendix 2, Item N, schedule the appointments using the previously completed Telephone Records from Task 4.3 and the appointment sheets in the software scheduling program.
2. Once all appointments have been scheduled, print an Appointment List for Drs. Bond, Adams, and Clark for those days with new appointments.
3. Place the Appointment List in your Completed Work folder behind Task 4.2.

TASK **4.4**

Records Management

SUPPLIES NEEDED (p. 427):

- 2 blank Patient Information forms (located in the Supplies section)
- 2 blank Subsequent Findings forms (located in the Supplies section)
- 2 file folder labels (located in the general *Practice Kit* box)
- 2 file folders (located in the general *Practice Kit* box)
- Telephone Records from Task 4.3

1. **You will now establish medical records for the two new patients from Task 4.3—Kristie Olson and Lilly Rice.**
   - Locate the file folders and the file labels in the packet.
   - Secure the labels for each patient to the file folders.

2. **Assemble the patient's medical record.**
   - Locate the Patient Information forms and complete the forms with only the information taken from the messages in Task 4.3 for Kristie Olson and Lilly Rice.
   - The order of the medical record for Kristie Olson and Lilly Rice should be:
     - Completed Patient Information form (first)
     - Subsequent Findings sheet (second)

3. **Once you have completed this task, place the forms in alphabetic order in the Completed Work folder directly behind Task 4.3.**

You have just finished Day Four; you're almost halfway through your internship. Good job! Let's go on to Day Five.

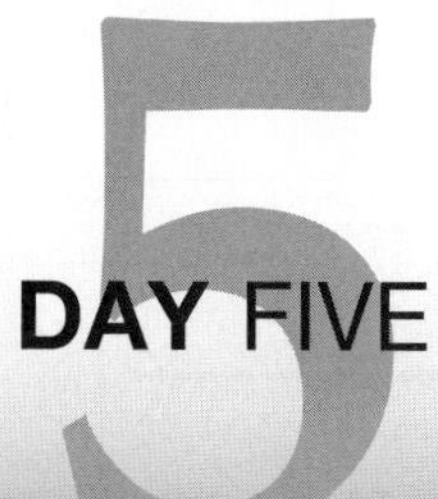

DAY FIVE

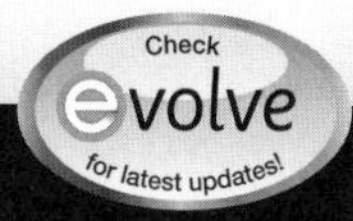
Check
evolve
for latest updates!

Friday, April 11, 2008

TASK **5.1**

Medical Transcription

SUPPLIES NEEDED (p. 435):

- 2 Operative Report forms **(Figure 5-1)** (located in the Supplies section and the Forms Library on the companion Evolve site)
- Companion Evolve site containing medical transcription from April 9 and 10, Task 5.1.

1. Locate the "Medical Transcription" area on the companion Evolve site (Task 5.1).
   - Today you will start your morning by completing the transcription. Gladys is going to cover the reception desk and you are to key in operative reports dictated by Dr. Bond and Dr. Clark.

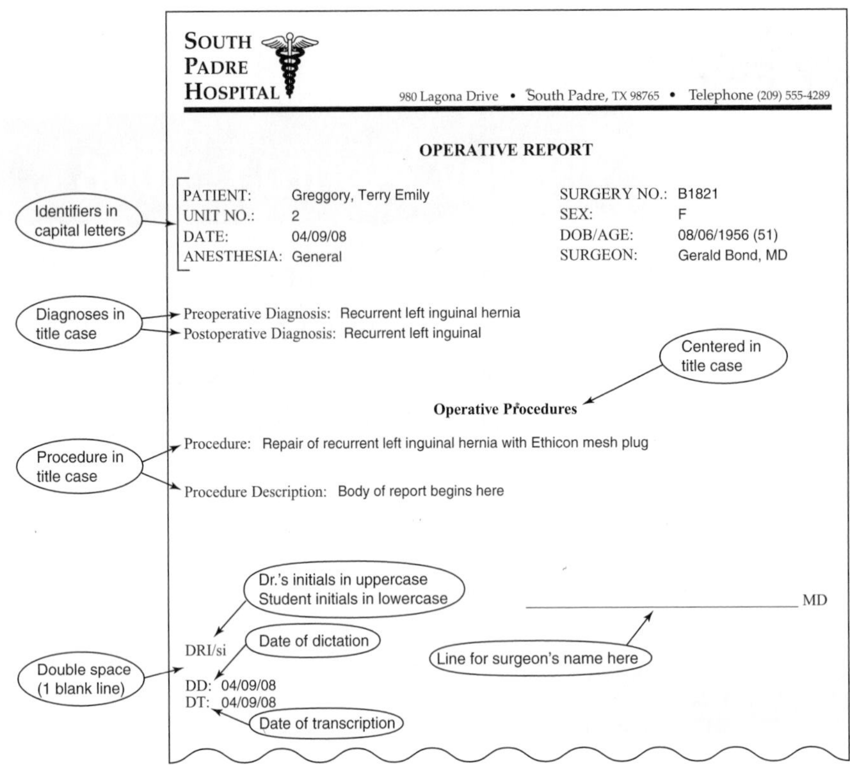
South Padre Hospital
980 Lagona Drive • South Padre, TX 98765 • Telephone (209) 555-4289

OPERATIVE REPORT

PATIENT: Greggory, Terry Emily
UNIT NO.: 2
DATE: 04/09/08
ANESTHESIA: General
SURGERY NO.: B1821
SEX: F
DOB/AGE: 08/06/1956 (51)
SURGEON: Gerald Bond, MD

Preoperative Diagnosis: Recurrent left inguinal hernia
Postoperative Diagnosis: Recurrent left inguinal

Operative Procedures

Procedure: Repair of recurrent left inguinal hernia with Ethicon mesh plug

Procedure Description: Body of report begins here

_____________________ MD

DRI/si

DD: 04/09/08
DT: 04/09/08

Figure **5-1** **Operative Report form with explanations.**

2. On completion of the medical transcription, place it in the Completed Work folder directly behind Task 4.4.
   - From this point on, no directions will be provided for the location of forms. It will be assumed that you will get the forms from the Supplies section of this text, Appendix 4, or the Evolve site.

TASK **5.2**

Posting Charges to a Superbill

SUPPLIES NEEDED:

- 6 superbills from Completed Task folder from Task 3.5
- Fee Schedule (displayed in **Figure 5-2**)

1. Gladys has asked you to post charges for the patients seen yesterday. Normally the diagnosis codes and services provided during the patients' visits would already be entered either by provider or clinical staff; however, in order to assist you in becoming more familiar with the superbill, you will be entering the service(s) provided for these patients, and completing the requested future appointments area if indicated. You are **not** to schedule the appointments indicated; just enter any future appointment onto the superbill in the "Return Appointment" area. Using the superbills completed in Task 3.5, indicate the following services and diagnosis codes for these patients:

Patient	Service	Diagnosis Code
a. Mary Bogert Dr. Adams has requested a return visit in 10 days	99213	599.0
b. Elizabeth Fenton	99387	V70.0
c. Amanda Foster Dr. Adams has requested a return visit in 1 month	99213	V22.2
d. Jack Masci Dr. Clark has requested a return visit in 10 days	99214	531.0
e. Jean Olson Dr. Clark has requested a return visit in 15 days	99205	278.00
f. Lori Whittaker Physician requesting consultation was Dr. Blackburn	99244	455.9

2. **Figure 5-2** illustrates the office visit area of the superbill. For your use, Gladys has written the fee schedule on a superbill. You will be using these amounts to post the charges for the patient services to each of the superbills you have just completed. You are not to total the balance due yet. You will be instructed to do that in Task 5.3. However, be certain to enter "Today's Total" in the appropriate box on the form.

√	DESCRIPTION	CPT	Diag.	FEE
	OFFICE VISIT			
	NEW PATIENT			
	Problem Focused			
	Exp Problem Focused	99202		75.00
	Detailed	99203		95.00
	Comp/ Mod MDM	99204		105.00
	Comp/ High MDM	99205		120.00
	ESTABLISHED PATIENT			
	Minimal/Nurse Visit	99211		45.00
	Problem Focused	99212		55.00
	Exp Problem Focused	99213		65.00
	Detailed	99214		85.00
	Comprehensive	99215		105.00
	CONSULTATION			
	Problem Focused	99241		120.00
	Exp Problem Focused	99242		140.00
	Detailed	99243		160.00
	Comp/ Mod MDM	99244		200.00
	Comp/High MDM	99245		250.00
	Requesting Provider ________			
	Post-op Exam	99024		0.00
	PREVENTIVE MEDICINE			
	NEW PATIENT			
	Infant – 1 yr	99381		95.00
	1 yr – 4 yr	99382		110.00
	5 yr – 11 yr	99383		110.00
	12 yr – 17 yr	99384		135.00
	18 yr – 39 yr	99385		150.00
	40 yr – 64 yr	99386		170.00
	65 yr and over	99387		200.00
	ESTABLISHED PATIENT			
	Infant – 1 yr	99391		80.00
	1 yr – 4 yr	99392		80.00
	5 yr – 11 yr	99393		80.00
	12 yr – 17 yr	99394		100.00
	18 yr – 39 yr	99395		120.00
	40 yr – 64 yr	99396		140.00
	65 yr and over	99397		160.00

Figure **5-2** **Fee schedule.**

3. Once you have completed all six superbills, place them in alphabetic order and go on to Task 5.3, where you will enter further information onto these superbills.

Billing and Banking Procedures

SUPPLIES NEEDED (p. 439):

- 6 superbills completed in Task 5.2
- 1 Journal of Daily Charges and Payments (located in the Supplies section)
- 6 blank patient statements (located in the Supplies section)
- 7 partially completed patient statements (located in the Supplies section)
- 1 deposit ticket (located in the Supplies section)

1. Gladys asks you to post payments to the superbills for some of the patients seen yesterday. Usually, Kerri Marshall, the insurance specialist, would post payments the day the payments were received, but Gladys wanted you to have an opportunity to process the payments as a part of your internship experience. **Figure 5-3** illustrates the blocks where payment information is to be entered on the superbill. The following are checks received from the patients represented on the superbills. Be certain to calculate the Balance Due and place your initials on the line next to the "Rec'd by." If the patient pays nothing, initial and enter zero in the amount paid.

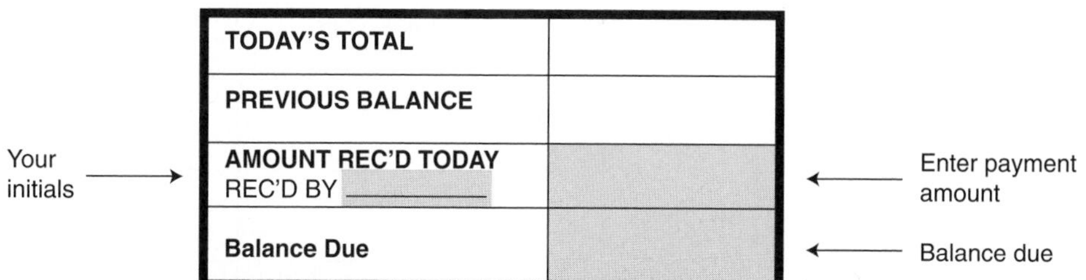

Figure **5-3** **Superbill payment placement area to be completed.**

Patient	Payment
a. Mary Bogert, 2502 32nd Avenue South, South Padre, Texas 98765	$25.00
b. Elizabeth Fenton, 201 2nd Avenue North, South Padre, Texas 98765	$125.00
c. Amanda Foster, 1603 Todd Avenue, South Padre, Texas 98765	$0
d. Jack Masci, 809 Heights Drive, South Padre, Texas 98765	$75.00
e. Jean Olson, 2405 Elm Way Drive, South Padre, Texas 98765	$50.00
f. Lori Whittaker, 3204 34th Avenue South, South Padre, Texas 98765	$100.00

2. Next, you are to enter the above payments two more times: once onto a statement for the patient and once onto the Journal of Daily Charges and Payments. **Figure 5-4** illustrates the placement of the payment data on Mary Bogert's patient statement. Note that the "DATE" is the date the service was provided to the patient, not the date the charges and payments were posted. **Figure 5-5** illustrates the Journal of Daily Charges and Payments areas that you will be completing for the patient Mary Bogert. You will enter the payments on the patient statement and the Journal of Daily Charges and Payments.

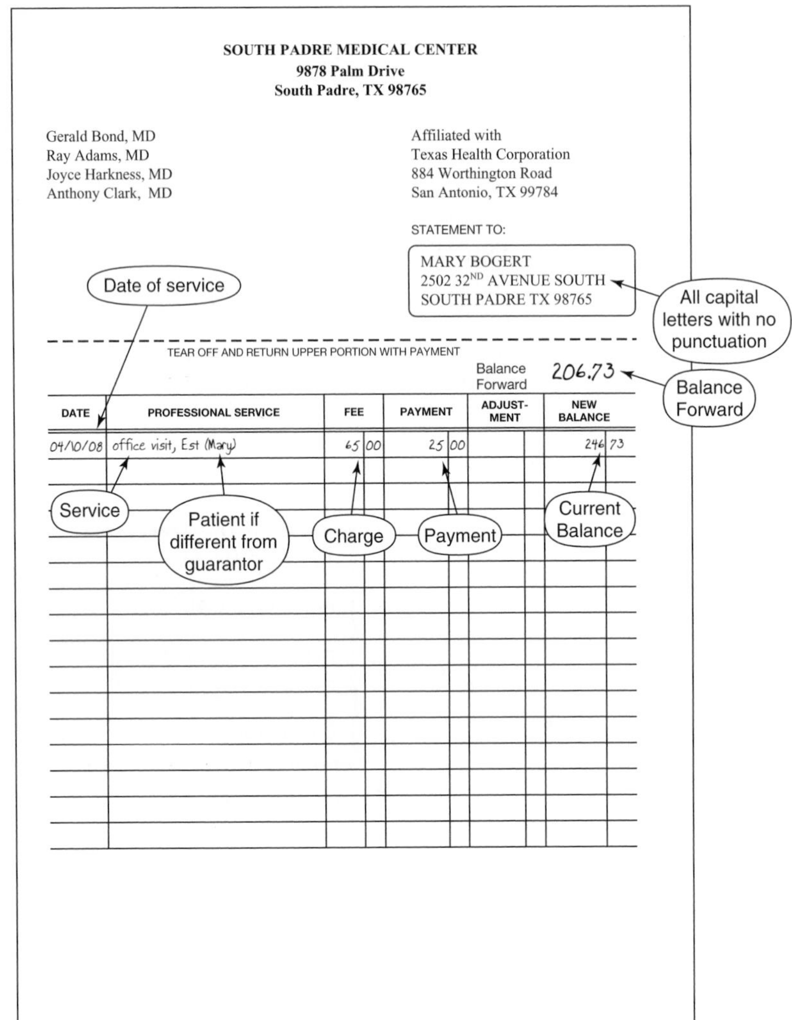

SOUTH PADRE MEDICAL CENTER
9878 Palm Drive
South Padre, TX 98765

Gerald Bond, MD
Ray Adams, MD
Joyce Harkness, MD
Anthony Clark, MD

Affiliated with
Texas Health Corporation
884 Worthington Road
San Antonio, TX 99784

STATEMENT TO:

MARY BOGERT
2502 32ND AVENUE SOUTH
SOUTH PADRE TX 98765

TEAR OFF AND RETURN UPPER PORTION WITH PAYMENT

Balance Forward 206.73

DATE	PROFESSIONAL SERVICE	FEE	PAYMENT	ADJUST-MENT	NEW BALANCE
04/10/08	office visit, Est (Mary)	65 00	25 00		246 73

Figure **5-4** **Patient statement for Mary Bogert.**

JOURNAL OF DAILY CHARGES & PAYMENTS

	DATE	PROFESSIONAL SERVICE	FEE	PAYMENT	ADJUST-MENT	NEW BALANCE	OLD BALANCE	PATIENT'S NAME	
1	04/10/08	office visit, Est (Mary)	65 00	25 00		246 73	206 73	Bogert, Mary	1
2									2

Figure **5-5** **Journal of Daily Charges and Payments.**

Complete the patient statements as follows:

Statement to:	Patient's name and address in capital letters with no punctuation
Balance Forward:	The previous amount from the last statement
Date:	Date the service was provided
Professional Service:	The type of service, such as "office visit," and if the patient is an established patient ("Est") or new patient ("New"). Also the name of the patient if it is different from the guarantor (the person responsible for paying the bill).
Fee:	The charge for the service
Payment:	The payment made to the account
New Balance:	The amount due after adding charges and subtracting payments

3. Now record the following payments made today onto the Journal of Daily Charges and Payments and also onto the patient statements. The partially completed statements for these patients are located in the Supplies section. Use today's date in the DATE column of the Journal of Daily Charges and Payments.

a. Thomas Blair	$26.00	Check number 890
b. Maynard Hovlett	$150.00	Cash
c. Larry Smith	$35.00	Check number 15346
d. Anne Meires	$55.00	Cash
e. Edward Goldman	$50.00	Check number 90001
f. Jasper Hunt	$100.00	Check number 236
g. Lewis Rock	$200.00	Check number 101011

4. Now that you have entered all payment information onto the Journal of Daily Charges and Payments, you are ready to proof the posting. You do this by adding up columns A through E (illustrated in **Figure 5-6**) and placing the totals on line 31 of the journal sheet under the bold line (see Figure 5-6).

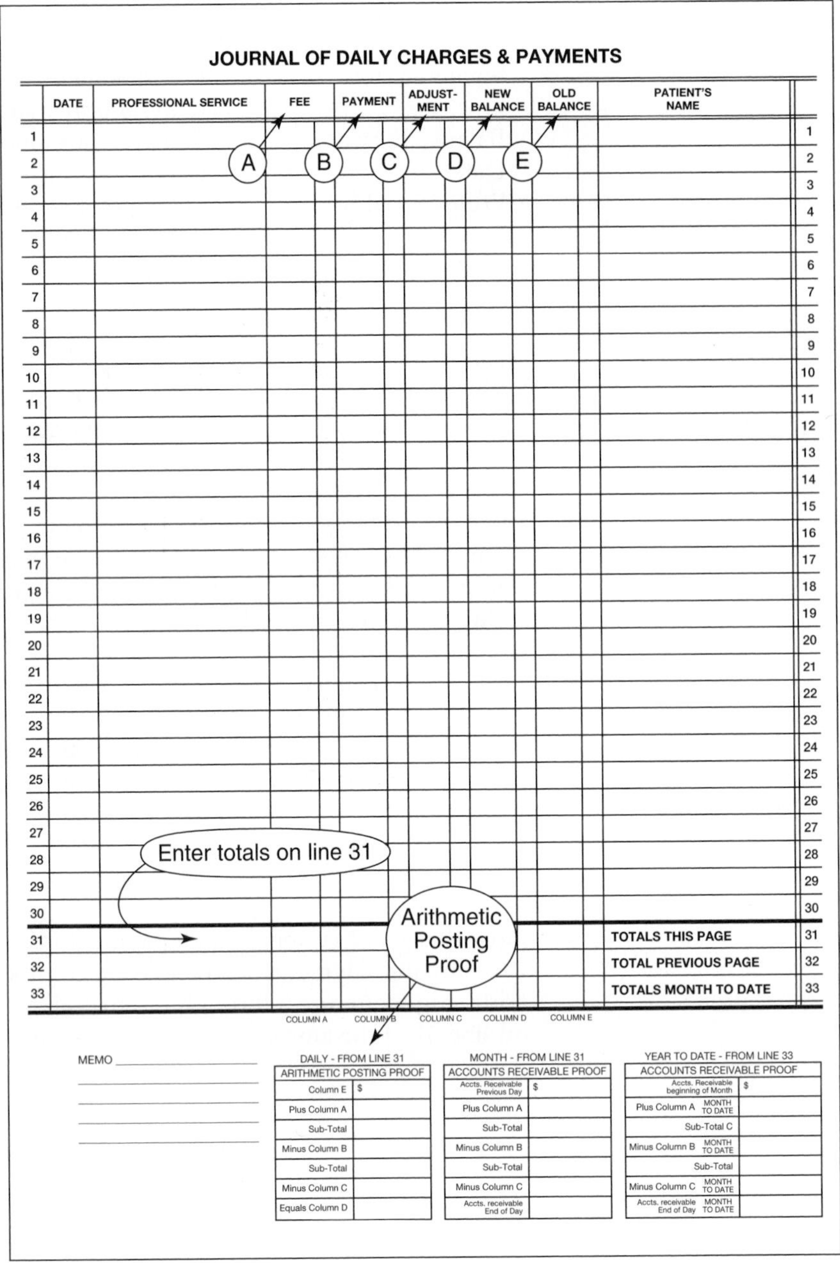

JOURNAL OF DAILY CHARGES & PAYMENTS
DATE
PROFESSIONAL SERVICE
FEE
PAYMENT
ADJUST-MENT
NEW BALANCE
OLD BALANCE
PATIENT'S NAME
A
B
C
D
E
Enter totals on line 31
Arithmetic Posting Proof
TOTALS THIS PAGE
TOTAL PREVIOUS PAGE
TOTALS MONTH TO DATE
COLUMN A
COLUMN B
COLUMN C
COLUMN D
COLUMN E
MEMO
DAILY - FROM LINE 31
ARITHMETIC POSTING PROOF
Column E $
Plus Column A
Sub-Total
Minus Column B
Sub-Total
Minus Column C
Equals Column D
MONTH - FROM LINE 31
ACCOUNTS RECEIVABLE PROOF
Accts. Receivable Previous Day $
Plus Column A
Sub-Total
Minus Column B
Sub-Total
Minus Column C
Accts. receivable End of Day
YEAR TO DATE - FROM LINE 33
ACCOUNTS RECEIVABLE PROOF
Accts. Receivable beginning of Month $
Plus Column A MONTH TO DATE
Sub-Total C
Minus Column B MONTH TO DATE
Sub-Total
Minus Column C MONTH TO DATE
Accts. receivable End of Day MONTH TO DATE

Figure **5-6** **Columns A-E, totals on line 31 for proof of posting.**

Complete the Journal of Daily Charges and Payments as follows:

Date:	The date of the service was provided
Professional Service:	The type of service, such as "office visit," and if the patient is an established patient ("Est") or a new patient ("New"). Also include the name of the patient if it is different from the guarantor (the person responsible for paying the bill).
Fee:	The charge for the service
Payment:	The payment made to the account
New Balance:	The amount due after adding charges and subtracting payments
Old Balance:	The amount brought forward from last month
Patient's Name:	Last name, comma, first name

These totals are then transferred to the "Arithmetic Posting Proof" [illegible]he form (see Figure 5-6). Your entries are correct when the resulting nu[illegible] from the proofing equals the number in column D ("New Balance") on the journal form.

5. Gladys has asked that you prepare a deposit ticket **(Figure 5-7)** for all the cash and checks you have posted to the journal sheet. Complete the deposit ticket now. The total of the bank deposit should be the same as the total in column B ("Payments") of the journal.

DEPOSIT TICKET

SOUTH PADRE MEDICAL CENTER
9878 PALM DRIVE
SOUTH PADRE, TX 98765

FIRST NATIONAL BANK
100 FIRST STREET
SOUTH PADRE, TX 98765

DATE ____________________

DEPOSITS MAY NOT BE AVAILABLE FOR IMMEDIATE WITHDRAWAL

00001001002005

	DOLLARS	CENTS
CURRENCY		
COIN		
CHECKS LIST EACH SEPARATELY		
1 2		
3 4		
5 6		
7 8		
9 10		
11 12		
13 14		
15 16		
17 18		
19 20		
21 22		
23 24		
25 26		
27 28		
TOTAL FROM OTHER SIDE OR ATTACHED LIST		
PLEASE RE-ENTER TOTAL HERE — TOTAL		

$

Total

Checks and other items are received for deposit subject to the provisions of the Uniform Commercial Code or any applicable collection agreement.

Figure **5-7** **Deposit ticket entry of total.**

DAY FIVE TASK 5.3

6. When you have finished entering all the information for this task, place all the documentation in the Completed Work folder after Task 5.1.

1. Using the completed superbills from Task 5.3, Gladys wants you to enter the charges and payments for each patient into the new software system. She has given you step-by-step instructions for entry of both charges and payments in Software Instructions, Items G through H.

2. Once you have entered the charges and payments for all the superbills, print a Patient Ledger for each of these patient accounts. Directions on how to print these are located in Software Instructions, Item I.

3. Next, print a Patient Day Sheet User Match Report for April 11. Directions on how to print the report are in Software Instructions, Item J.

4. Place the Patient Ledgers and Patient Day Sheet User Match Report in your Completed Work folder behind Task 5.2.

TASK 5.4

Petty Cash and Checking

SUPPLIES NEEDED (p. 469):

- 1 letterhead form (located in the Supplies section and on the companion Evolve site)
- 2 checks (located in the Supplies section)
- 1 petty cash journal form (located in the Supplies section)
- 1 check register (located in the general *Practice Kit* box)
- 2 completed statements (Field and Zacharizison) (located in the Supplies section)
- Patient statement for Jack Masci from Task 5.3.

1. Today Gladys has requested that you write a letter (use letterhead) to Jack Masci regarding his account, on which $509 is in the 90 days aged category. Prepare the letter for Gladys to sign. Although Mr. Masci has made a payment, he has not sufficiently paid down the balance. Messages requesting payment on the account have been sent to Mr. Masci on three previous occasions. Inform Mr. Masci that he should contact Kerri Marshall to make arrangements for payment of the account or the account will be turned over to the collection agency. A $75 payment was posted to Mr. Masci's account in Task 5.3.

2. Gladys has asked you to write a check for $100 to be used to set up a petty cash fund for the office. The check is to be written paid to the order of the "First National Bank—Cash" and recorded on the check register. The address of the bank is to be listed on lines 2 and 3 of the "TO THE ORDER OF" area on the sample check as illustrated in **Figure 5-8.** When you have the check prepared, you are to begin the journal that Gladys drafted that will be used to keep track of how the petty cash funds are spent by entering the beginning balance at the top right-hand corner of the petty cash journal.

South Padre Medical Center
9878 Palm Drive
SOUTH PADRE, TX 98765

FIRST NATIONAL BANK
100 FIRST STREET
SOUTH PADRE, TX 98765

98-95/1251

NO 872

PAY Fifty Dollars and no/100 DOLLARS

DATE	CHECK NO.	AMOUNT
10/30/01	872	50 00

TO THE ORDER OF First National Bank
100 First Street
South Padre, TX 98765

⑈0⑆0123⑈ ⑆4567⑈8901⑆ ⑈1234567890⑈

Figure **5-8 Sample check.**

3. You are now to write a check to reimburse a patient for a credit balance, post a nonsufficient fund check, and post a collection agency payment. You will record each transaction on the check register. The following is the information to perform these tasks:
   - Write a check to Gloria Hydorn for $26.89 to reimburse her for a credit balance on her account. Her address is 862 Oceanside Way, South Padre, TX 98765. Kerri has already recorded the refund on Gloria's account. Enter this check information on the check register.
   - A check deposited last week has been returned for nonsufficient funds (NSF). The check is from David Oakland for $56.00. Kerri has made the notation of NSF check on the patient statement. You are to record the NSF check on the check register by writing "David Oakland" in the "Paid To" column, using today's date in the "Date" column, NSF in the "Check Number" and "Description" columns, and deducting the $56.00 from the balance in the check register.
   - Record a check on the check register that was received from the Island Collection Agency today in the amount of $309.32. Kerri has already credited the various patients' accounts represented by this check. In the "Description" column indicate "Collections" and record the $309.32 in the deposit column.

4. Kerri has asked you to post a credit to Norma Field's patient statement in the amount of $100 and to make an adjustment to the account for $80 because today Kerri received an explanation of benefits (EOB, an explanation of the payments and adjustments), number 2001134. Kerri explained to you that the $80 was the amount that Medicare would not pay and that we cannot charge the patient this amount because our physicians participate in the Medicare program. The $80 becomes a write-off to the clinic, which means that the amount is deducted from the patient's account as if it were never charged. Post the $100 Medicare payment to the "Payment" column, and the EOB adjustment to the "Adjustment" column.

5. Kerri has asked that you reconcile the clinic's bank statement for her. Reconciliation of a bank statement is a procedure in which the balance from a bank statement, as illustrated in **Figure 5-9**, is compared with the customer's checkbook balance with the addition of any deposits and/or deductions since the bank statement was issued. Kerri provides a bank statement that indicates the balance was $21,028.02 as of April 9. Since then, Kerri deposited checks in the amount of $5,020.69 on April 10. Using the check register you used earlier today, determine if the clinic's check register balance is the same as the bank's balance using the following formula:

A. Bank statement balance	$21,028.02
a. Less outstanding checks (there are 3, from check register)	176.89
b. Plus deposits not shown (there are 2)	5330.01
B. Corrected bank balance	26181.14
a. Less any NSF or bank charges (there is 1)	56.00
C. Corrected checkbook balance	26,125.14

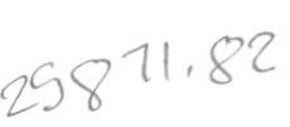

The checkbook balances when the amount on line C of the formula is the same as the last balance in the check register.

0821-402054

#821

N
2

CALL (888) 555-2932
24 HOURS/DAY, 7 DAYS/WEEK
FOR ASSISTANCE WITH
YOUR ACCOUNT.

PAGE 1 OF 2 THIS STATEMENT COVERS: 6/22/XX THROUGH 7/22/XX

INTEREST CHECKING 0821-402054

SUMMARY

PREVIOUS BALANCE	252.10	MINIMUM BALANCE	142.55
DEPOSITS	68.74+	AVERAGE BALANCE	220.00
INTEREST EARNED	.18+	ANNUAL PERCENTAGE YIELD EARNED	.96%
WITHDRAWALS	109.55−		
CUSTOMER SERVICE CALLS	.00−		
INTERLINK/PURCHASE FEE	.00−	INTEREST EARNED 1994	2.23
MONTHLY CHECKING FEE AND OTHER CHARGES	.00−		
► **NEW BALANCE**	**211.47**		

USE YOUR EXPRESS CARD TO MAKE UNLIMITED PURCHASES AT RETAILERS DISPLAYING THE INTERLINK SYMBOL. (A $1 MONTHLY FEE MAY APPLY.)

CHECKS AND WITHDRAWALS

CHECK	DATE PAID	AMOUNT	CHECK	DATE PAID	AMOUNT
202	7/05	15.05	203	7/15	94.50

DEPOSITS

	DATE POSTED	AMOUNT
CUSTOMER DEPOSIT	7/22	68.74
INTEREST PAYMENT THIS PERIOD	7/22	.18

BALANCE INFORMATION

DATE	BALANCE	DATE	BALANCE	DATE	BALANCE
6/22	252.10	7/05	237.05	7/15	142.55
				7/22	211.47

24 HOUR CUSTOMER SERVICE

EACH ACCOUNT COMES WITH 3 COMPLIMENTARY CALLS PER STATEMENT PERIOD.

CALLS TO 24 HOUR CUSTOMER SERVICE THIS STATEMENT PERIOD: 0

INTEREST INFORMATION

FROM	THROUGH	INTEREST RATE	ANNUAL PERCENTAGE YIELD (APY)
6/22	7/22	1.00%	1.01%

INTEREST RATE/APY AS OF 7/22/XX IF YOUR BALANCE IS

$ 0 - 4,999	1.00%	1.01%
$ 5,000 - 9,999	1.00%	1.01%
$ 10,000 AND OVER	1.00%	1.01%

MEMBER FDIC

STATEMENT

Figure **5-9** **Example of bank statement.** *(From Young AP, Proctor DB:* Kinn's the medical assistant: an applied learning approach, *ed 11, St. Louis, 2011, Saunders.)*

6. Kerri asked that you post a $37.50 credit to Maynard Zacharizison's account based on a check received from the Island Collection Agency. Mr. Zacharizison's account balance was $200 and the collection agency made an agreement with him that if he would pay $75 total on the account, the remainder of the bill would be removed, which he has now done. You are to credit the account with the second payment of $37.50 and adjust the account (enter $125.00 in the "Adjustment" column). Mr. Zacharizison's balance will now be zero.

7. You will place all work in the Completed Work folder directly behind Task 5.3.

Well, you're over halfway there. Great job so far! Now let's move on to Day Six.

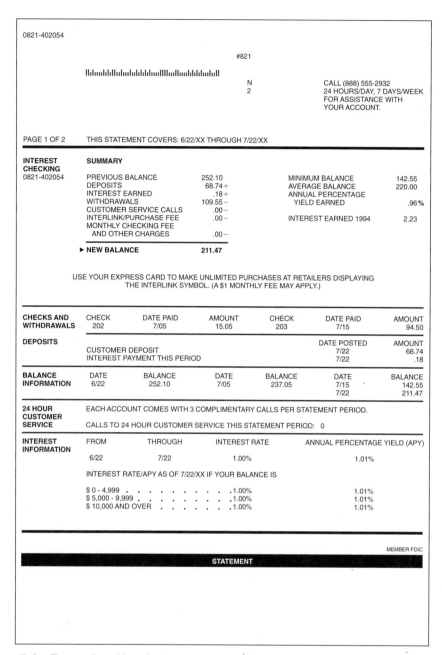

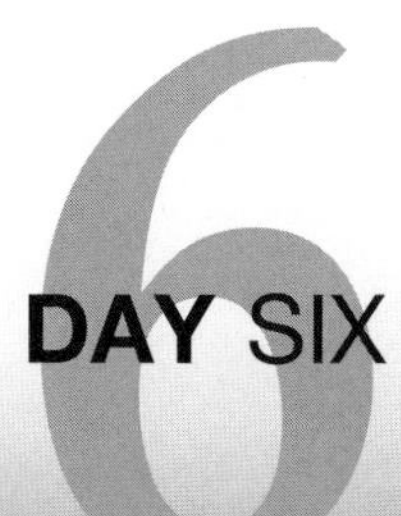

DAY SIX

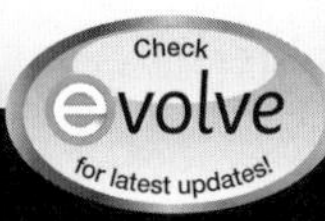
Check
evolve
for latest updates!

Monday, April 14, 2008

TASK **6.1**

Internet Research

SUPPLIES NEEDED:

- Computer with access to the Internet
- 1 file folder
- 1 file folder label

1. Research "Incident To"
   - This morning Gladys has a special project for you to do. You will be going onto the Internet and researching "Incident To" for the physicians. "Incident to" services are those that are furnished at the same time as the physician's professional service.

2. Work from a computer with Internet access.
   - Do a search by typing in the words "incident to" using a search engine such as www.google.com or www.yahoo.com. Place quotation marks at the beginning and end of the entry to ensure that you locate the entire statement, not just one of the two words of the search. You are looking for information on "Incident To" as it relates to billing requirements for Medicare patients. Locate what you think is the best information on the subject and print five copies.

3. Prepare a file folder with file folder label.
   - Locate the file folder and file label. Type or write "INCIDENT TO" in capital letters on the label. Secure the label to the file folder.
   - Place the research papers in the folder and file in the Completed Work folder.

TASK **6.2**

Establishing a Meeting

SUPPLIES NEEDED (p. 481):

- Patient appointment sheet for Wednesday, April 16, from your Completed Work folder
- 5 memo forms (located in the Supplies section and the Forms Library on the companion Evolve site)

1. Assist Gladys with establishing a meeting.
- You will be assisting Gladys with establishing a meeting with the information you researched on "Incident To" in Task 6.1. The physicians requested the information on "Incident To" and would like Gladys to present the information researched at a meeting of all clinic physicians. The meeting is to be scheduled for Wednesday, April 16, from 12 PM to 1 PM.
- First, you will need to review the appointment schedule for Wednesday, April 16, to determine if each physician is available at the time indicated. Once you have established that all physicians are available, mark the schedule for the meeting by placing an X though the time block of 12 PM though 1 PM and noting "Office Meeting" on each physician's schedule.
- You will need 5 memo forms. Gladys has asked you to prepare a memo to each of the physicians (Drs. Bond, Adams, Harkness, and Clark) and one for Gladys as a reminder.

2. What to include in the memo.
- The memo will include today's date and all physicians' complete names followed by "MD." Be sure to **bold** each name that pertains to the physician it is sent to (as illustrated in **Figure 6-1**). The memo will also state the date and time of the meeting, the place where the meeting will be held (Conference Room), and the topic to be discussed.

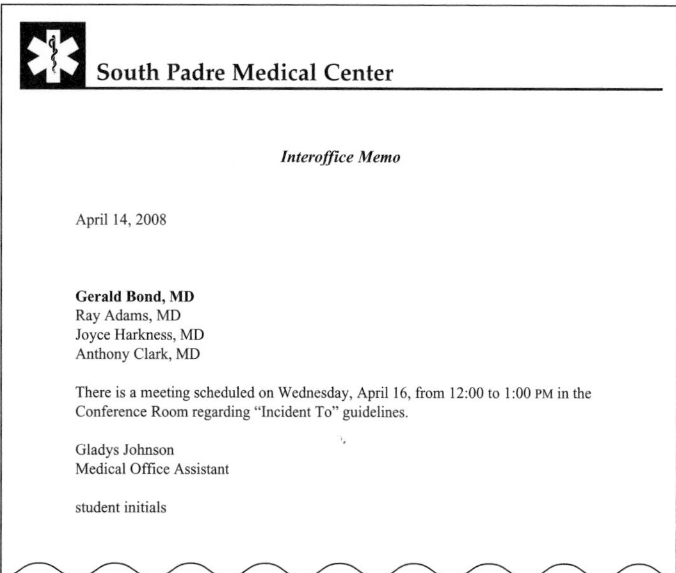

South Padre Medical Center

Interoffice Memo

April 14, 2008

Gerald Bond, MD
Ray Adams, MD
Joyce Harkness, MD
Anthony Clark, MD

There is a meeting scheduled on Wednesday, April 16, from 12:00 to 1:00 PM in the Conference Room regarding "Incident To" guidelines.

Gladys Johnson
Medical Office Assistant

student initials

Figure **6-1** **Interoffice memo.**

3. Once you have completed all memos, place them in the folder you prepared and then in the Completed Work folder directly behind Task 6.1.

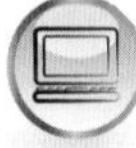

1. Enter the "Incident To" meeting into the software for all Center physicians.

TASK **6.3**

Telephone Messages

SUPPLIES NEEDED (p. 491):

- Companion Evolve site containing the telephone messages for Task 6.3
- 5 blank Telephone Records (located in the Supplies section)

1. Locate the "Telephone Messages" area on the companion Evolve site (Task 6.3).
    - Telephone messages came into the office during the lunch hour. Gladys has asked you to listen to the voice mail of the calls and complete a Telephone Record for each call.
    - If a patient requests an appointment, you will be completing the request in Task 6.4.

Gerald Bond, MD
Ray Adams, MD
Joyce Harkness, MD
Anthony Clark, MD

South Padre Medical Center

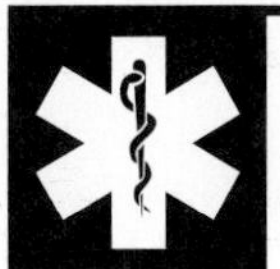

9878 Palm Drive
South Padre, TX 98765
Telephone (209) 555-3356

TASK **6.4**

Scheduling Appointments

SUPPLIES NEEDED (p. 495):

- 10 previously dated appointment sheets for Monday, April 7, to Friday, April 18, from your Completed Work file
- 2 file folders
- 2 preprinted file labels
- 2 blank Patient Information forms (located in the Supplies section)
- Telephone Records from Task 6.3

1. Assemble the patient's medical record.
   - Locate the file folders and the file labels in the packet. Using the Telephone Records from Task 6.3, locate the labels for the two new patients that are requesting appointments. Secure the label to each file folder.
   - For each new patient, fill out the Patient Information form that is supplied for you with data from the Telephone Record. Place the form for each patient into the correct patient file folder.
2. Schedule appointments.
   - Finish this task by scheduling the two new and one established patient appointments as requested from the Telephone Records.
   - Once you have scheduled the appointment that is indicated on the Telephone Record, indicate the appointment date and time on the Telephone Record in the "Response" block.
3. Once you have finished this task, place the Telephone Records (Task 6.3) directly behind Task 6.2, and place the file folders with the Patient Information forms inside each folder into the Completed Work folder directly behind Task 6.3.

1. Schedule appointments using the Telephone Records from Task 6.3 and the appointment sheets in the software scheduling program.
2. Once all appointments have been scheduled, print an Appointment List for all providers for each day an appointment was scheduled during this task.
3. Place the Appointment Lists in your Completed Work folder behind Task 6.3.

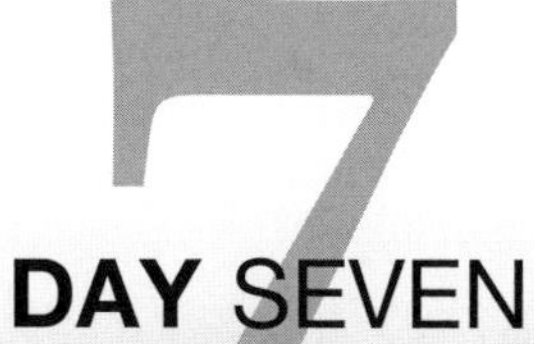

DAY SEVEN

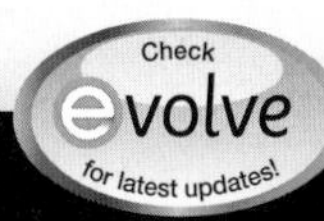

Tuesday, April 15, 2008

TASK **7.1**

Insurance Claim Forms

SUPPLIES NEEDED (p. 499):

- 6 blank CMS-1500 health insurance forms (located in the Supplies section)
- 6 Patient Face Sheets from Completed Work folder from Task 3.5
- 6 completed superbills from Completed Work folder from Task 5.2 (used again in Task 5.3)

1. Prepare CMS-1500 health insurance forms.
   - This morning Gladys has asked you to complete CMS-1500 health insurance forms using the information from the Patient Face Sheet and the completed superbills from Task 5.2 and used in Task 5.3.
   - Included on the CMS-1500 health insurance forms will be the patient information, date of service, and type of insurance.
   - See Appendix 3 for detailed directions on completing the CMS-1500.

2. The employment and marital status of each patient is:
   Mary Bogert is married.
   Elizabeth Fenton is married.
   Amanda Foster is married and employed.
   Jack Masci is married and employed.
   Jean Olson is single and employed.
   Lori Whittaker is single and was referred by Theodore Blackburn, MD.

Gladys has also requested that no "Amount Paid" be recorded on the CMS-1500.

3. Once you have completed all the information for each patient on the CMS-1500 health insurance forms, place them in alphabetic order in the Completed Work folder directly behind Task 6.4. Return to their correct locations in the Completed Work folder the Patient List (behind Task 3.4) and superbills (behind Task 5.2).

TASK **7.2**

Patient Reception

SUPPLIES NEEDED (p. 511):

- Appointment schedule for April 15 and 16 from your Completed Work file
- 3 file folders
- 3 preprinted file labels
- 3 blank Patient Information forms (located in the Supplies section)
- 3 blank Subsequent Findings forms (located in the Supplies section)

The remainder of the morning will be spent working at the reception desk. Gladys has asked you to prepare a new patient file folder for three of the new patients who are scheduled on Tuesday, April 15, and Wednesday, April 16.

1. **Assemble the patient's medical record.**
   - Locate the file folders and the file labels in the packet. On the appointment schedule for April 15 you will see that Li Wong and Lillian Schultz are new patients scheduled with Dr. Adams, and on April 16 George Jones has been scheduled with Dr. Harkness. Prepare a medical record for each of these three new patients. Gladys has already prepared the record for Fred Peterson.

2. **Patient Information forms.**
   - Prepare a Patient Information form for each patient. Once you have completed the Patient Information form with as much information as possible, place each form into the patient's folder.
   - Next, prepare a Subsequent Findings form to be placed into the patient's folder as the second sheet in the folder.
   - Once you have completed this task, place all your work in the Completed Work folder directly behind Task 7.1.

TASK **7.3**

Scheduling Nursing Home Services

SUPPLIES NEEDED:

- Appointment schedules for April 16 and April 17 from the Completed Work folder

Once a month Gladys schedules appointments for the physicians to see their patients at the South Padre Nursing Home. Today Gladys will have you perform this duty. Dr. Adams, Dr. Harkness, and Dr. Clark have stated that they would like to have a full morning or afternoon to go to the nursing home. If a full morning or afternoon is not available, schedule as much time as possible for the nursing home visit. They all also have requested that they see patients at the nursing home on either Wednesday, April 16, or Thursday, April 17.

The travel time will not be scheduled separately. For example, Dr. Harkness has lunch from 1–2 PM and 2–6 PM is marked off for the nursing home visit.

1. You will check the appointment schedule for each of these two days indicated and block off either a morning or afternoon for each of the three physicians. You will do this by placing an X through the time period that is open for each physician. Indicate "Nursing Home" on the blocked-off time.

2. Once you have completed this task, place the appointment schedule back in your Completed Work folder.

1. Using the step-by-step instructions for matrixing the schedule located in Software Instructions, Item A, block off time for nursing home visits for Dr. Adams, Dr. Harkness, and Dr. Clark. Follow the guidelines for time requested as in Task 7.3.

2. Print an Appointment List for each provider for April 17.

3. Place the Appointment List in your Completed Work folder behind Task 7.2.

TASK **7.4**

Telephone Messages

SUPPLIES NEEDED (p. 523):

- Companion Evolve site containing the telephone messages for April 15 (Task 7.4)
- 5 blank Telephone Records (located in the Supplies section)

1. Locate the "Telephone Messages" area on the companion Evolve site (Task 7.4)
    - Telephone messages came into the office during the time the clinic was closed. Gladys has asked you to listen to the voice mail and complete a Telephone Record for each call.
    - If a message is left for a member of the clinic staff, you are to write the message for the appropriate person indicated in the telephone message.
    - For patients who requested appointments for today, set those messages aside because you will be scheduling these appointments in Task 7.5.
    - Refer patients who are calling regarding laboratory results to Gladys.

TASK **7.5**

Scheduling Appointments

SUPPLIES NEEDED:

- Appointment schedule for Tuesday, April 15, 2008
- Completed Telephone Records from Task 7.4

1. Scheduling appointments from the telephone records.
    - Now that you have received the messages from the voice mail, you need to schedule any requests for appointments with Dr. Adams; all other physicians are unavailable today. All of the information needed to schedule the appointments is taken from the Telephone Record from Task 7.4. Once you have scheduled the appointments, indicate the appointment date and time on the Telephone Record in the "Response" section.

2. Gladys informs you that Dr. Bond was called out of town on a family emergency and will not be in the office today and asks you to mark this on his schedule.

3. Once you have scheduled the appointments requested from the messages, place the appointment schedule back in your Completed Work folder and return the Telephone Record (Task 7.4) to the correct location in the Completed Work folder.

1. Using the Telephone Record from Task 7.4, schedule the requested appointments with Dr. Adams. All of the appointments are to be scheduled for today.

2. Print an Appointment List for April 15 and place it in your Completed Work folder behind Task 7.4.

TASK **7.6**

Scheduling Surgeries

SUPPLIES NEEDED (p. 527):

- Appointment schedule for April 16 and April 17 from your Completed Work file
- 6 Preauthorization forms (as illustrated in **Figure 7-1**) (located in the Supplies section)
- 6 physician-completed Surgical Request and Information forms (a blank form is illustrated in **Figure 7-2**)
- 6 completed Patient Information forms

This afternoon you will be working with Joan Bothum, a medical assistant who schedules surgeries for the surgeons and obtains preauthorizations for those surgeries scheduled. All surgeries are performed at the South Padre Hospital.

1. **Complete the Request for Preauthorization for Surgery forms.**
   - Using the Surgical Request and Information forms and the Patient Information forms, complete a Request for Preauthorization for Surgery form for each patient. Be sure to fill out the Preauthorization form as completely as possible as illustrated in **Figure 7-3**. Use 04/16/08 or 04/17/08 as the "Admit Date."

REQUEST FOR PREAUTHORIZATION FOR SURGERY

Surgeon: (circle one) Gerald Bond, MD / Ray Adams, MD / Joyce Harkness, MD / Anthony Clark, MD

PATIENT NAME: ____________ FACILITY: ____________

DATE OF BIRTH: ____________ ADMIT DATE: ____________

ACCOUNT #: ____________ SURGERY DATE: ____________

INSURANCE: ____________ POLICY#: ____________

PROCEDURE: ____________

DIAGNOSIS: ____________

AUTHORIZATION: ____________

COMPLETED BY: ____________

DATE COMPLETED: ____________

Figure **7-1** **Request for Preauthorization for Surgery form.**

DAY SEVEN TASK 7.6

South Padre Medical Center

SURGICAL REQUEST AND INFORMATION

This portion is to be completed by requesting surgeon.

Surgeon: ❑ Gerald Bond, MD
❑ Ray Adams, MD
❑ Joyce Harkness, MD
❑ Anthony Clark, MD

Schedule: ❑ URGENT ❑ IMMEDIATE ❑ PATIENT CONVENIENCE

Date Requested: ______________ Time Requested: ______________

Patient Name: ______________

Procedure: ______________

Procedure Code(s): ______________

Diagnosis(es): ______________

Diagnosis(es) Code(s): ______________

Estimated Surgery Time: ______________

Surgical Assistant Requested: ______________

Additional Information: ______________

This portion is to be completed by scheduling personnel.

Surgery Date: ______________ Time: ______________
Day Date

Authorization Obtained: ❑ YES ❑ NO ❑ REQUESTED

If authorization has been requested and response is pending, list date and contact information from the initial request.

Requested From: ______________ Date: ______________
(Carrier and person)

Telephone: ______________ Ext: ______________

Completed By: ______________

Date Completed: ______________

Figure **7-2 Blank Surgical Request and Information form.**

REQUEST FOR PREAUTHORIZATION FOR SURGERY

Surgeon: (circle one) Gerald Bond, MD (circled)
Ray Adams, MD
Joyce Harkness, MD
Anthony Clark, MD

Date of surgery unless otherwise specified

PATIENT NAME: Sam Klint FACILITY: S. Padre Hospital

DATE OF BIRTH: 02/11/46 (62) ADMIT DATE: 04/16/08

ACCOUNT #: 00000-0012 SURGERY DATE: 04/16/08

INSURANCE: BC/BS of Texas POLICY#: MKL2211

PROCEDURE: Kidney BX 50200

DIAGNOSIS: Renal Failure 586

AUTHORIZATION: BC/BS of Texas

COMPLETED BY: Student's name

DATE COMPLETED: 04/15/08

Figure **7-3 Completed Request for Preauthorization for Surgery form.**

2. **Schedule surgery times for each physician.**
   - Using the appointment schedule for Wednesday, April 16, and Thursday, April 17, and the Surgical Request and Information forms that were previously completed, schedule each patient with the appropriate physician on the Center's appointment schedule. On the first line of the schedule, write the patient's last name, followed by the first name and any initials. The next line will be the type of surgery to be performed (such as "Kidney Biopsy"). The last line will be the diagnosis for which the surgery is being performed (such as "Dx: Renal Failure). The length of time for each surgery is located in Appendix 2, Item N. If the patient information does not fill in the lines for the allotted time, block the remaining time frame with Xs (as illustrated in **Figure 7-4**).

3:00	Klint, Sam J.
3:15	Kidney Bx
3:30	Dx: Renal Failure
3:45	X X X X X
4:00	
4:15	

Figure **7-4** **Example of matrixing appointment time for surgery.**

Schedule the surgeries in the following order:
Klint, Sam J.
Adams, Tony W.
Harkland, Emmy L.
Bates, Michelle L.
Anderson, Charlie M.
Wood, Tina J.

Once you have entered the surgeries onto the schedule, complete the bottom portion of the Surgical Request and Information form by entering the date and time the surgery has been scheduled as illustrated in **Figure 7-5.** Also indicate that insurance authorization has been received for all six patients by placing an X in the box next to "YES" on the Authorization Obtained line. Sign your name and date the form.

South Padre Medical Center

SURGICAL REQUEST AND INFORMATION

This portion is to be completed by requesting surgeon.

Surgeon: ☒ Gerald Bond, MD
☐ Ray Adams, MD
☐ Joyce Harkness, MD
☐ Anthony Clark, MD

Schedule: ☐ URGENT ☒ IMMEDIATE ☐ PATIENT CONVENIENCE

Date Requested: 04-15-08 Time Requested: 8:10 AM

Patient Name: KLINT, SAM J. ACCOUNT #: 00000-0012

Procedure: BIOPSY OF KIDNEY

Procedure Code(s): 50200

Diagnosis(es): RENAL FAILURE

Diagnosis(es) Code(s): 586

Estimated Surgery Time: 1 HOUR OUTPATIENT

Surgical Assistant Requested: —

Additional Information: —

This portion is to be completed by scheduling personnel.

Surgery Date: Wednesday (Day) 04/16/08 (Date) Time: 3:00 pm

Authorization Obtained: ☒ YES ☐ NO ☐ REQUESTED

If authorization has been requested and response is pending, list date and contact information from the initial request.

Requested From: ______ (Carrier and person) Date: ______

Telephone: ______ Ext: ______

Completed By: Student's Name

Date Completed: 04/15/08

Figure **7-5** **Surgical Request and Information form.**

- Using the Surgical Request and Information forms you just completed, you would schedule the inpatient and outpatient surgeries with the hospital. You are to assume that the staff member whom you called at the hospital approved all of the procedure times as requested and scheduled.

3. **Once you have completed this task, place all of your completed work and the appointment schedule in the Completed Work folder after Task 7.5.**

1. Using the completed Surgical Request and Information forms from Task 7.6, schedule the inpatient and outpatient surgeries in the software scheduling program.
2. Print an Appointment List for each provider for April 16 and April 17, and place it in your Completed Work folder behind Task 7.6.

TASK 7.7

Medical Records

SUPPLIES NEEDED (p. 563):

- 6 file folders
- 6 preprinted file labels
- 6 completed Patient Information sheets from Task 7.6 supplies
- 6 blank Subsequent Findings forms (located in the Supplies section)

This afternoon you will be responsible for assembling patient files for each patient who is scheduled for surgery on Wednesday, April 16, and Thursday, April 17. All of these patients will be coming in for postoperative visits and will need a patient file.

1. Assemble the patient medical record.
    - Locate the file folders and file labels in the packet. The patient's name is in capital letters on each label, with last name first followed by the patient's first name and middle initial. The patients are from are Task 7.6. Secure the labels to each file folder.

2. Place each Patient Information sheet in the patient's file folder, making sure the Patient Information sheet is placed first in the correct file folder.

3. Subsequent Findings form.
    - You will also need to place a Subsequent Findings form in each of the file folders. Using the information from the Patient Information forms from Task 7.6, complete the information on the top of each Subsequent Findings form. This will be the second page to be placed in the patient's file folder.

4. Once you have completed this task, place the file folders with both of the completed forms in the proper file folders in your Completed Work folder.

1. Enter into the new software program the demographic information from the completed Patient Information forms for each patient from Task 7.6. The step-by-step instruction for entering patient information is located in Software Instructions, Item E. Once all the demographic information has been entered, print a Patient Face Sheet for each patient and review the information for errors. The instructions for printing the Patient Face Sheet are located in Software Instructions, Item F.

2. Place the printed Patient Face Sheets in the Completed Work folder.

This completes your tasks for Day Seven. On to Day Eight. You're doing a great job!

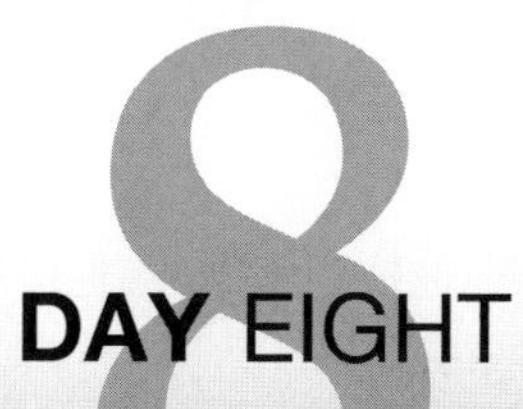

DAY EIGHT

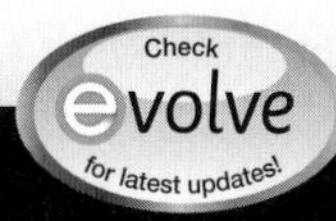
Check
evolve
for latest updates!

Wednesday, April 16, 2008

TASK **8.1**	Arranging for Physician Travel
TASK **8.2**	Inventory Management
TASK **8.3**	Telephone Messages
TASK **8.4**	Medical Transcription

TASK 8.1

Arranging for Physician Travel

SUPPLIES NEEDED (p. 575):

- Travel schedule for Dr. Harkness (located in the Supplies section)
- Blank piece of paper

1. Gladys has supplied you with a handwritten itinerary from which you will prepare an itinerary (as illustrated in **Figure 8-1**) for Dr. Harkness's overnight trip. Once you have completed Dr. Harkness's itinerary, place it in your Completed Work folder behind Task 7.7.

Itinerary for Dr. Joyce Harkness
New York City Cardiac Conference

4:45 am	Friday, April 18, arrive at South Padre Airport
5:30 am	Flight 19 leaves South Padre, destination New York City

Figure **8-1** **Travel schedule for Dr. Harkness.**

TASK 8.2

Inventory Management

SUPPLIES NEEDED (p. 577):

- Reception inventory sheet (located in the Supplies section)

1. Complete an inventory sheet.
    - Gladys has asked you to inventory the furniture in the patient waiting room after office hours today. She refers you to Appendix 2, Policies and Procedures, Item R, for details on how to complete the inventory sheet. Inventory the items in the office reception photo **(Figure 8-2)** with the inventory sheet in the Supplies Section for this task.
    - Place the work in the Completed Work folder.

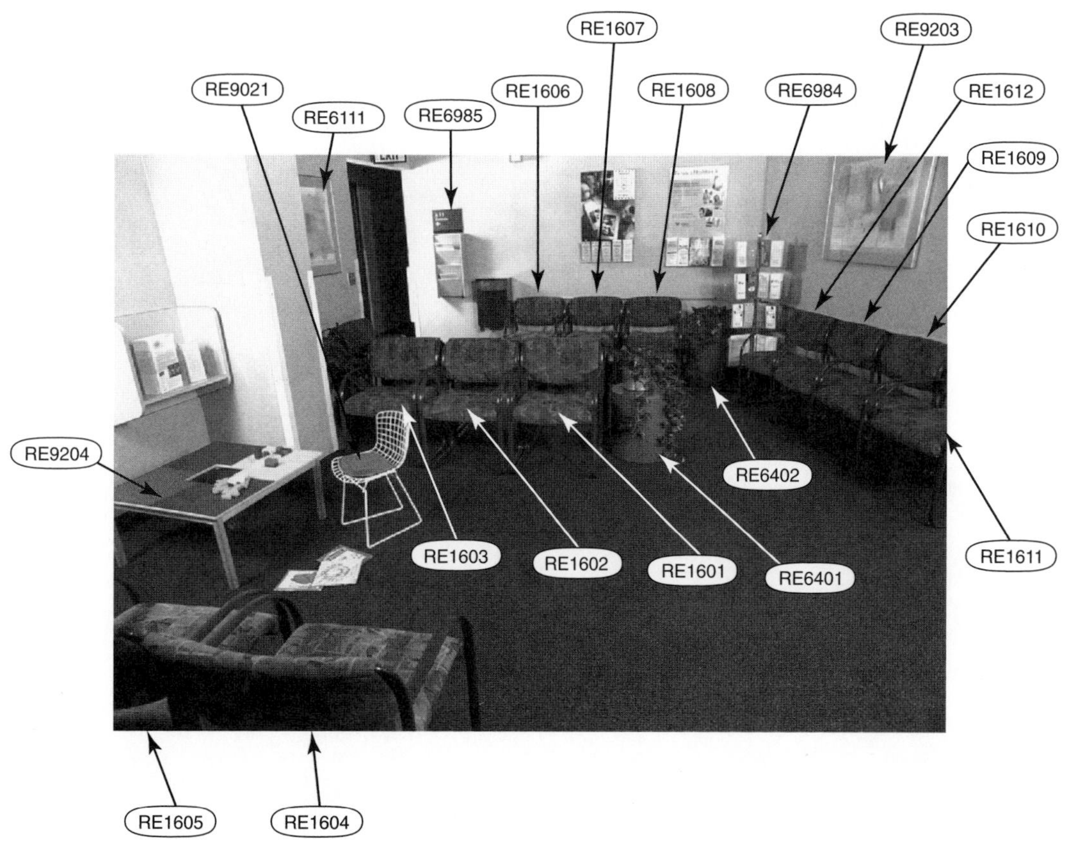

Figure **8-2** **Office inventory.** *(From Potter BP:* Medical office administration: a worktext, *ed 2, St. Louis, 2010, Saunders.)*

TASK 8.3

Telephone Messages

SUPPLIES NEEDED (p. 579):

- Companion Evolve site containing the telephone messages for April 16 (Task 8.3)
- Answer sheet for Task 8.3 (located in the Supplies section)

1. Locate the "Telephone Messages" area on the companion Evolve site (Task 8.3).
   - Telephone messages came into the office during the time the clinic was closed. Gladys has asked you to listen to the voice mail and complete the Answer Sheet with the correct response to each call.
   - Place in your Completed Work folder.

TASK **8.4**

Medical Transcription

SUPPLIES NEEDED **(p. 581)****:**

- Companion Evolve site containing the medical transcription from April 16
- 2 Operative Report forms (located in the Supplies section and in the Forms Library on the companion Evolve site)

1. Locate the "Medical Transcription" area on the companion Evolve site.
   - This afternoon Gladys will cover the reception desk while you transcribe the medical dictation for surgeries performed earlier today.
   - Two operative reports were dictated. You are to key each dictation as indicated on the Evolve site.

2. Once you have completed this task, place all of the reports in your Completed Work folder.

That's it for Day Eight. Great work! You have learned so much so far, so let's learn a little more. On to Day Nine.

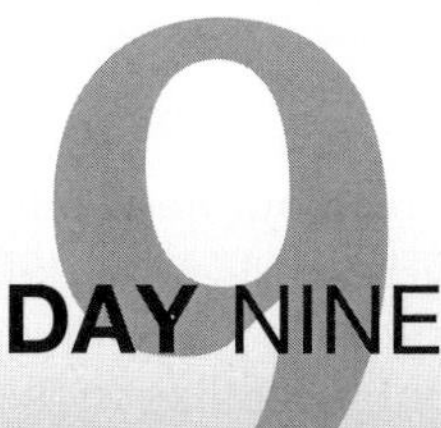

DAY NINE

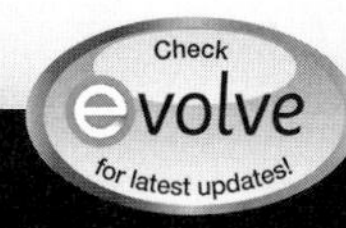

Thursday, April 17, 2008

TASK **9.1**	Software Installation
TASK **9.2**	Dashboard Functions
TASK **9.3**	Patient Registration Record
TASK **9.4**	Health History Form

TASK **9.1**

Software Installation

SUPPLIES NEEDED:

- Computer
- Practice Partner software (CD in the envelope at the back of the book)

Today, you are going to begin your electronic health record (EHR) training experience. An EHR system in health care settings is fast becoming standard, so over the next two days you will be introduced to Practice Partner EHR software. The software includes a versatile medical record that makes accessing medical information fast and easy.

You will be working with the Employee Software Training System (ESTS) in a mock medical clinic, Constant Family Care. Do not worry that you might do something incorrectly while learning about the software; the ESTS has been configured to allow you access to a closed training system that uses a limited number of EHRs specifically designed for training purposes. When you have completed this training, you will receive your user name and password to the "live" system. Let's get started. First, you need to load the software onto the trainee computer using the directions that follow. If you set the date on your computer to April 2008 for the Medisoft activities in Days One through Eight, please reset it to the current date. After you have loaded the software, you will manipulate data in the electronic environment. Now, it is time to load the software and get going on your training!

You will now focus your attention on becoming familiar with Practice Partner EHR software. We will begin by guiding you through the installation of this software.

Note: Instructions for printing and archiving data using Practice Partner EHR software are available on the Evolve site. These instructions will be needed in a classroom environment.

STEP-BY-STEP DIRECTIONS 1-9:

1. Insert Practice Partner Sales Demo Version 9.3.2 into the computer and a dialog box will automatically open to notify you that software is going to be installed on the computer. Click "Next."

2. On the second screen, a dialog box will notify you that you are about to install the software. Click "Install" to begin installation.

3. When prompted, click "OK" and allow the software to run until installation is finished. This will take several minutes.

4. A dialog box will open that states the installation is complete. Click the "Finish" button.

5. Click the Start button in the lower left corner of your screen. "Practice Partner EMR" should appear in the list of options or under All Programs>Interactive Sales Demo>Practice Partner EMR. Click on it to start the program.

6. Practice Partner will launch with the screen in **Figure 9-1**. Enter the user name "pmsi" and password "master," then click "OK" on the two following dialog boxes to launch the software. Accept as default each box and the software will open to the Dashboard.

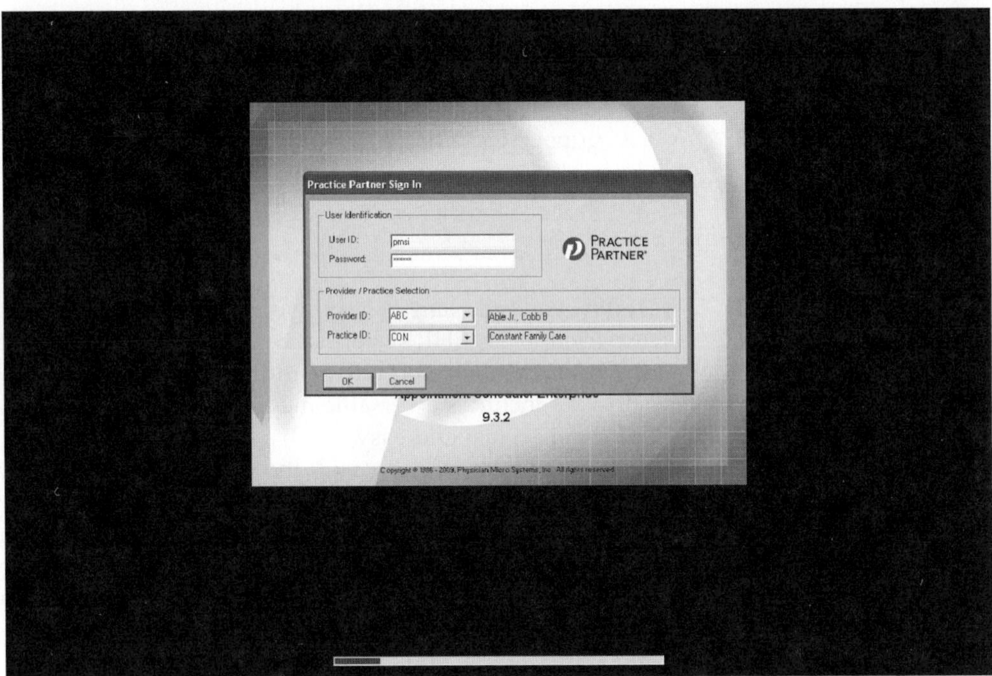

Figure **9-1** **Practice Partner User ID and Password dialog box.** *Practice Partner® is a registered trademark of McKesson Corporation and/or one of its subsidiaries. Practice Partner® screen shots and materials used with the permission of McKesson Corporation. © 2010 McKesson Corporation. All rights reserved.*

7. A Disclaimer Notice will open, as displayed in **Figure 9-2**, to inform you of the proprietary material bundled into the software. Click "OK" to continue launching the software.

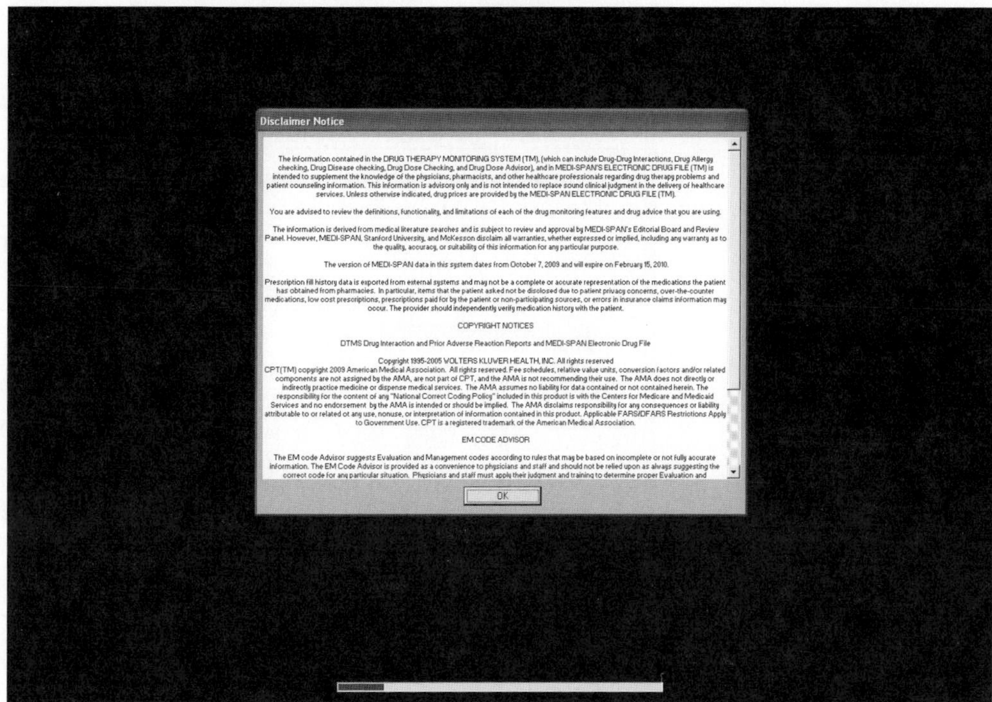

Figure **9-2** **Disclaimer Notice.** *Practice Partner® is a registered trademark of McKesson Corporation and/or one of its subsidiaries. Practice Partner® screen shots and materials used with the permission of McKesson Corporation. © 2010 McKesson Corporation. All rights reserved.*

8. A dialog box will open that states that the Drug Interaction or Allergy Checking database has expired. Click "OK."

9. Practice Partner opens with the Dashboard screen as shown in **Figure 9-3**.

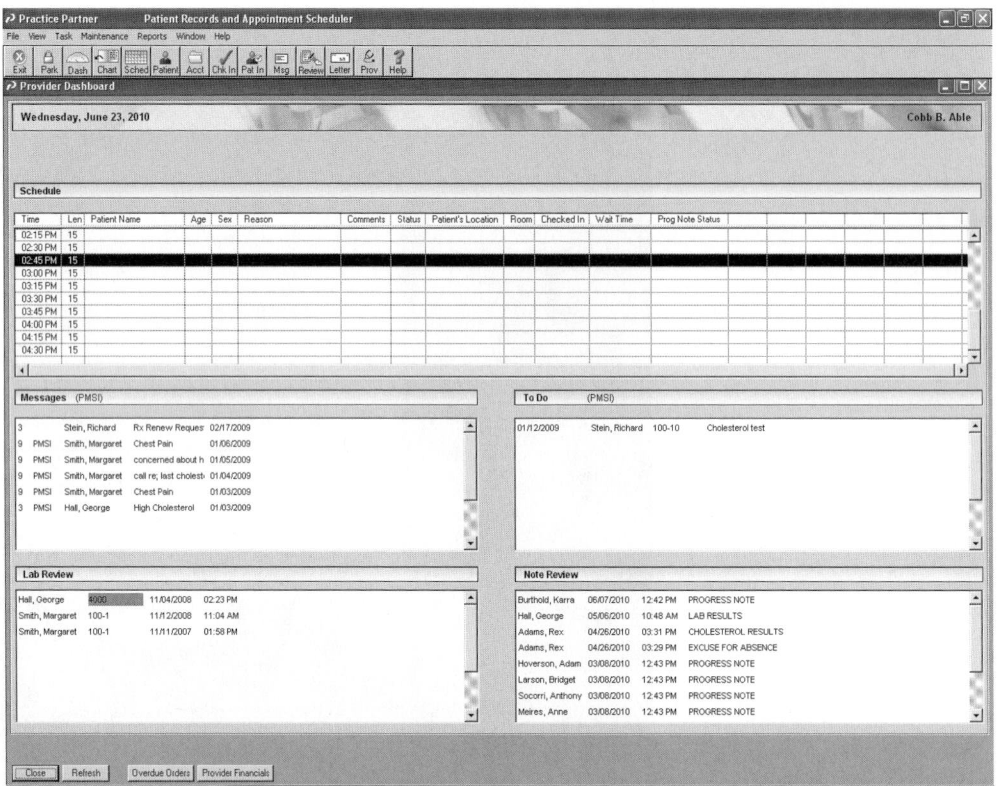

Figure **9-3** **Dashboard opens with Dr. Cobb B. Able's information.** *Practice Partner® is a registered trademark of McKesson Corporation and/or one of its subsidiaries. Practice Partner® screen shots and materials used with the permission of McKesson Corporation. © 2010 McKesson Corporation. All rights reserved.*

Your Practice Partner software is now loaded on the trainee computer and you are ready to begin learning about all the great features of this EHR software in Task 9-2.

TASK **9.2**

Dashboard Functions

SUPPLIES NEEDED:

- Practice Partner software

The Dashboard is the central hub of the software—the place to which you will return to access the functions of the software. Let's take a closer look at the Dashboard features. For now, you won't be learning about how each of these functions works; rather, you are learning where each of the buttons is located. **Figure 9-4** illustrates each of the Dashboard features. The Exit button closes the software. Park is a feature that is very helpful when you are leaving the computer area or protecting the privacy of information that is displayed on your desktop (computer screen). Within the Health Insurance Portability and Accountability Act of 1996, there are privacy requirements that closely govern disclosure of patients' protected health information (PHI). The contents of the EHR are protected information, so develop a habit of using the Park feature. When you click the "Park" button, the User ID and Password dialog box appears and covers the monitor surface with the Practice Partner background. To return to the Dashboard, enter the user name and password again. The screen then opens to the Dashboard you were on before you parked. The Dash button returns you to the Dashboard (software central). For example, click the "Sched" button next to the Dash button to open the schedule. Click the "Dash" button to return to the Dashboard and close the schedule.

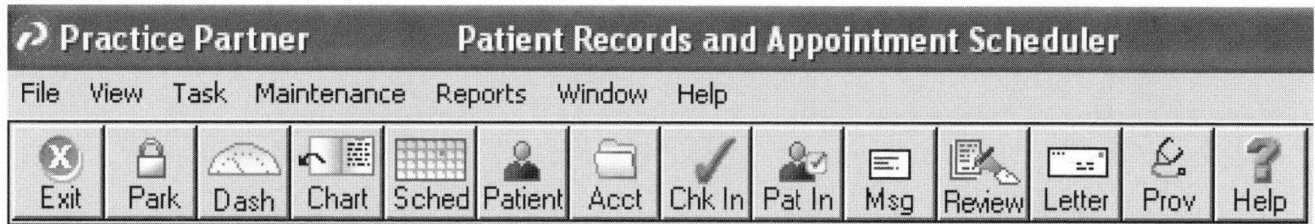

Figure **9-4** **Dashboard buttons.** *Practice Partner® is a registered trademark of McKesson Corporation and/or one of its subsidiaries. Practice Partner® screen shots and materials used with the permission of McKesson Corporation. © 2010 McKesson Corporation. All rights reserved.*

The Chart button displays the Patient Information dialog box used to locate the EHR for any patient. The Sched button enables the scheduling feature of the software. You will not use the Sched feature for these activities. The Patient button displays the Patient Information dialog box.

The Acct button opens the Medical Billing component of the software; however, for these activities you will not be using this feature. The Chk In button opens the Patient Look Up dialog box of the software that allows you to locate and check a patient in for an appointment. The Pat In button opens the Patients In feature to access various functions of the software that will be reviewed later. The Msg feature opens e-mail; from here you manage your e-mail by receiving, sending, and deleting messages. Review opens the messages on the Dashboard that require review. The Letter button opens the Patients Lookup dialog box, enabling you to identify the patient to whom or about whom a letter is going to be written. The software assists you by automatically inserting patient information into the documents being prepared.

There are only two more buttons in this quick review of the Dashboard; after reviewing these you will be ready to get started using the features of this dynamic EHR software. The Prov feature opens a dialog box that allows you to identify the provider or physician information that will be displayed on the Dashboard. With this feature you can switch between the various Dashboard screens. In the medical office, your Dashboard can only be accessed by entering your user name and password. The system manager can also access any Dashboard, but only for technical assistance. For the purposes of the ESTS, you are allowed to access other Dashboards for educational purposes only, but on the live system you can only access your Dashboard. It is your responsibility to safeguard your user name and password to protect the security of your Dashboard.

The Help feature is a useful tool as you learn about the Practice Partner software. When you click the "Help" button, a search feature appears. The search feature is similar to those used in word processing software, and allows you to search for information by topics, terms, or favorites.

Note that the default (automatically displayed) screen for the software opens the Dashboard for Cobb B. Able (indicated by an arrow); the date is the date (indicated by an arrow) on which you are opening the software.

The tasks you will complete are set in the fictional Constant Family Care clinic, located in the state of Washington. The practice includes a variety of health care professionals, but for this training activity, you will be logged in as Cobb B. Able, Jr., MD. His provider ID is ABC.

TASK 9.3

Patient Registration Record

SUPPLIES NEEDED (p. 585):

- 12 Patient Information forms from the Supplies section
- Practice Partner software

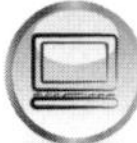

Today, you are going to use various features of the Practice Partner software. There are step-by-step directions throughout the ESTS, so just follow along and soon you will be accessing information quickly. You will find that the software is very user-friendly.

Begin by opening the software to display the Dashboard as illustrated in **Figure 9-5**.

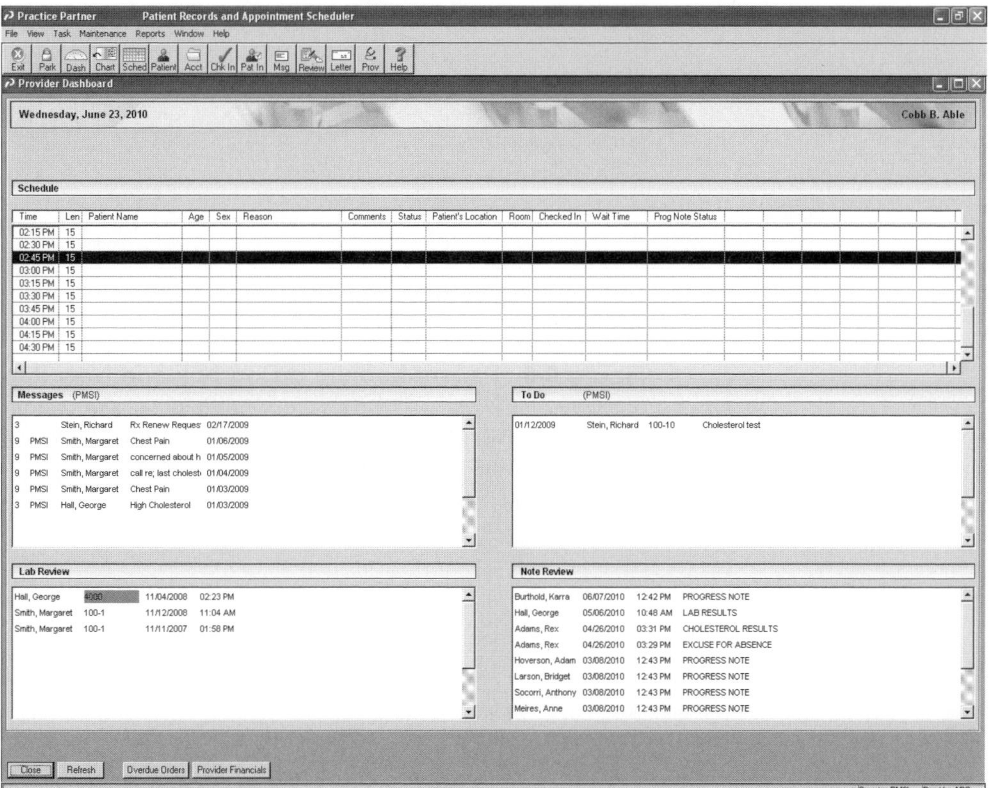

Figure **9-5** **Dashboard of EHR.** *Practice Partner® is a registered trademark of McKesson Corporation and/or one of its subsidiaries. Practice Partner® screen shots and materials used with the permission of McKesson Corporation. © 2010 McKesson Corporation. All rights reserved.*

Next, click the "Chart" button (refer to Figure 9-4) to display the Patient Lookup dialog box as illustrated in **Figure 9-6**. At the bottom of the Patient Lookup dialog box, click the "New Patient" button.

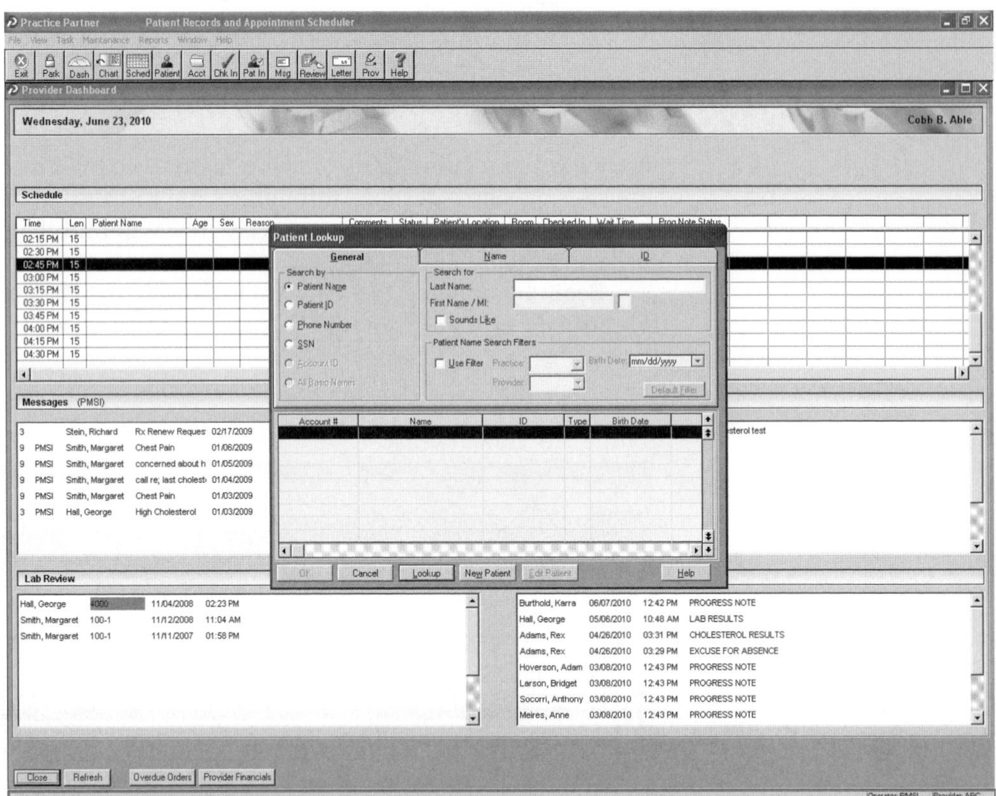

Figure **9-6** **Patient Lookup dialog box and New Patient tab.** *Practice Partner® is a registered trademark of McKesson Corporation and/or one of its subsidiaries. Practice Partner® screen shots and materials used with the permission of McKesson Corporation. © 2010 McKesson Corporation. All rights reserved.*

The "Patient <New>" dialog box is displayed. The screen opens to the General tab, as shown by the arrow in **Figure 9-7**.

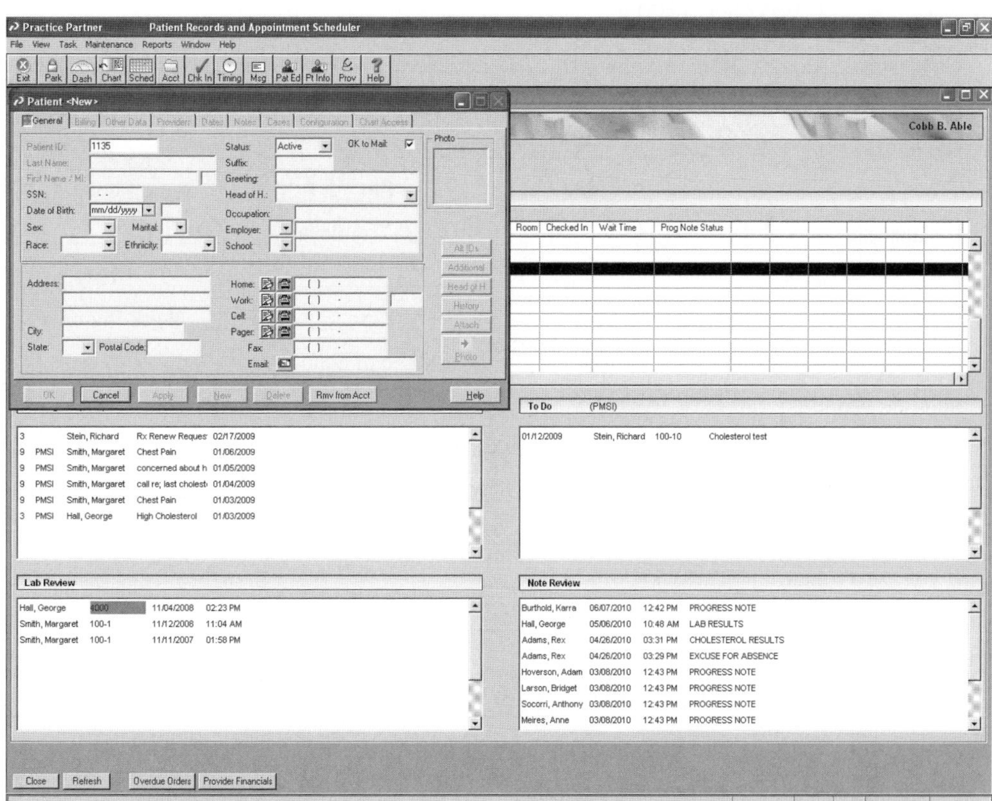

Figure **9-7** **Patient <New> dialog box.** *Practice Partner® is a registered trademark of McKesson Corporation and/or one of its subsidiaries. Practice Partner® screen shots and materials used with the permission of McKesson Corporation. © 2010 McKesson Corporation. All rights reserved.*

Figure 9-8 displays the Patient Information form completed by Joe P. Carlson. You are going to input the information from Joe's form into the computer.

Constant Family Care

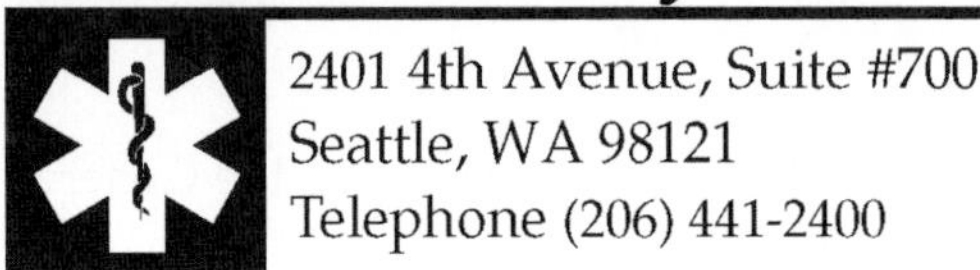

2401 4th Avenue, Suite #700
Seattle, WA 98121
Telephone (206) 441-2400

PATIENT INFORMATION

Please Print

Today's Date Current Date

Last Name Carlson First Name Joe Initial P

Date of Birth 6/23/65 Age ______ Sex M SS# 621-84-9898

Home Address Street 60 Moss Avenue City South Padre

State WA Zip 98765 Home Phone (209) 555-6400

Occupation Plumber Employer Self

Employer Address Street Same City ______

State ______ Zip ______ Work Phone (____) ______

Are you currently a student? Yes (No) Name of School ______

Spouse's Name none Marital Status M (S) D W SEP

Spouse's SS# ___-___-___ Spouse's Employer ______

In case of emergency, notify Susan Carlson Relationship sister

Home Phone (209) 555-4211 Work Phone (____) none

If you are a minor: Parent's ______ SS# ___-___-___

Street ______ City ______ State ______ Zip ______

Home Phone (____) ______ Work Phone (____) ______

Reason for Visit Headaches

Work related injury? Yes (No) Date of injury ______

Automobile accident? Yes (No) Date of injury ______

Other injury? Yes (No) Date of injury ______

Insurance (Primary) Company Name: Washington Health Corporation

Street 1756 56th Ave City Houston State WA Zip 99881

Subscriber's Name self

Relationship to Subscriber: ______

Policy # DCR6341 Group # ______

Insurance (Secondary) Company Name: ______

Street ______ City ______ State ______ Zip ______

Subscriber's Name ______

Relationship to Subscriber: ______

Policy # ______ Group # ______

Assignment of Benefits:

I directly assign all medical/surgical benefits, including major medical benefits and Medicare, to Central Medical Partners. I understand that this authorization for assignment remains in effect until I revoke it in writing. A photocopy of this assignment will be considered as valid as this original assignment. I further understand that I am responsible for my indebtedness no matter what charges the insurance pays for.

Insured or Guardian's Signature Joe P Carlson Date Current Date

Figure **9-8** **Joe P. Carlson's completed Patient Information form.** *Practice Partner® is a registered trademark of McKesson Corporation and/or one of its subsidiaries. Practice Partner® screen shots and materials used with the permission of McKesson Corporation. © 2010 McKesson Corporation. All rights reserved.*

1. Place your cursor in the white space to the right of the Last Name line in the Patient <New> dialog box.

2. Key in the last name of the patient ("Carlson"), then hit the Tab key to move to the First Name, and enter "Joe."

3. Hit the Tab key again and move to the box to type the patient's middle initial ("P").

4. Tab again to move to the Social Security number (SSN) box and enter the number for this patient ("621-84-9898"). Hyphens are not necessary when you enter the SSN because the software will automatically move the cursor to the next space for you.

5. Tab to the Date of Birth space and enter the birth date as stated on the Patient Information form. Enter a zero for single-numbered days, months, or years. For example, June is entered as "06." Enter the patient's birthday ("06/23/1965"). Note that when you tab forward to the next data entry block, the patient's age automatically appears.

6. Tab forward to enter the sex of the patient. Click the arrow to the left of the data entry block and a drop-down menu will appear. Scroll down to the "M" to identify this patient as male.

7. Tab to the Marital data block and, using the drop-down menu located to the right of the box, select "S" to identify the patient as single.

8. The patient information does not indicate Race or Ethnicity, so leave those two data blocks blank and continue to tab forward to the Status data block. The default is "Active," which is correctly checked for this patient.

9. Tab forward to the "OK to mail" data block, which is checked by default and is correct for this patient because the patient registration form does not indicate any mailing status. Leave the default check mark as it appears.

10. Tab forward to the Suffix data block, which is left blank unless the patient lists a suffix such as "Sr.," "Jr.," or "III."

11. Tab forward to the Greeting data block, which is used to indicate the salutation line when addressing a letter to the patient. In this case, the default is "Dear."

12. Tab forward to the Head of H (Head of Household) data block, which has a drop-down arrow to the right of the box. Click the arrow, scroll down to "Self," and highlight it so the term "Self" is in the box on the patient registration form. If the patient is a married female or a child, leave this box blank, and if the patient is a single or married male, enter "Self" in the box. (This is not meant to be sexist; it is just the technical categorization within the software.)

13. Tab forward to the Occupation box. Key in the occupation listed on the Patient Information form as "Plumber."

14. Tab forward to the Employer area and, using the drop-down menu, select the letter "Y."

15. Tab to the next block to enter the Employer, which in this case is "Self" because Joe is self-employed.

16. Tab forward to the School area. If the patient is a student, click on the "School" tab and select "P" for part time or "F" for full time. Leave this blank if the patient's student status is unknown. Since Joe is not a student, leave the area blank.

17. Tab forward to the next block. If the patient is a student at any school, enter the school if known. Since Joe is not a student, we will leave this blank.

18. Tab to the space next to Address and key in the address of the patient ("60 Moss Avenue"), tabbing or moving your curser as you also complete the City ("South Padre"), State ("WA"), and Zip Code ("98765") areas of the form.

19. Tab forward to the Home telephone number and enter "209-555-6400." Note that the software automatically moves forward to enter each digit of the telephone number, only requiring you to enter the digits and not the hyphens. Enter Work and Cell telephone numbers if listed on the Patient Information form. Joe did not indicate a work or cell telephone number.

20. The correctly entered patient information for Joe Carlson appears as illustrated in **Figure 9-9**. Click the "Apply" button at the bottom of the dialog box and the information you keyed in is saved to the software.

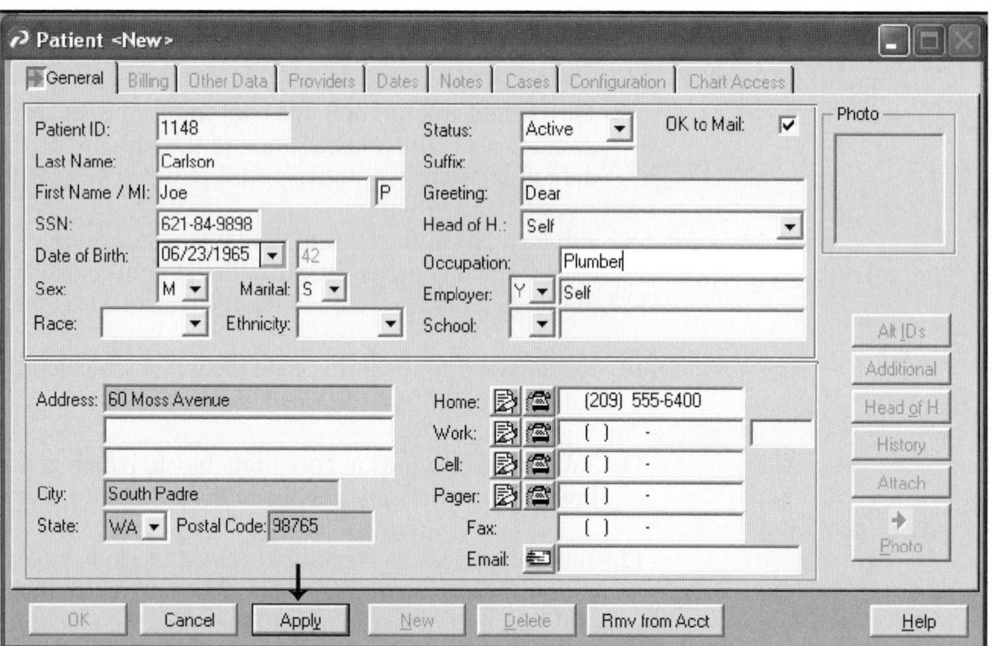

Figure **9-9 General tab of the Patient <New> dialog box with Joe Carlson's information.** *Practice Partner® is a registered trademark of McKesson Corporation and/or one of its subsidiaries. Practice Partner® screen shots and materials used with the permission of McKesson Corporation. © 2010 McKesson Corporation. All rights reserved.*

21. Continue entering information on the Patient <New> dialog box by clicking the "Additional" button (located to the right of Joe's home phone number) to display the screen shown in **Figure 9-10**.

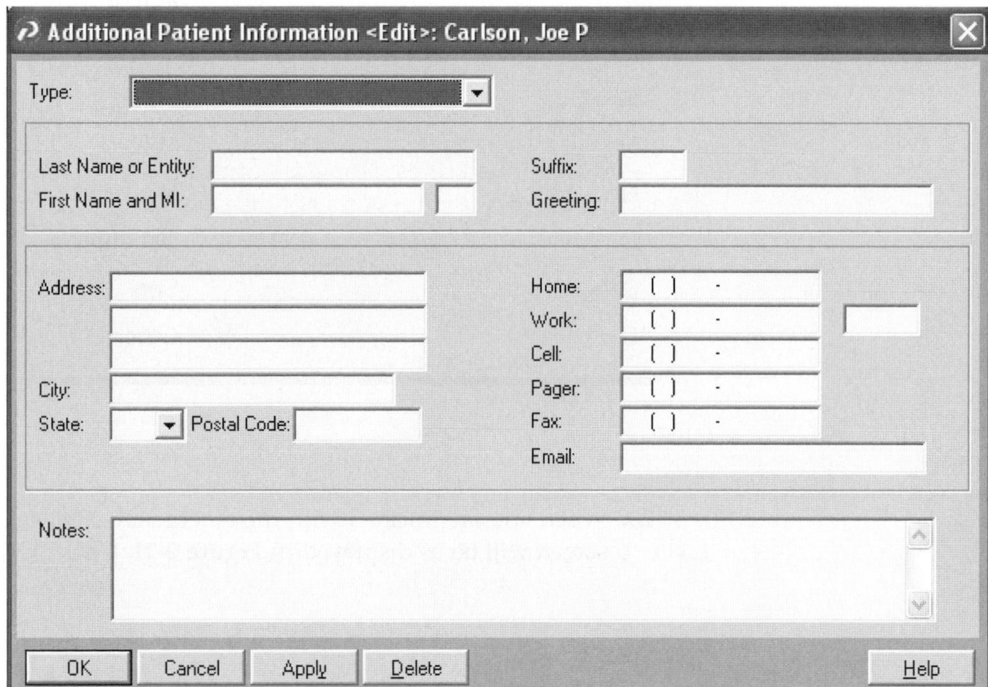

Figure **9-10** **Additional button in the Patient <New> dialog box.** *Practice Partner® is a registered trademark of McKesson Corporation and/or one of its subsidiaries. Practice Partner® screen shots and materials used with the permission of McKesson Corporation. © 2010 McKesson Corporation. All rights reserved.*

22. In the "Type" window, select "Emergency Conta" and key in the emergency contact's last name and first name in the appropriate boxes. Enter the emergency contact's home phone number. If the emergency contact has multiple phone numbers or offers an address, these can also be included in the additional fields. Since Joe's contact did not indicate another phone number or an address, we will leave them blank. In the notes box, type the relationship to patient using the abbreviations in **Table 9-1**. If the emergency contact has a Social Security number, you would also enter it into the notes box at this time.

TABLE **9-1:** Emergency Contact Relationship Abbreviations

BR	Brother
SS	Sister
M	Mother
F	Father
H	Husband
W	Wife
Ne	Niece
Nw	Nephew
D	Daughter
S	Son
O	Other

23. When you are finished with the emergency contact information for Joe, the screen will be as displayed in **Figure 9-11**. Click "OK" when you are finished.

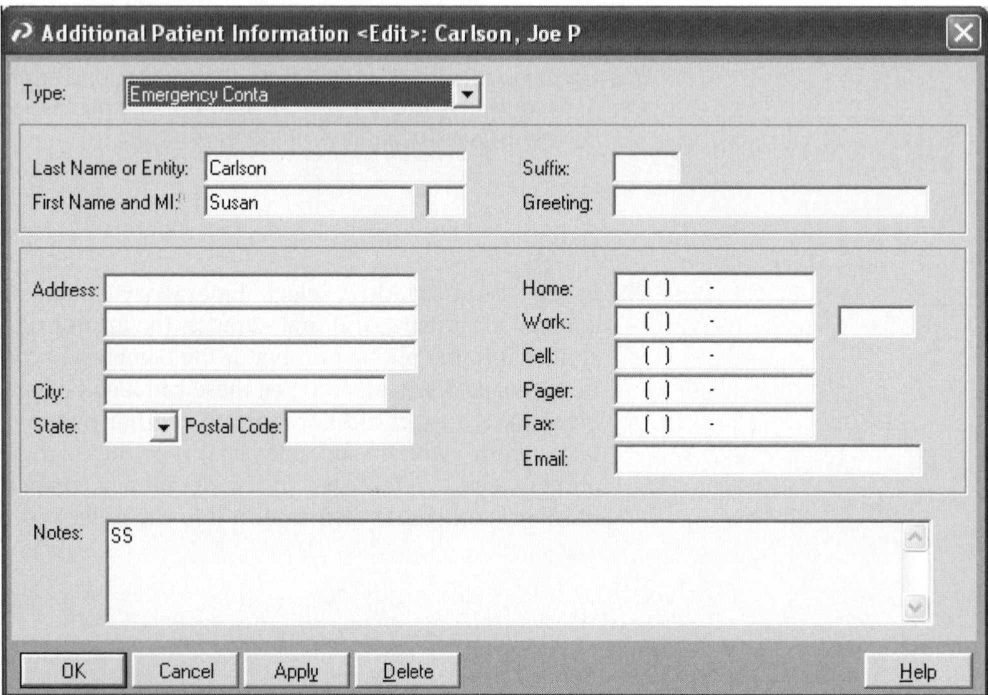

Figure **9-11** **Joe Carlson's completed Emergency Contact.** *Practice Partner® is a registered trademark of McKesson Corporation and/or one of its subsidiaries. Practice Partner® screen shots and materials used with the permission of McKesson Corporation. © 2010 McKesson Corporation. All rights reserved.*

24. Click the "Providers" tab to display the dialog box shown in **Figure 9-12**.

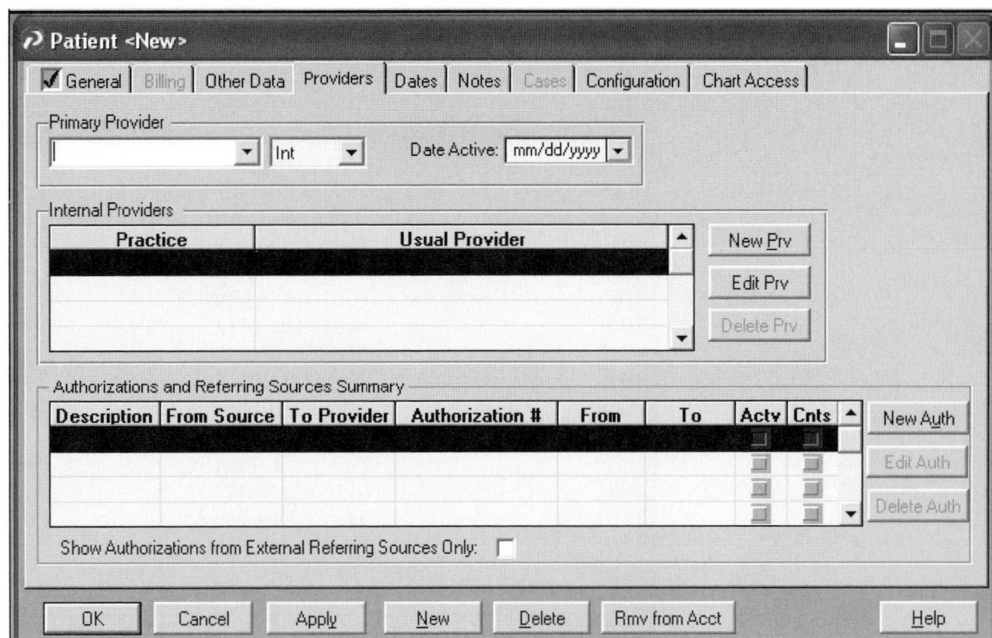

Figure **9-12 Providers tab of the Patient <New> dialog box.** *Practice Partner® is a registered trademark of McKesson Corporation and/or one of its subsidiaries. Practice Partner® screen shots and materials used with the permission of McKesson Corporation. © 2010 McKesson Corporation. All rights reserved.*

25. Click the drop-down arrow to the right of the Primary Provider box and the Provider Select dialog box will be displayed as shown in **Figure 9-13**. Joe is here today for an appointment with Dr. Able, whose provider initials are ABC. Double-click Dr. Able's name to automatically load the information into the Primary Provider area on the dialog box as shown in **Figure 9-14**. The "Date Active" automatically indicates the date you entered the information.

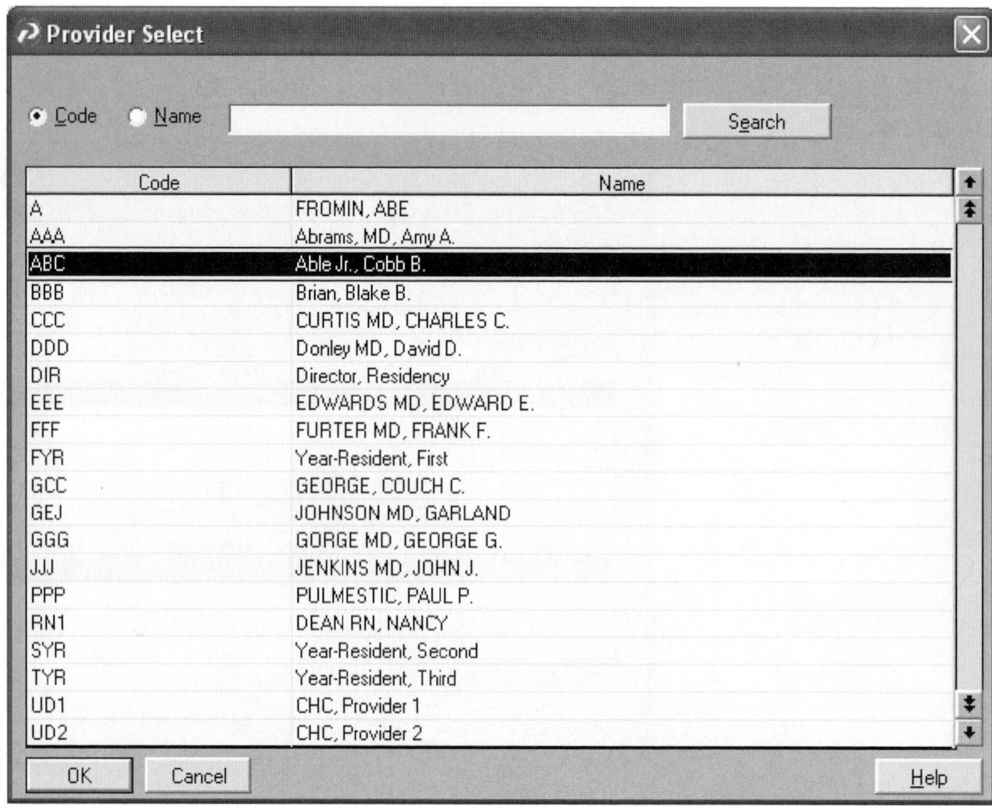

Figure **9-13** **Provider Select dialog box.** *Practice Partner® is a registered trademark of McKesson Corporation and/or one of its subsidiaries. Practice Partner® screen shots and materials used with the permission of McKesson Corporation. © 2010 McKesson Corporation. All rights reserved.*

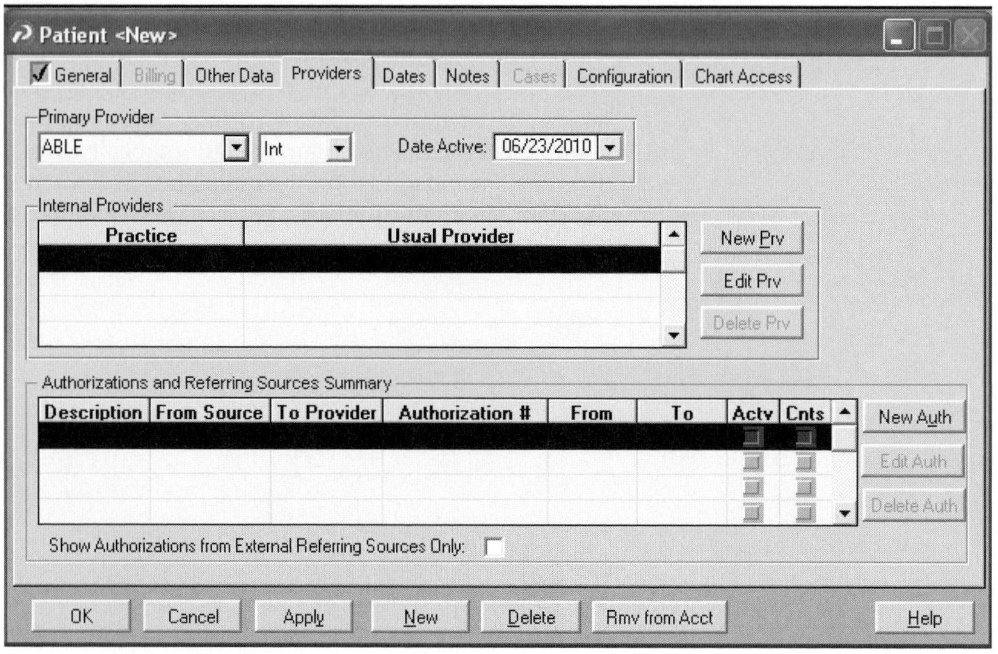

Figure **9-14** **Primary Provider automatically loads into dialog box.** *Practice Partner® is a registered trademark of McKesson Corporation and/or one of its subsidiaries. Practice Partner® screen shots and materials used with the permission of McKesson Corporation. © 2010 McKesson Corporation. All rights reserved.*

26. Next, click the "New Prv" button (new provider) as shown in **Figure 9-15** to indicate that Joe's usual provider is Dr. Able and the usual practice is Central Medical Partners.

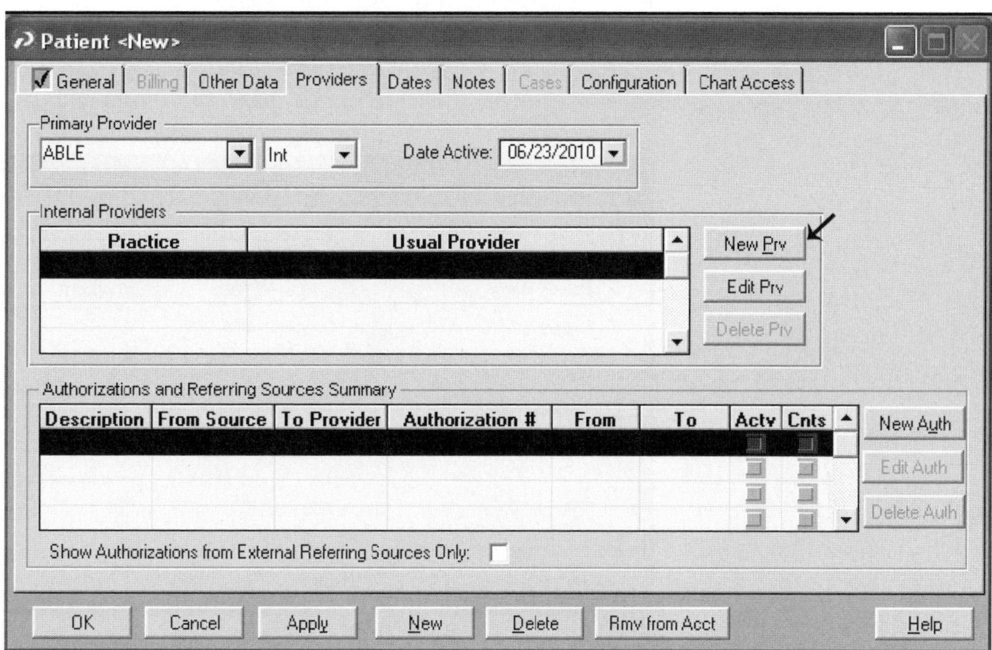

Figure **9-15** **Indicating the physician and practice defaults.** *Practice Partner® is a registered trademark of McKesson Corporation and/or one of its subsidiaries. Practice Partner® screen shots and materials used with the permission of McKesson Corporation. © 2010 McKesson Corporation. All rights reserved.*

27. A dialog box as illustrated in **Figure 9-16** will appear. Click on the down arrow next to the Usual Provider block; a list appears. Double-click Dr. Able's name. Note that the dialog box has a check next to "Default," (beneath "Other Provider"), which means that whenever Joe's medical record is accessed, Dr. Able will be the provider. Click the "OK" button to return to the "Patient <New>" dialog box; the provider information automatically inserts. Finish by clicking "OK" at the bottom of the "Patient <New>" dialog box to return to the Dashboard.

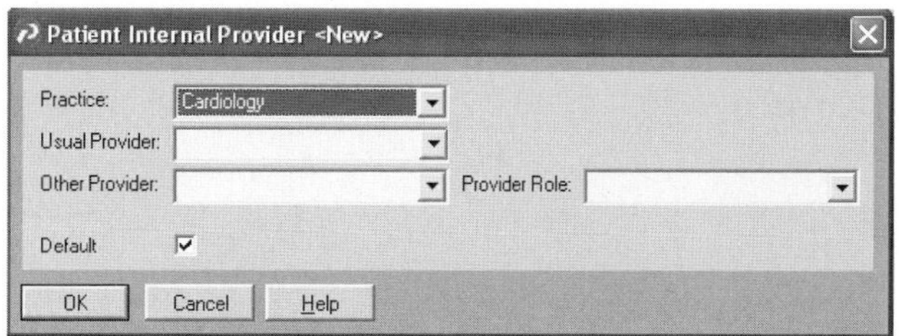

Figure **9-16** **Patient Internal Provider dialog box.** *Practice Partner® is a registered trademark of McKesson Corporation and/or one of its subsidiaries. Practice Partner® screen shots and materials used with the permission of McKesson Corporation. © 2010 McKesson Corporation. All rights reserved.*

You are now going to locate the patient record you just created. From the Dashboard, click the "Patient" button on the Dashboard that initiates the Patient Lookup dialog box (refer to Figure 9-6). In the box next to "Last Name," enter "carlson" and either press "Enter" on your keyboard or click the "Lookup" bottom at the bottom of the dialog box. Either method will display the screen in **Figure 9-17**. Note that the most probable name is highlighted in black.

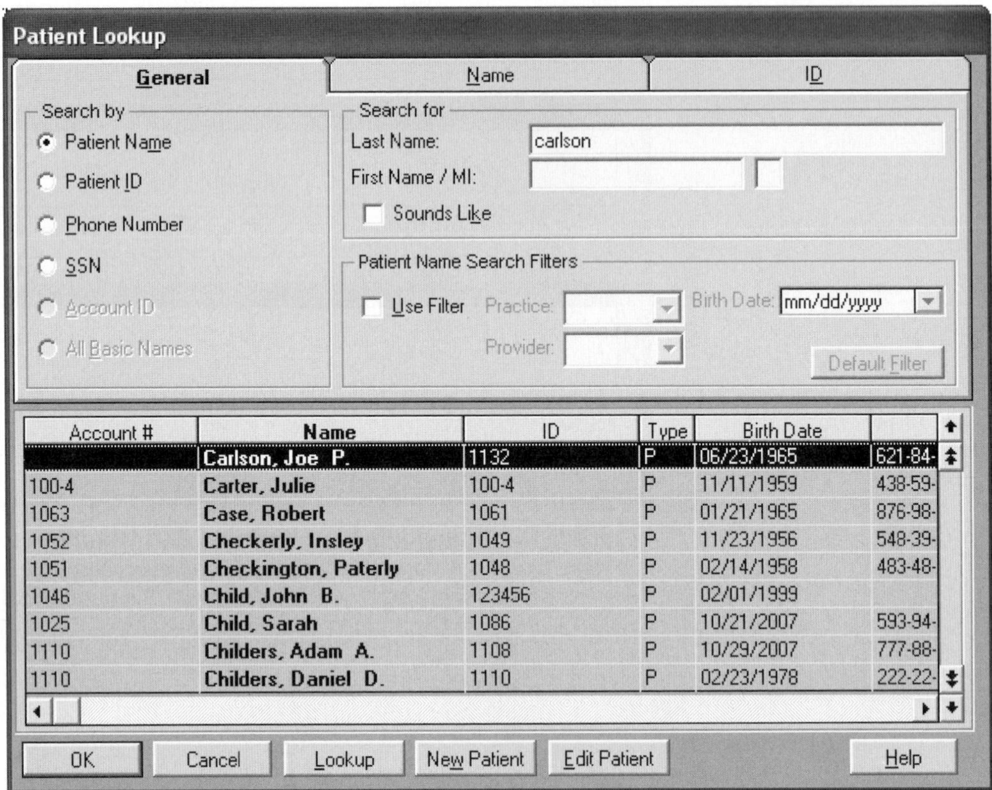

Figure **9-17** **Lookup screen search feature.** *Practice Partner® is a registered trademark of McKesson Corporation and/or one of its subsidiaries. Practice Partner® screen shots and materials used with the permission of McKesson Corporation. © 2010 McKesson Corporation. All rights reserved.*

Double-click the black entry (Carlson, Joe P.) and Joe's record will appear as shown in **Figure 9-18**. Click "OK" to return to the Dashboard.

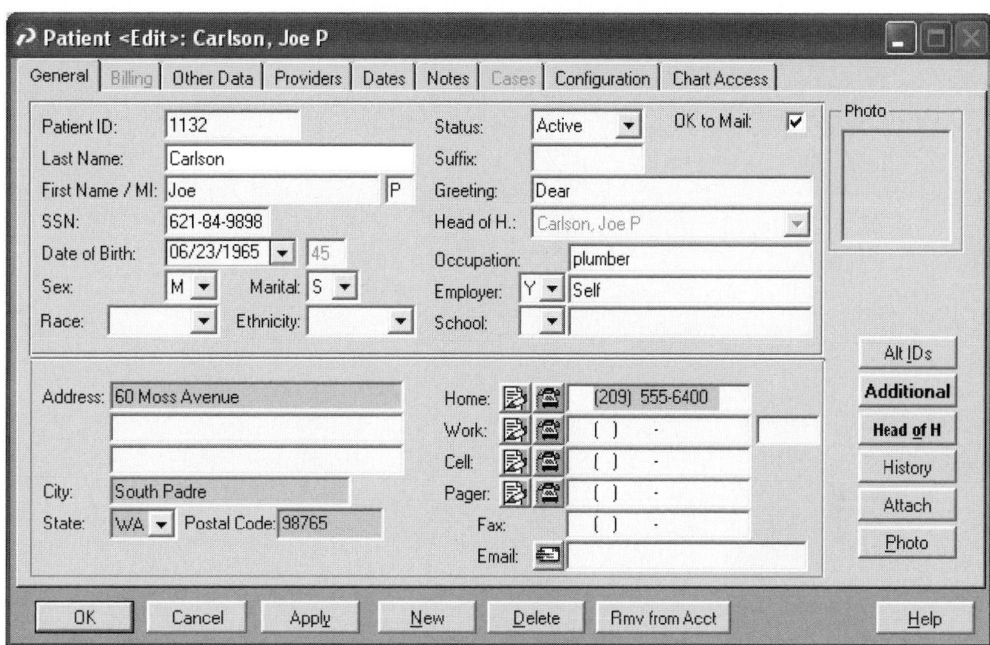

Figure **9-18 Returning to a newly entered patient record.** *Practice Partner® is a registered trademark of McKesson Corporation and/or one of its subsidiaries. Practice Partner® screen shots and materials used with the permission of McKesson Corporation. © 2010 McKesson Corporation. All rights reserved.*

You did a fine job of entering the information for Joe Carlson. The first time you enter information, it seems fairly complex, but now you are going to practice creating patient records for 11 new patients to ensure you are comfortable with the process. The patient names, including Joe Carlson, are as follows:

1. Joe P. Carlson
2. Carrie R. Anderson
3. David T. Oakland
4. Kathy F. Forest
5. Silvia S. Scott
6. Karra J. Burthold
7. Sylvia P. Kennedy
8. Aggy P. Carlisle
9. Anne R. Meires
10. Bridget G. Larson
11. Adam G. Hoverson
12. Anthony N. Socorri

Complete the patient records in the order listed and remember to complete the "Patient Information," "Emergency Conta," and "Provider" fields. All of the patients in this activity are being registered for Dr. Able.

TASK 9.4

Health History Form

SUPPLIES NEEDED:

- Companion Evolve site containing 10 electronic documents labeled Task 9.4.
- Practice Partner software

You are showing a real aptitude for working with the EHR and that is an excellent skill to have as you begin your new career in a medical setting. Today you are going to transfer documents into the patients' records that you created in the last task. Locate Task 9.4 on the Evolve site and click on it. The folder will open and 10 jpeg (picture) files will be displayed. Right-click on each jpeg and choose "Save Target As" from the drop-down menu. When the "Save As" dialog box opens, click on "Desktop" and then click "Save." You cannot place these jpeg files in a folder on your desktop, but only directly on your desktop. If you place the jpeg files in a folder, the software will not recognize the files. Download the files onto your desktop now.

With the 10 jpeg documents on your desktop, open the Practice Partner software to the Dashboard. Click "Task" on the toolbar as illustrated in **Figure 9-19**. On the drop-down menu, select "Scan."

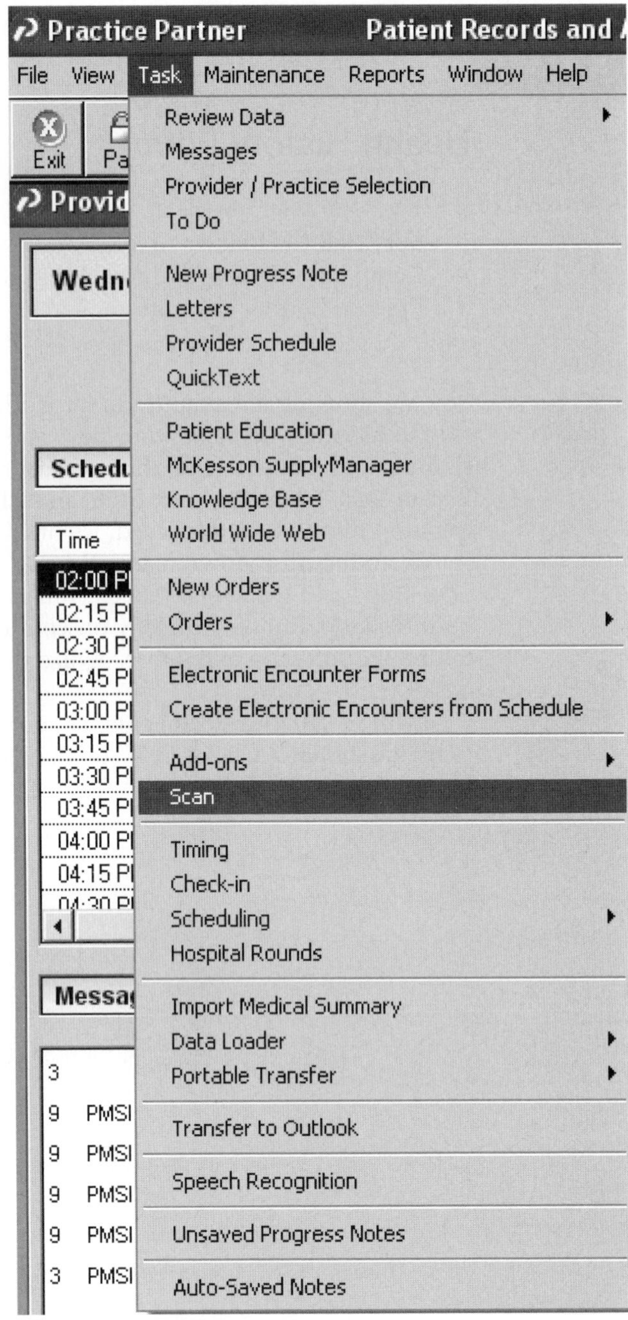

Figure **9-19** **Scanning Documents using the "Task" tab.** *Practice Partner® is a registered trademark of McKesson Corporation and/or one of its subsidiaries. Practice Partner® screen shots and materials used with the permission of McKesson Corporation. © 2010 McKesson Corporation. All rights reserved.*

This will open the Practice Partner Zoom program as shown in **Figure 9-20**. From here you will be able to import documents into patient records. In the medical setting that uses the EHR, documents are received from a variety of health care sources. These electronically transmitted documents are then stored in the EHRs. Also, in the transition from a paper-based medical setting to an EHR-based setting, many documents are scanned into an electronic format and then electronically filed into the EHR. The Zoom feature of the software assists you in the transfer task.

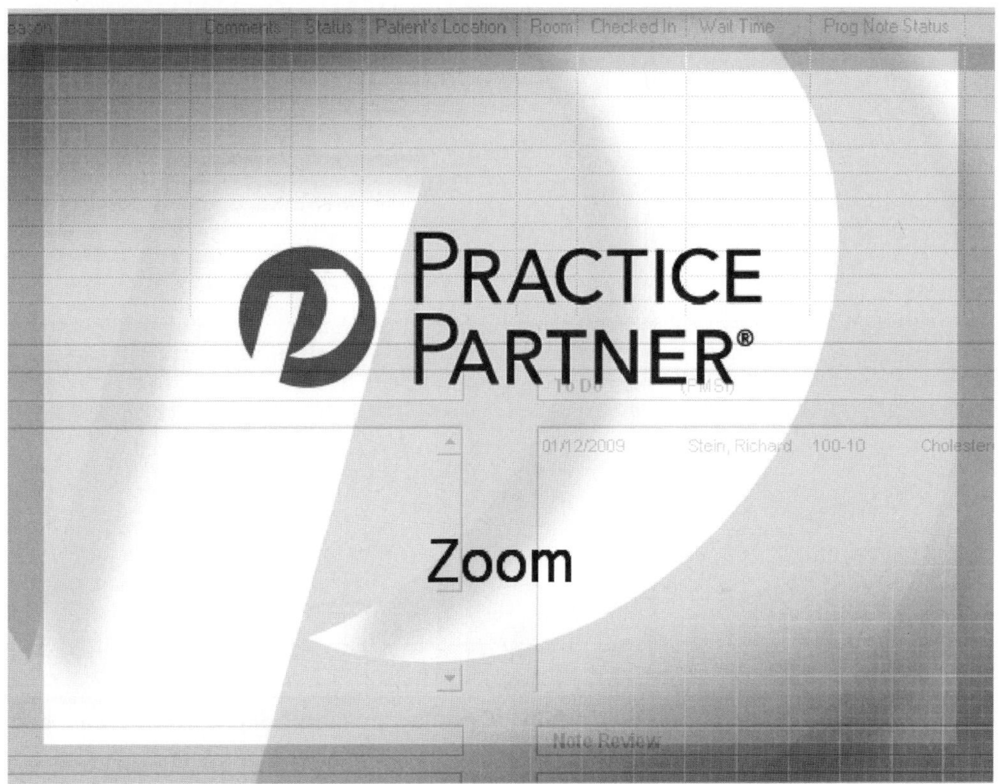

Figure **9-20** **Practice Partner Zoom.** *Practice Partner® is a registered trademark of McKesson Corporation and/or one of its subsidiaries. Practice Partner® screen shots and materials used with the permission of McKesson Corporation. © 2010 McKesson Corporation. All rights reserved.*

The Practice Partner Zoom window will open automatically. Click the "Browse" button as in **Figure 9-21**.

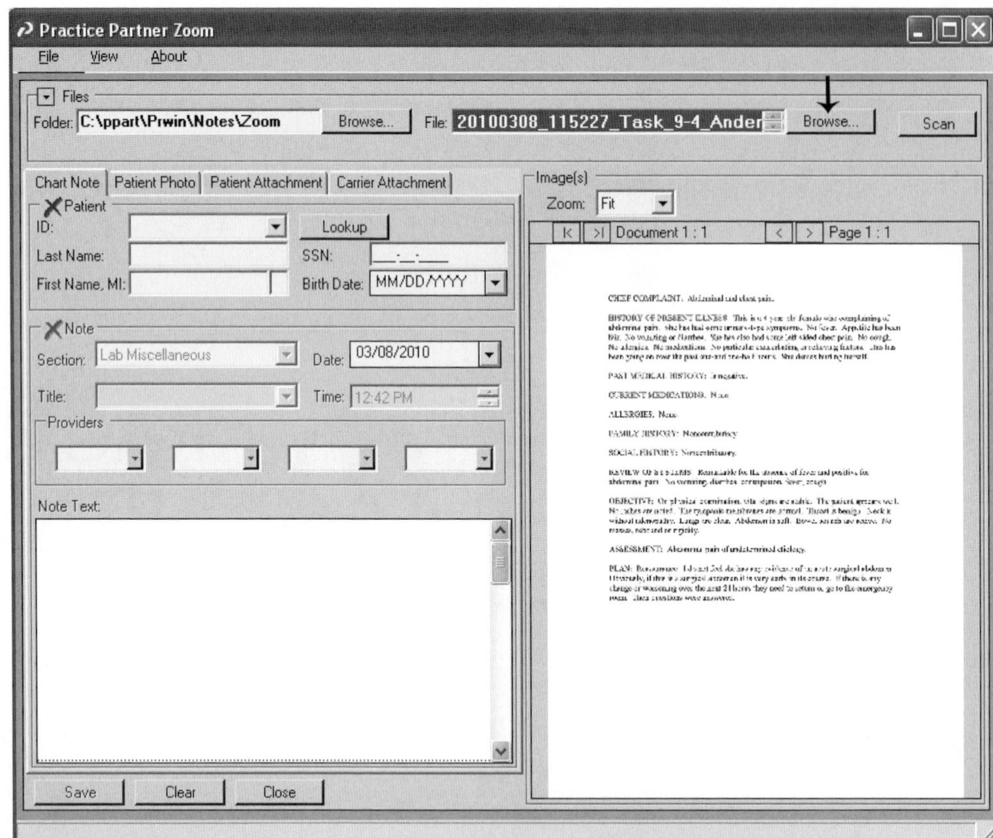

Figure **9-21** **Opening available files.** *Practice Partner® is a registered trademark of McKesson Corporation and/or one of its subsidiaries. Practice Partner® screen shots and materials used with the permission of McKesson Corporation. © 2010 McKesson Corporation. All rights reserved.*

A dialog box will open to prompt you to "Choose File." Click on the "Desktop" icon. A list of items on your desktop will be displayed when you click the "Desktop" icon as in **Figure 9-22**.

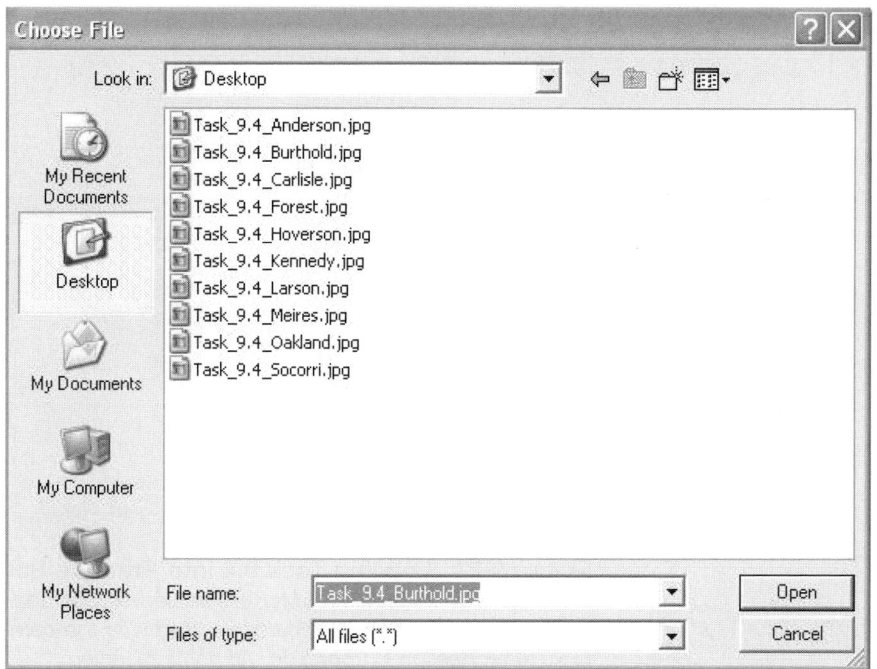

Figure **9-22 Selecting the downloaded jpeg from your Desktop.** *Practice Partner® is a registered trademark of McKesson Corporation and/or one of its subsidiaries. Practice Partner® screen shots and materials used with the permission of McKesson Corporation. © 2010 McKesson Corporation. All rights reserved.*

Double-click on the "Task 9.4_Burthold.jpg" and Practice Partner will load the document into the Practice Partner Zoom view as displayed in **Figure 9-23**. You can increase the size of the document by rolling your cursor over it.

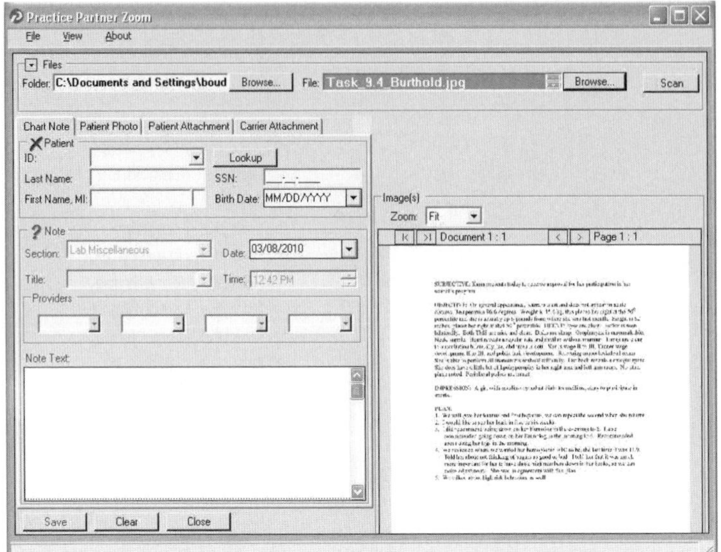

Figure **9-23** **Loading Task 9.4 into Practice Partner Zoom.** *Practice Partner® is a registered trademark of McKesson Corporation and/or one of its subsidiaries. Practice Partner® screen shots and materials used with the permission of McKesson Corporation. © 2010 McKesson Corporation. All rights reserved.*

Once the document is loaded into the Practice Partner Zoom view, you next need to place the document into the patient's chart. Enter "Burthold" into the Last Name box illustrated in **Figure 9-24**. Then click the "Lookup" button as shown in Figure 9-24.

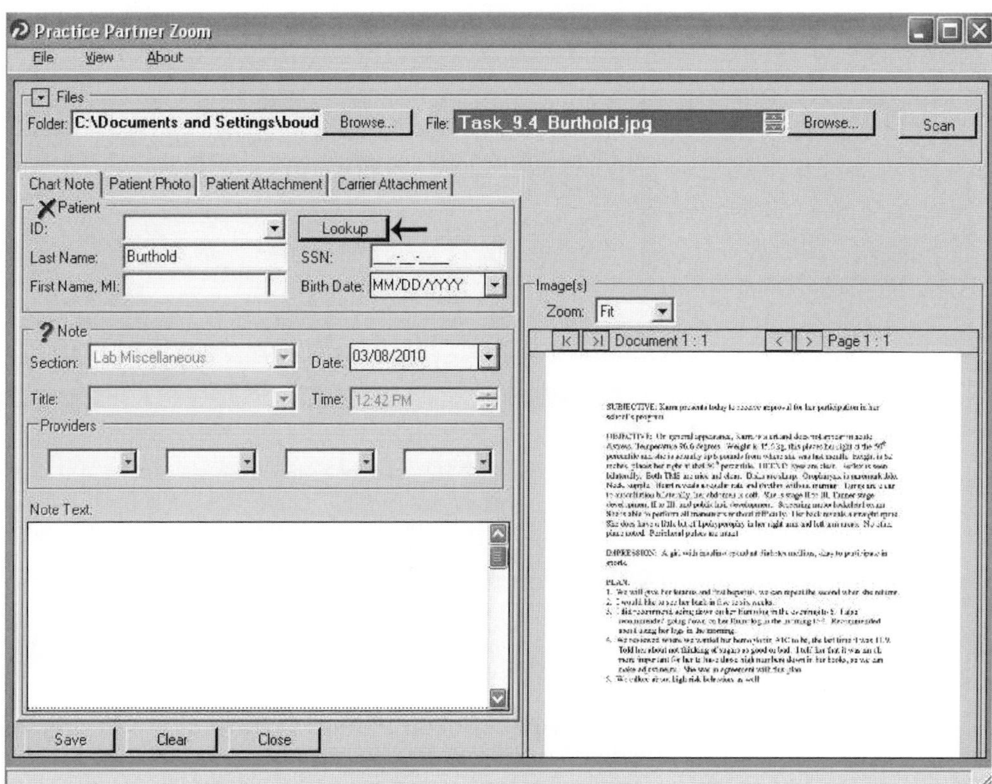

Figure **9-24** **Using the Last Name to locate the patient's chart.** *Practice Partner® is a registered trademark of McKesson Corporation and/or one of its subsidiaries. Practice Partner® screen shots and materials used with the permission of McKesson Corporation. © 2010 McKesson Corporation. All rights reserved.*

The software will display the Patient Lookup feature as shown in **Figure 9-25**. Double-click the Burthold entry.

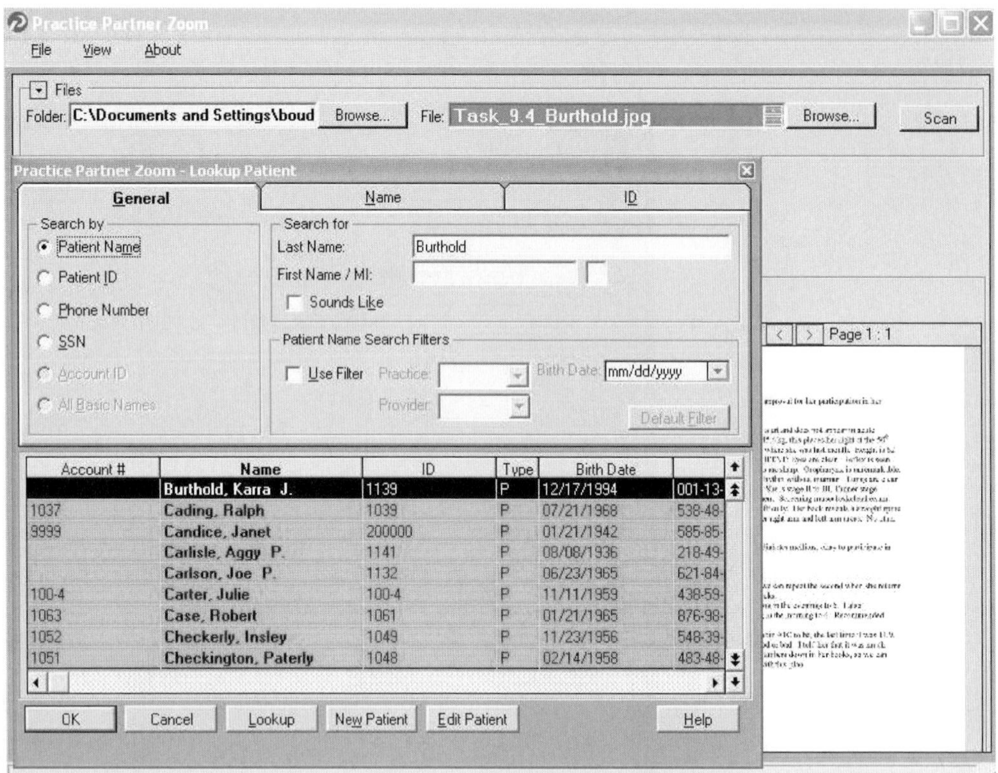

Figure **9-25 Lookup Patient feature of the Practice Partner Zoom.** *Practice Partner® is a registered trademark of McKesson Corporation and/or one of its subsidiaries. Practice Partner® screen shots and materials used with the permission of McKesson Corporation. © 2010 McKesson Corporation. All rights reserved.*

The Lookup feature locates the necessary data for Karra Burthold and automatically completes the information on the Practice Partner Zoom dialog box as shown in **Figure 9-26**. Note that there is a green check mark (✓) next to "Patient" indicating that all necessary information has been completed. There is a red X next to the Note section indicating that all necessary information has not been completed for that section. In the Note section, the default is "Lab Miscellaneous" with an arrow to the right. Click the arrow and select "Progress Notes" from the drop-down menu. In the Title box, click the arrow to the right and from the drop-down menu choose "Progress Notes."

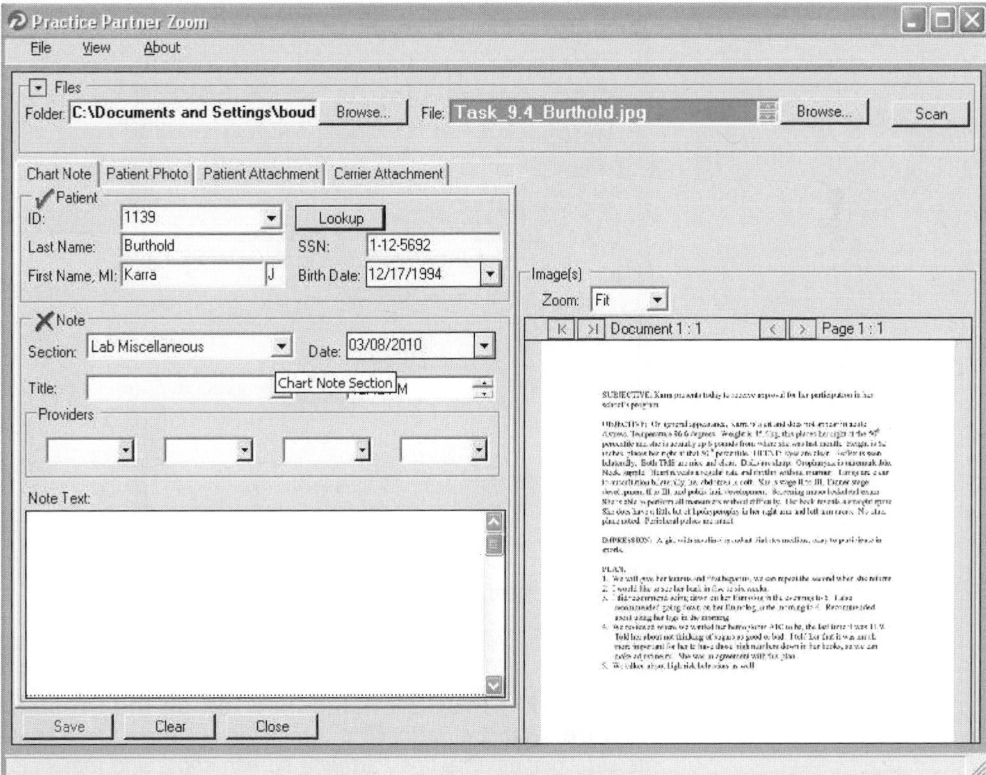

Figure **9-26** **Selecting information in the Practice Partner Zoom "Note" section.** *Practice Partner® is a registered trademark of McKesson Corporation and/or one of its subsidiaries. Practice Partner® screen shots and materials used with the permission of McKesson Corporation. © 2010 McKesson Corporation. All rights reserved.*

The Provider must now be identified by clicking the arrow to the right of the first box under the Provider section. When the arrow is clicked, a Provider Selection dialog box will appear from which you can select the physician—in this case, the physician is Cobb B. Able. In the *Date* field, enter 04/17/2008.

Dr. Able's name will automatically be placed in the Provider box as illustrated in **Figure 9-27**. Note that the red X has become a green check mark indicating that all the Note information has been correctly entered.

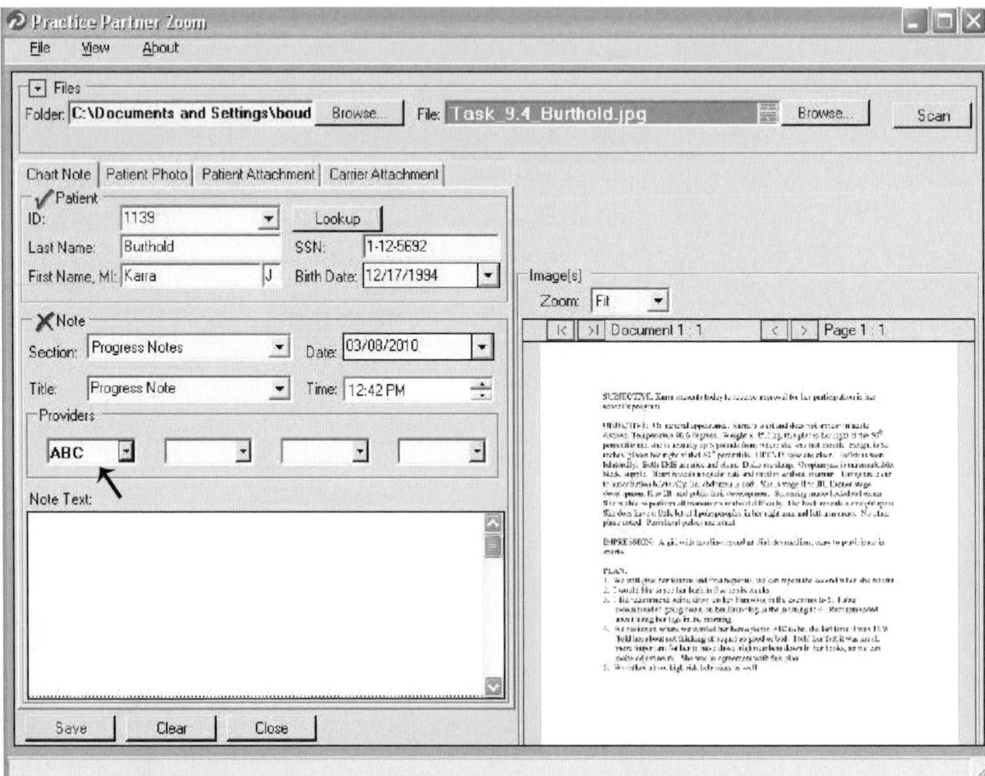

Figure **9-27 Provider name inserted on the Practice Partner Zoom feature.** *Practice Partner® is a registered trademark of McKesson Corporation and/or one of its subsidiaries. Practice Partner® screen shots and materials used with the permission of McKesson Corporation. © 2010 McKesson Corporation. All rights reserved.*

Click the "Save" button on the bottom left corner of the Practice Partner Zoom feature to place the document into Karra Burthold's chart as a progress note. You know the note was correctly saved because the "Note Saved" dialog box appears after you have pressed the "Save" button, as shown in **Figure 9-28**.

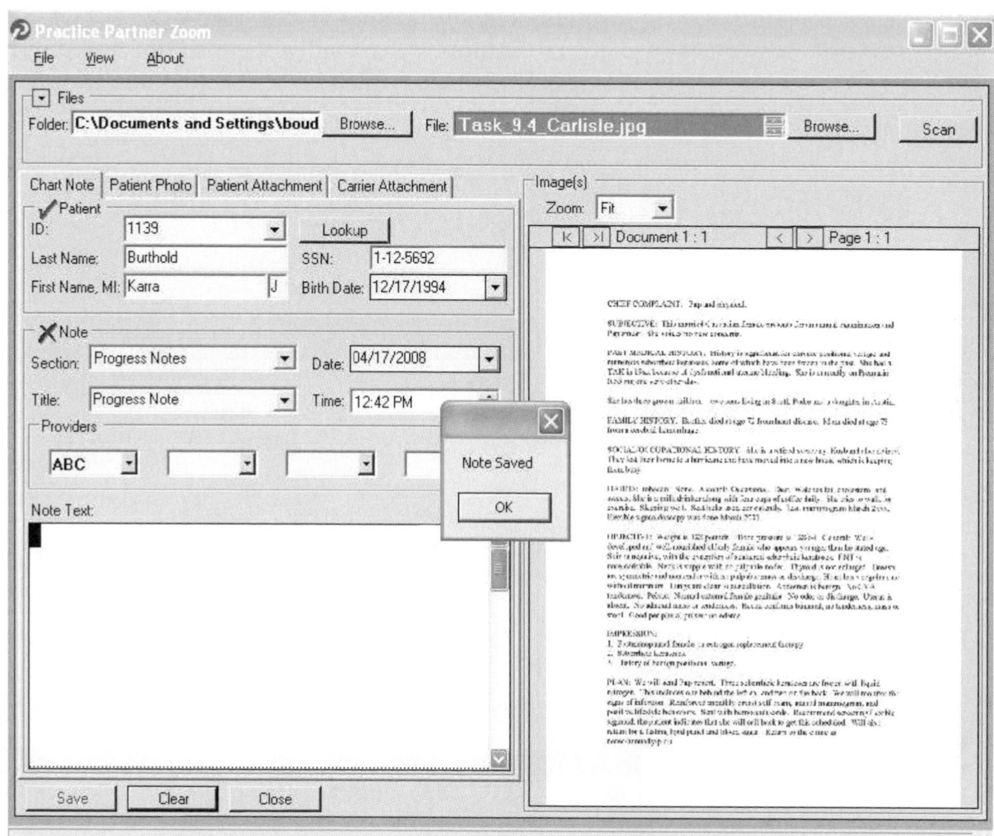

Figure **9-28** **Note Saved feature of the Practice Partner Zoom feature.** *Practice Partner® is a registered trademark of McKesson Corporation and/or one of its subsidiaries. Practice Partner® screen shots and materials used with the permission of McKesson Corporation. © 2010 McKesson Corporation. All rights reserved.*

Click "OK" on the Note Saved dialog box and the Practice Partner Zoom returns to the screen with all the information on Karra Burthold removed. At this point you could place the other patient records, but for right now, let's go check Karra Burthold's chart to make certain the note is correctly placed. Close the Zoom feature by clicking the "Close" button on the bottom of the Zoom dialog box and you are returned to the Dashboard.

Click the "Chart" button on the top toolbar of the Dashboard and a Patient Lookup dialog box appears. Type in "Burthold" in the Last Name area and a list of patient names will automatically populate the patient area. Double-click on "Burthold, Karra J." as shown in **Figure 9-29**.

Karra Burthold's chart will appear as illustrated in **Figure 9-30**. Click on the "Progress Notes" tab, which is the location you transferred the document into, and click "OK."

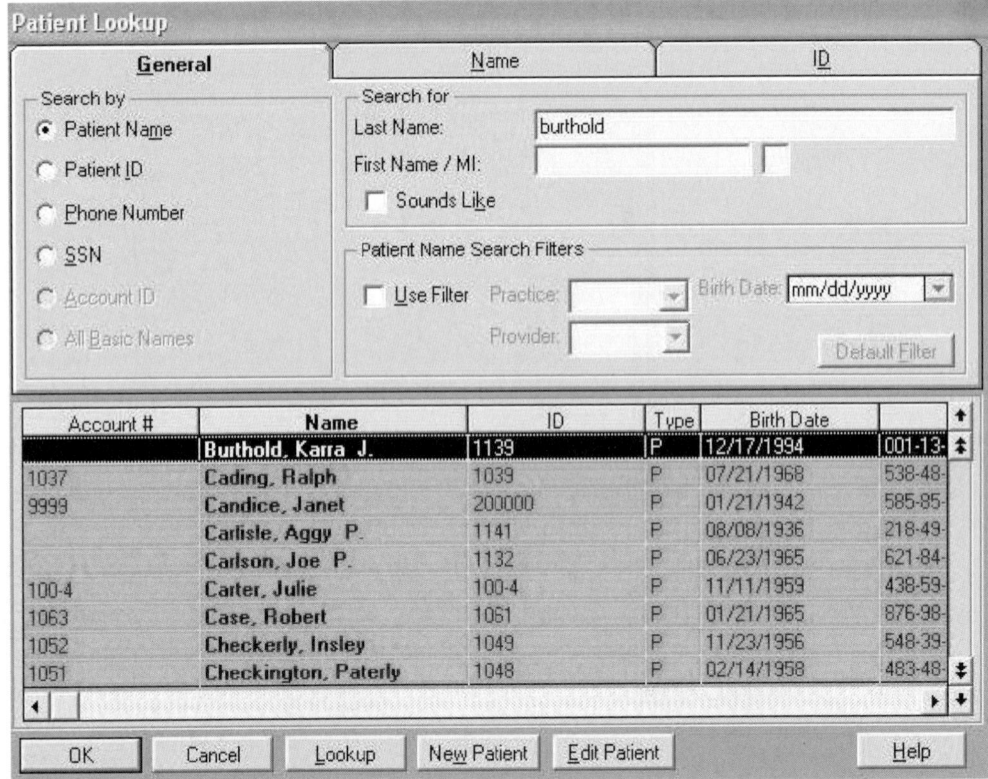

Figure **9-29** **Patient Lookup dialog box.** *Practice Partner® is a registered trademark of McKesson Corporation and/or one of its subsidiaries. Practice Partner® screen shots and materials used with the permission of McKesson Corporation. © 2010 McKesson Corporation. All rights reserved.*

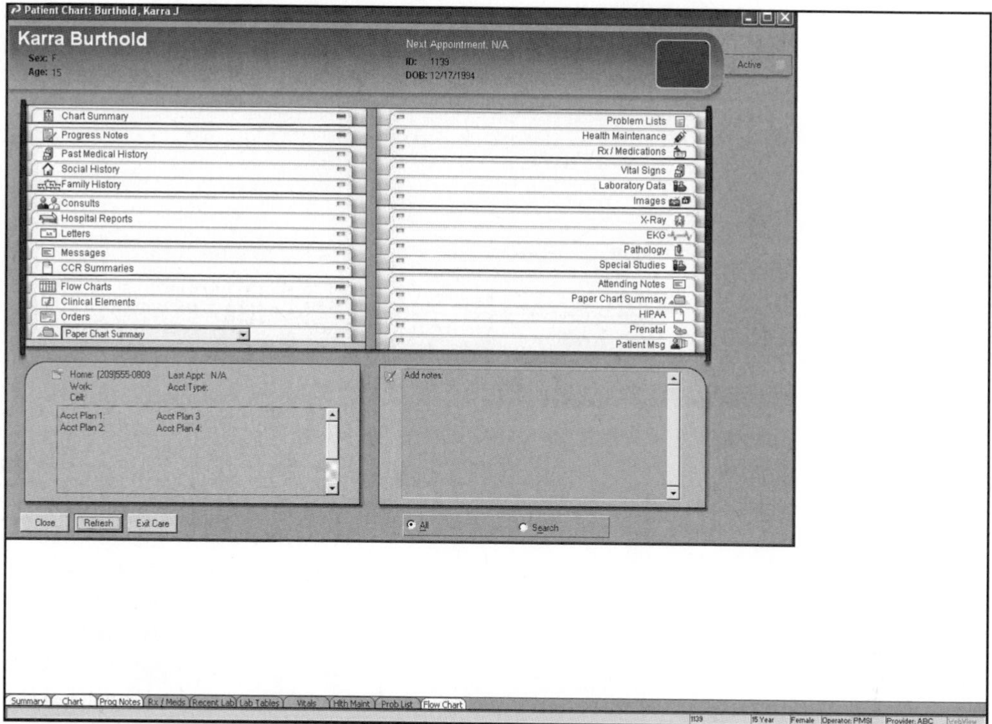

Figure **9-30** **Karra Burthold's chart.** *Practice Partner® is a registered trademark of McKesson Corporation and/or one of its subsidiaries. Practice Partner® screen shots and materials used with the permission of McKesson Corporation. © 2010 McKesson Corporation. All rights reserved.*

In the Progress Notes section of Karra's chart, you will see the information shown in **Figure 9-31**. Click on the link for Task 9.4_Burthold located in this Progress Notes area.

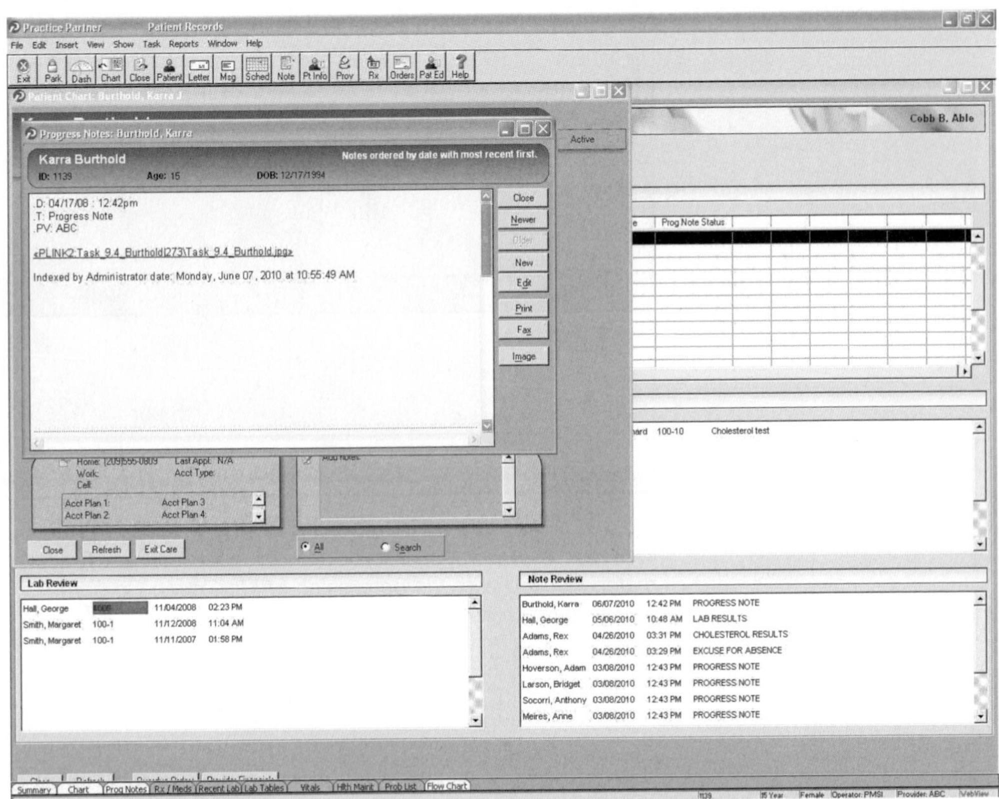

Figure **9-31** **Karra Burthold's Progress Notes.** *Practice Partner® is a registered trademark of McKesson Corporation and/or one of its subsidiaries. Practice Partner® screen shots and materials used with the permission of McKesson Corporation. © 2010 McKesson Corporation. All rights reserved.*

The document that you transferred into the chart will appear as in **Figure 9-32**.

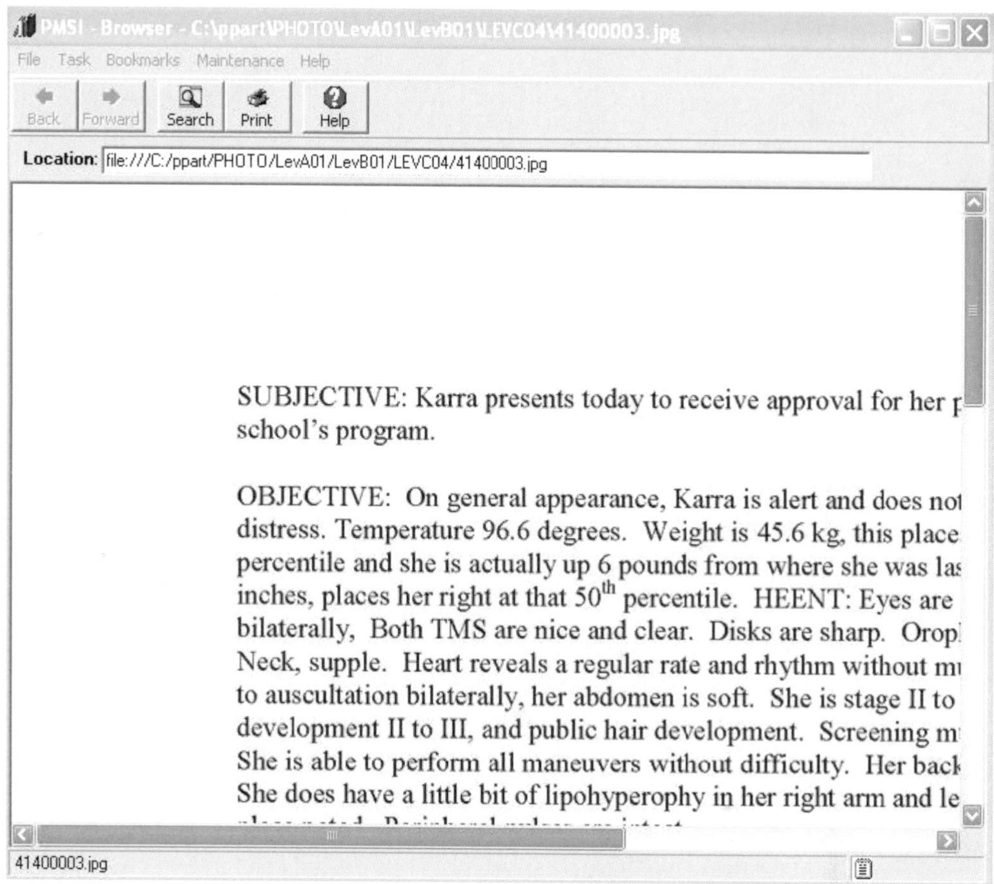

Figure **9-32** **Transferred document in Karra Burthold's chart.** *Practice Partner® is a registered trademark of McKesson Corporation and/or one of its subsidiaries. Practice Partner® screen shots and materials used with the permission of McKesson Corporation. © 2010 McKesson Corporation. All rights reserved.*

From this screen you can Print the document, should that be necessary.

You now need to continue this task by transferring the remaining 9 patient information jpegs into the remaining patient charts:

1. David T. Oakland
2. Kathy F. Forest
3. Carrie R. Anderson
4. Sylvia P. Kennedy
5. Aggy P. Carlisle
6. Anne R. Meires
7. Anthony N. Socorri
8. Bridget G. Larson
9. Adam G. Hoverson

This completes Day Nine; one more day to go.

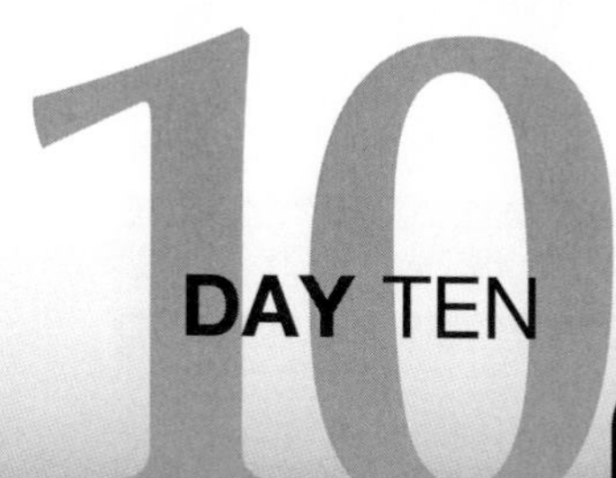

DAY TEN

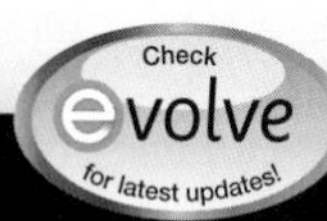

Friday, April 18, 2008

TASK **10.1**

Obtaining Information from the EHR

SUPPLIES NEEDED:

- Computer and Practice Partner software

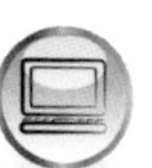

It is now time to learn about abstracting information from existing health records. To begin, open the software to the Dashboard.

Note that the Dashboard displays the physician's Schedule, Messages, Lab Reviews, To Do, and Note Reviews. In this example, "(PMSI)" is displayed where the employee's name would be displayed if this were an actual record. When you have completed your training, your name will be displayed where "(PMSI)" is currently displayed.

In the Message area, the third message is regarding "Smith, Margaret." Click the message and the message will open in the View Message dialog box as illustrated in **Figure 10-1**. Note the two buttons on the dialog box that are identified by the arrows—one for the telephone number and one for allergies. When you click either of these buttons a new dialog box opens displaying the patient's telephone number and any noted allergies.

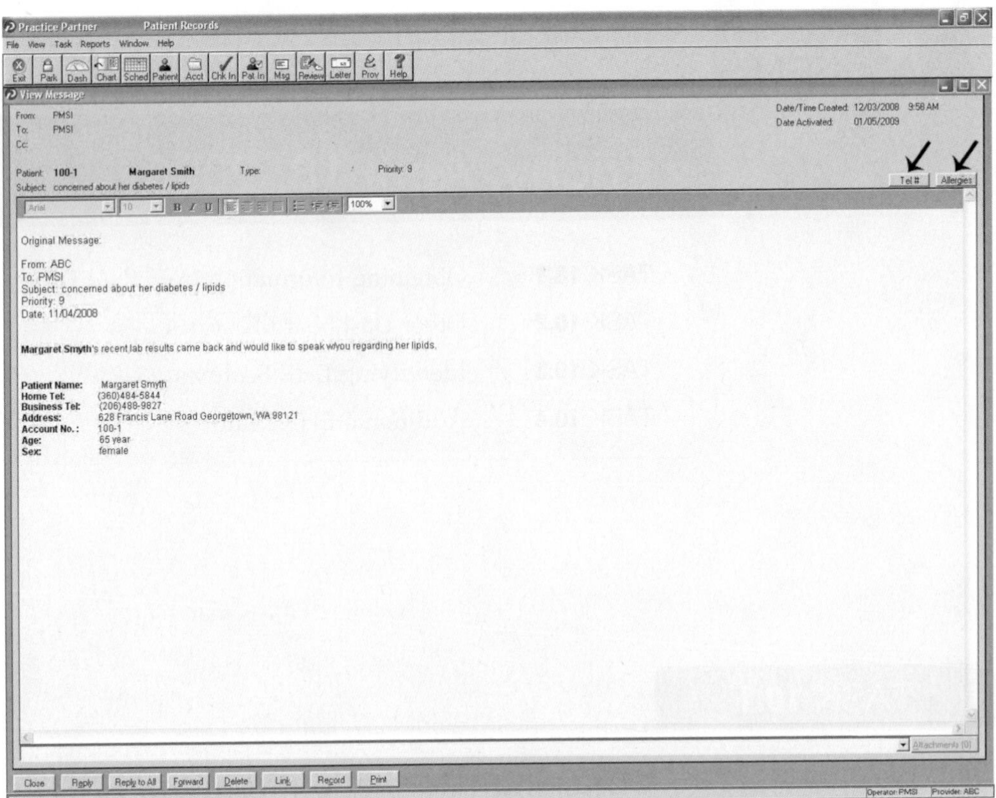

Figure **10-1** **View Message dialog box.** *Practice Partner® is a registered trademark of McKesson Corporation and/or one of its subsidiaries. Practice Partner® screen shots and materials used with the permission of McKesson Corporation. © 2010 McKesson Corporation. All rights reserved.*

You may now close Margaret Smith's message and return to the Dashboard.

TASK **10.2**

Other Dashboard Features

SUPPLIES NEEDED:

- Computer and Practice Partner software

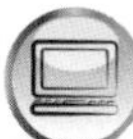

There are many other features in the Practice Partner software. For example, now you are going to learn about the message feature. Click the "Msg" button as illustrated in **Figure 10-2**.

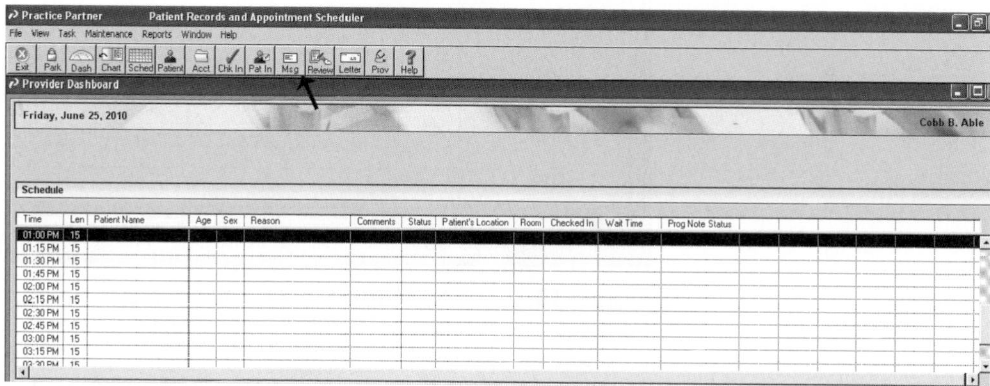

Figure **10-2** **Message feature.** *Practice Partner® is a registered trademark of McKesson Corporation and/or one of its subsidiaries. Practice Partner® screen shots and materials used with the permission of McKesson Corporation. © 2010 McKesson Corporation. All rights reserved.*

The message feature opens to the Inbox, as illustrated in **Figure 10-3**. There are also files for messages that have been archived, deleted, are pending, selected, and sent. Take a moment to click into each of the files and then return to the Inbox.

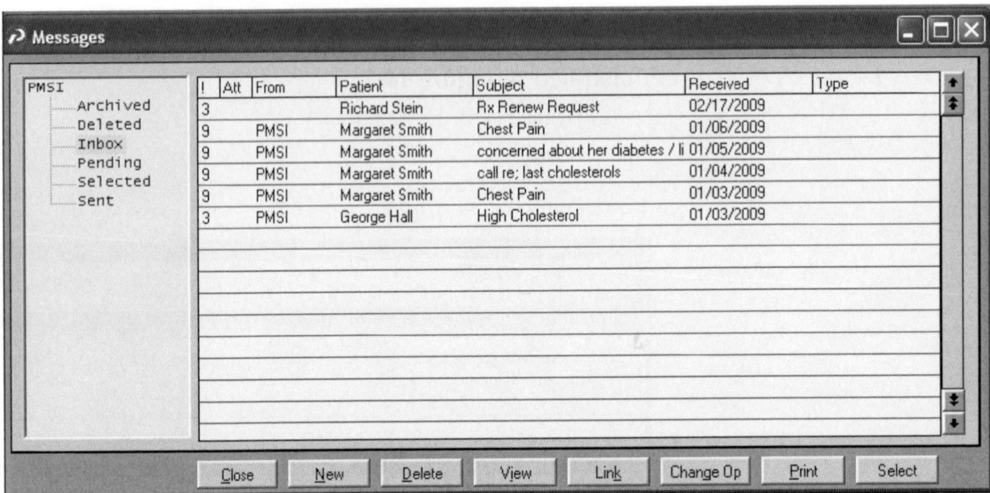

Figure **10-3** **Inbox feature.** *Practice Partner® is a registered trademark of McKesson Corporation and/or one of its subsidiaries. Practice Partner® screen shots and materials used with the permission of McKesson Corporation. © 2010 McKesson Corporation. All rights reserved.*

Documents often arrive in the medical office as attachments to an email. These documents can then be saved into the patient's EHR or printed. Open the "Deleted" file in the Messages area, scroll all the way to the bottom, and note that there is a document attached to a deleted email for Julie Carter, as illustrated in **Figure 10-4**.

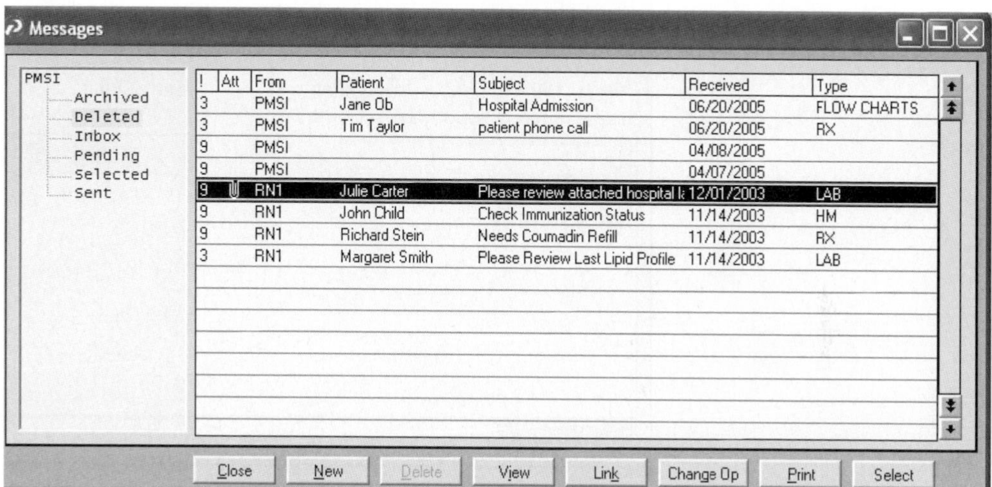

Figure **10-4** **Attachment in Julie Carter's message.** *Practice Partner® is a registered trademark of McKesson Corporation and/or one of its subsidiaries. Practice Partner® screen shots and materials used with the permission of McKesson Corporation. © 2010 McKesson Corporation. All rights reserved.*

Double-click on the message for Julie Carter; a dialog box appears as shown in **Figure 10-5** indicating that there is an attachment on the message that can be accessed by clicking on the "Attachments" button in the lower right.

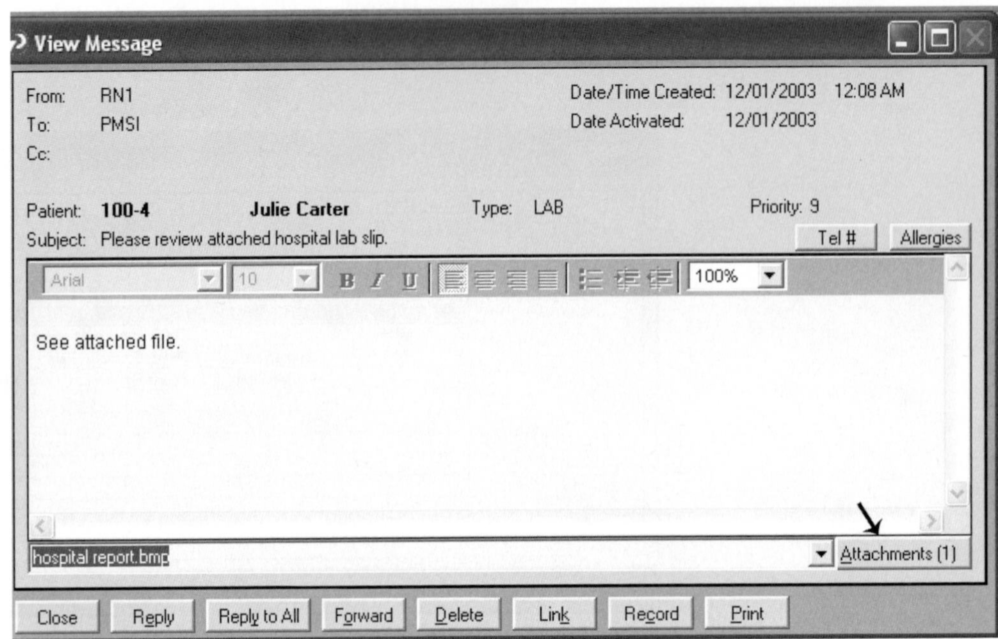

Figure **10-5** **Accessing attachments in e-mail.** *Practice Partner® is a registered trademark of McKesson Corporation and/or one of its subsidiaries. Practice Partner® screen shots and materials used with the permission of McKesson Corporation. © 2010 McKesson Corporation. All rights reserved.*

After clicking on "Attachments," another dialog box opens as shown in **Figure 10-6**, giving you the option to close, view, or save the message. Click on the "View" button in the dialog box; the attachment opens.

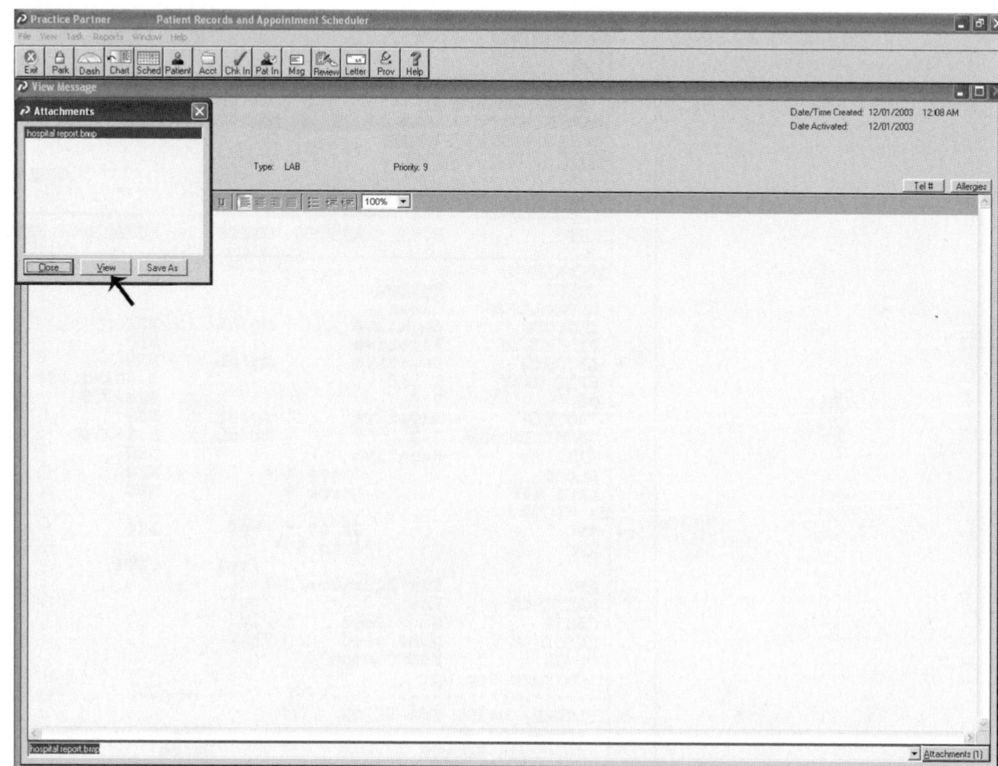

Figure **10-6** **Viewing attachments of an e-mail.** *Practice Partner® is a registered trademark of McKesson Corporation and/or one of its subsidiaries. Practice Partner® screen shots and materials used with the permission of McKesson Corporation. © 2010 McKesson Corporation. All rights reserved.*

Figure 10-7 reveals that the attachment is an image (picture) that has been scanned into the computer. The information is a "flat document," meaning that it cannot be edited, but the image can be printed.

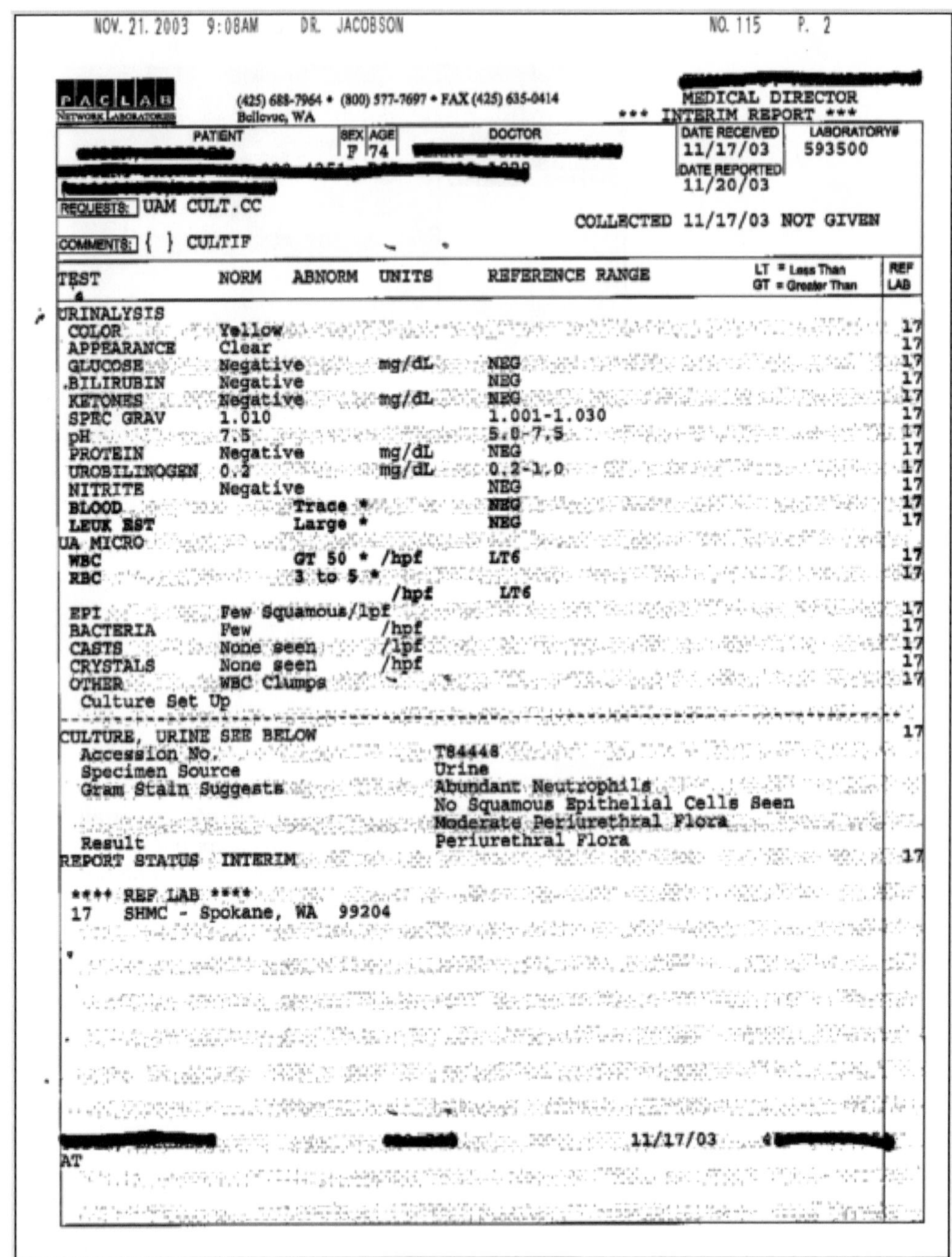

NOV. 21. 2003 9:08AM DR. JACOBSON NO. 115 P. 2

PACLAB NETWORK LABORATORIES (425) 688-7964 • (800) 577-7697 • FAX (425) 635-0414 Bellevue, WA

MEDICAL DIRECTOR
*** INTERIM REPORT ***

PATIENT | SEX F | AGE 74 | DOCTOR | DATE RECEIVED 11/17/03 | LABORATORY# 593500 | DATE REPORTED 11/20/03

REQUESTS: UAM CULT.CC

COLLECTED 11/17/03 NOT GIVEN

COMMENTS: { } CULTIF

TEST	NORM	ABNORM	UNITS	REFERENCE RANGE	REF LAB
URINALYSIS					
COLOR	Yellow				17
APPEARANCE	Clear				17
GLUCOSE	Negative		mg/dL	NEG	17
BILIRUBIN	Negative			NEG	17
KETONES	Negative		mg/dL	NEG	17
SPEC GRAV	1.010			1.001-1.030	17
pH	7.5			5.0-7.5	17
PROTEIN	Negative		mg/dL	NEG	17
UROBILINOGEN	0.2		mg/dL	0.2-1.0	17
NITRITE	Negative			NEG	17
BLOOD		Trace *		NEG	17
LEUK EST		Large *		NEG	17
UA MICRO					
WBC		GT 50 *	/hpf	LT6	17
RBC		3 to 5 *	/hpf	LT6	17
EPI	Few Squamous/lpf				17
BACTERIA	Few		/hpf		17
CASTS	None seen		/lpf		17
CRYSTALS	None seen		/hpf		17
OTHER	WBC Clumps				17

Culture Set Up

CULTURE, URINE SEE BELOW 17
Accession No. T84448
Specimen Source Urine
Gram Stain Suggests Abundant Neutrophils
No Squamous Epithelial Cells Seen
Moderate Periurethral Flora
Result Periurethral Flora
REPORT STATUS INTERIM 17

**** REF LAB ****
17 SHMC - Spokane, WA 99204

11/17/03
AT

Figure **10-7 Julie Carter's urinalysis report.** *Practice Partner® is a registered trademark of McKesson Corporation and/or one of its subsidiaries. Practice Partner® screen shots and materials used with the permission of McKesson Corporation. © 2010 McKesson Corporation. All rights reserved.*

Return to the Dashboard with the Messages feature open. Open the third message in the Inbox file—Margaret Smith—and locate the Link on the bottom toolbar as illustrated in **Figure 10-8**. Click on "Link" and the patient's EHR is displayed. Now, close the EHR and the message is still displayed.

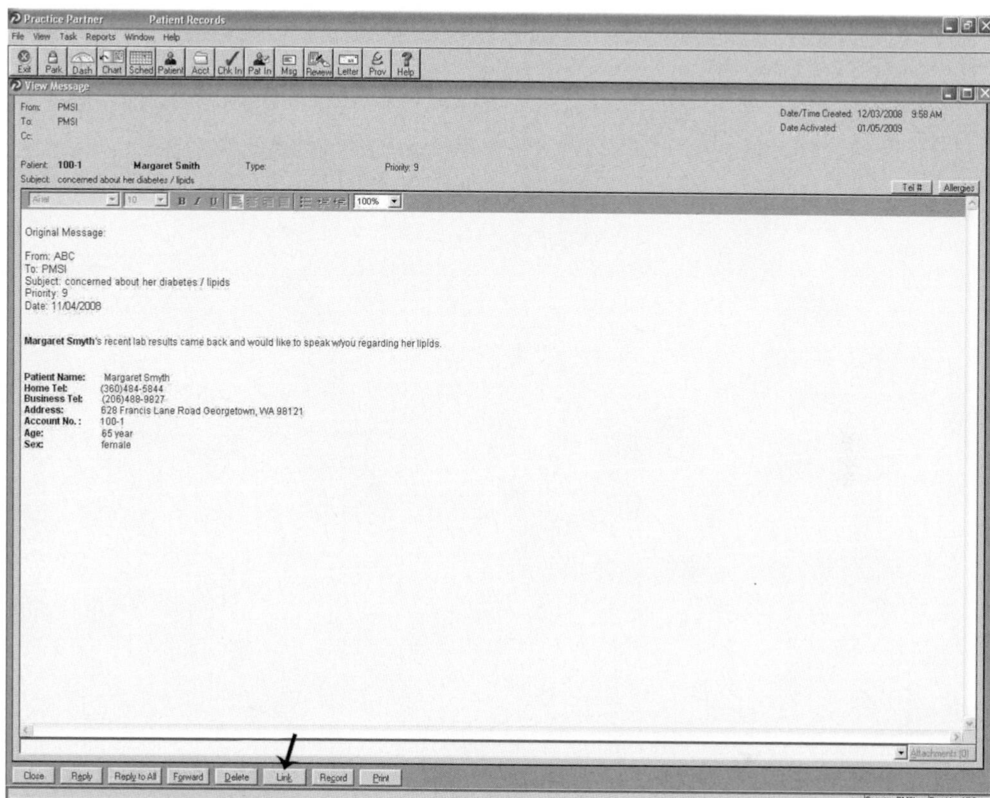

Figure **10-8** **Link feature opens the patient's chart.** *Practice Partner® is a registered trademark of McKesson Corporation and/or one of its subsidiaries. Practice Partner® screen shots and materials used with the permission of McKesson Corporation. © 2010 McKesson Corporation. All rights reserved.*

From this message screen the staff of the medical center can communicate with one another. For example, note that at the bottom of an open message you can reply, reply to all, forward, delete, record (append to the message), or print. Close the Message feature and return to the Dashboard.

There will be times in your office that an employee or other individual may approach your workstation at an angle that would make it possible to view the documents open on your computer screen. As stated earlier, you are responsible for protecting all health information; you can hide the contents of the screen by clicking on the "Park" button on the toolbar at the upper-left corner. Click the "Park" button now; a dialog box appears on the screen that requires you to re-enter the user name and password. All the contents of the screen are discreetly hidden from view. If someone approaches your desk at an angle that would allow viewing—even another employee—always Park the software. Also Park your software when you leave your desk. Remember that no one is to have access to confidential patient information—that includes viewing your computer screen.

You have done a great deal of hard work to get to this part of the activities and you have a basic understanding of the EHR. It is now time to answer more questions that will demonstrate your ability to access EHR information.

TASK 10.3

Identifying EHR Features

SUPPLIES NEEDED:

- Computer and Practice Partner software

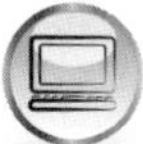

With the software open on the Dashboard, click the "Review" button on the toolbar at the top (next to the "Msg" button). When you click the "Review" button, the notes on the Dashboard will open, listing the Note most recently entered. Click the "Older" button on the right side of the screen until you reach the EKG report for Richard Stein, as seen in **Figure 10-9**. This will be the third note listed for Richard Stein. Scroll down using the scroll bar on the right side of the screen. Move the scroll bar all the way to the end of the report. From the Review screen, the physician or staff can access the patient's chart by clicking the "Open Chart" on the right side of the screen. A note will appear, notifying you that this patient is hard of hearing; click OK to continue to Richard's chart.

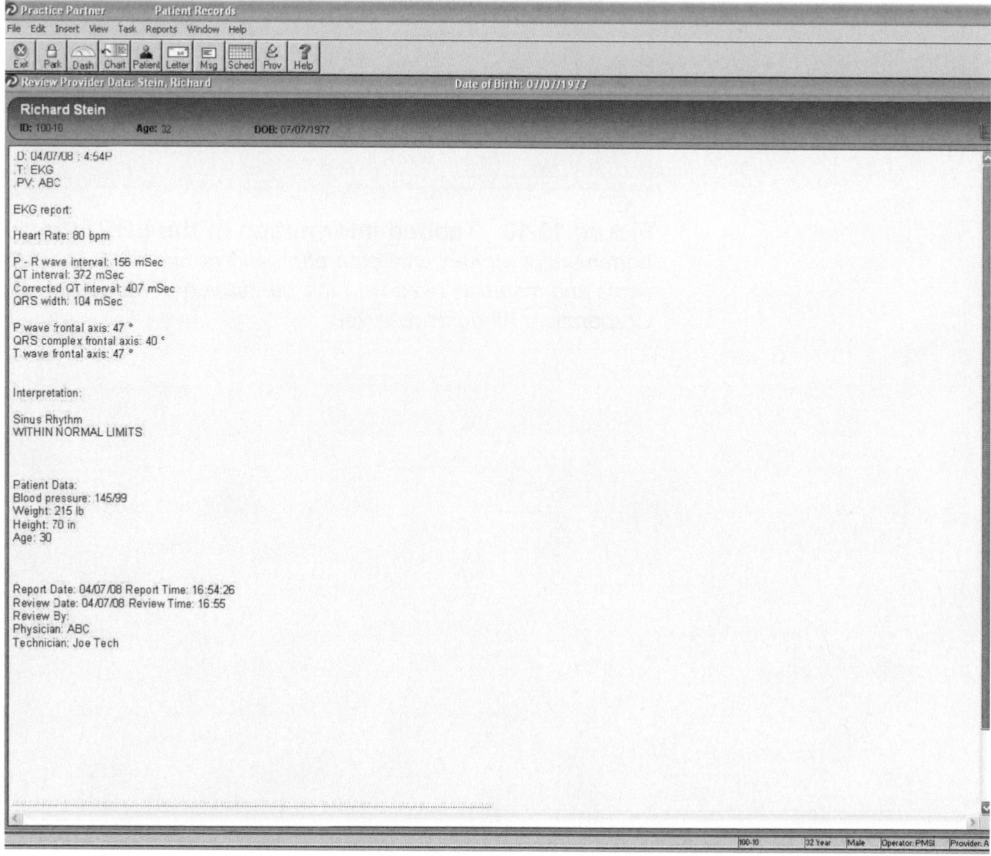

Figure **10-9** **Open Review section in Richard Stein's chart.** *Practice Partner® is a registered trademark of McKesson Corporation and/or one of its subsidiaries. Practice Partner® screen shots and materials used with the permission of McKesson Corporation. © 2010 McKesson Corporation. All rights reserved.*

With the chart open on the Dashboard, you can then open other data within the EHR. Click on the "Prog Notes" tab on the lower toolbar as shown in **Figure 10-10**.

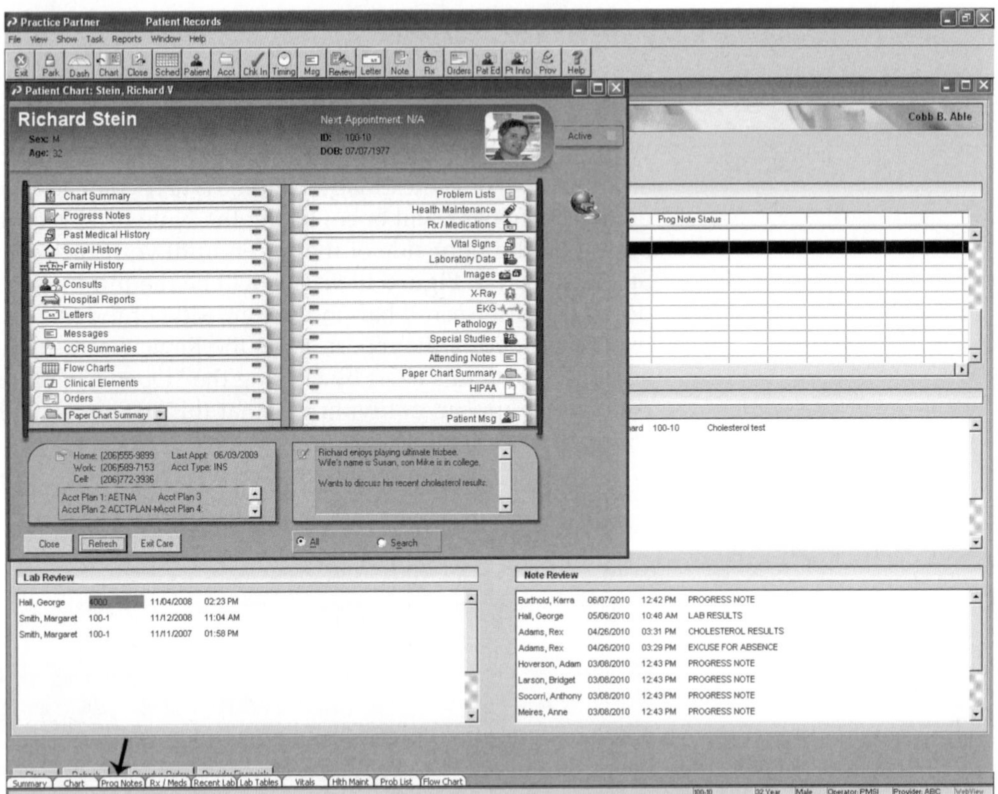

Figure **10-10** **Tabbed information in the EHR.** *Practice Partner® is a registered trademark of McKesson Corporation and/or one of its subsidiaries. Practice Partner® screen shots and materials used with the permission of McKesson Corporation. © 2010 McKesson Corporation. All rights reserved.*

The tabs are:

1. Summary
2. Chart
3. Prog Notes
4. Rx/Meds
5. Recent Lab
6. Lab Tables
7. Vitals
8. Hlth Maint
9. Prob List
10. Flow Chart

Access each of these tabs and subtabs on Richard's chart, so you are familiar with how to quickly view the information in the EHR.

There are also subtabs in the Prob List tab, as illustrated in **Figure 10-11**, which contain further information on the patient. You may now close Richard Stein's chart and return to the Dashboard.

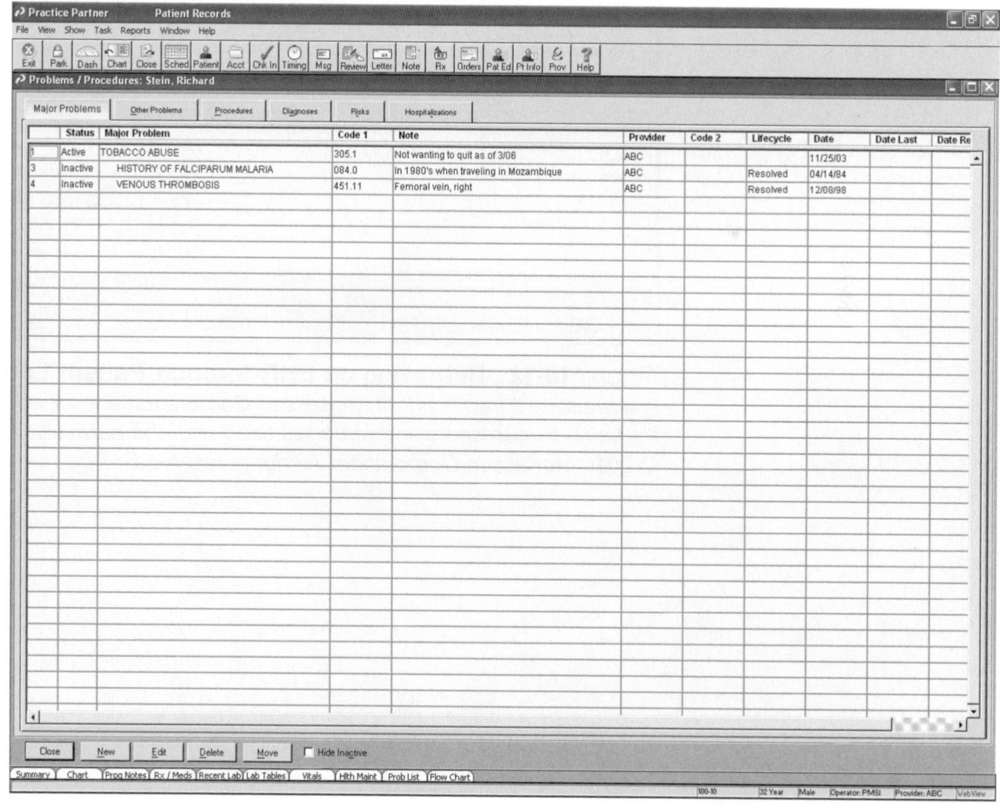

Figure **10-11 Subtabs in the EHR.** *Practice Partner® is a registered trademark of McKesson Corporation and/or one of its subsidiaries. Practice Partner® screen shots and materials used with the permission of McKesson Corporation. © 2010 McKesson Corporation. All rights reserved.*

The fastest way to search for a particular patient's EHR is by clicking the "Chart" button on the Dashboard toolbar, which opens the Patient Lookup box. From there you can type in the last name of a patient and search for them, as shown in **Figure 10-12**.

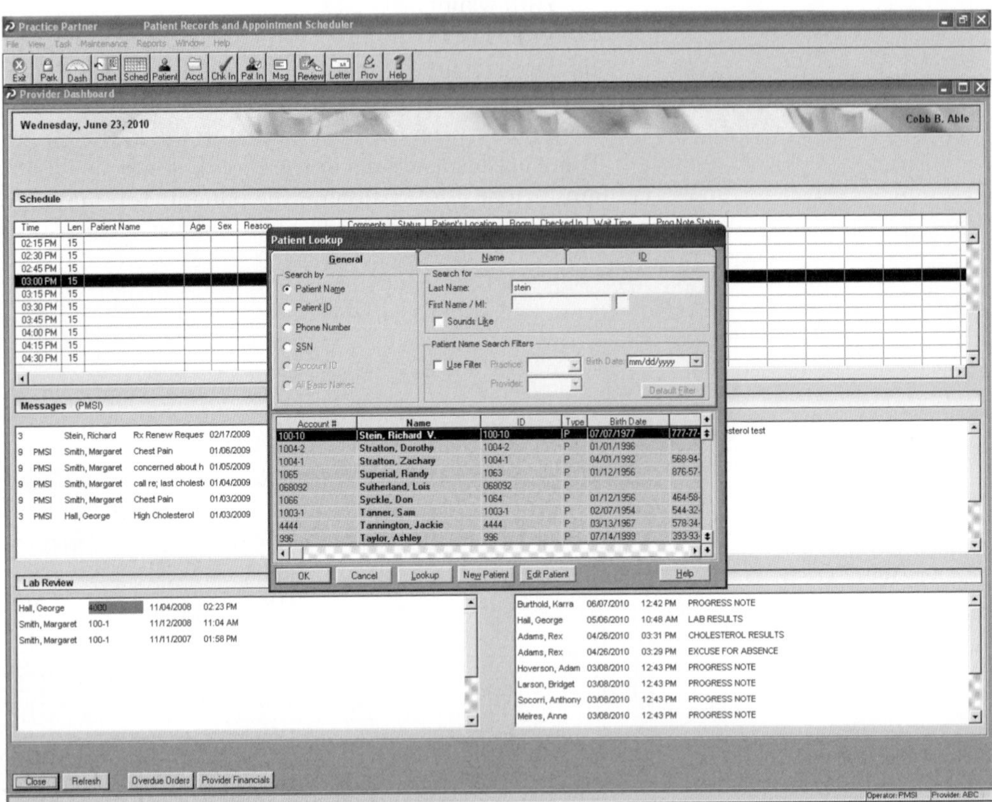

Figure **10-12 Retrieving an EHR through Patient Lookup.** *Practice Partner® is a registered trademark of McKesson Corporation and/or one of its subsidiaries. Practice Partner® screen shots and materials used with the permission of McKesson Corporation. © 2010 McKesson Corporation. All rights reserved.*

TASK 10.4

Additional EHR Features

SUPPLIES NEEDED:

- Computer and Practice Partner software

When a physician reviews laboratory data regarding a patient, the physician signs the data after it has been reviewed. The signature verifies the physician has reviewed the data and the data are then stored in the patient's EHR. The signature is also stored. For example, Margaret Smith's name appears on the Lab Review section of the Dashboard. When you click on her lab review from 11/12/08, a Lab Table Review dialog box is displayed. Click the "Lab Table" tab at the bottom of the dialog box and click on the entry "207" next to cholesterol on the 11/12/08 entry as shown in **Figure 10-13**. When you do this, the electronic signature appears at the bottom of the dialog box with "*CHOLESTEROL:* 11:04AM **High** <1-200> ABC," indicating that Dr. Able reviewed and signed off (reviewed and initialed) the laboratory results. Laboratory data are not stored in the EHR until the physician has signed off.

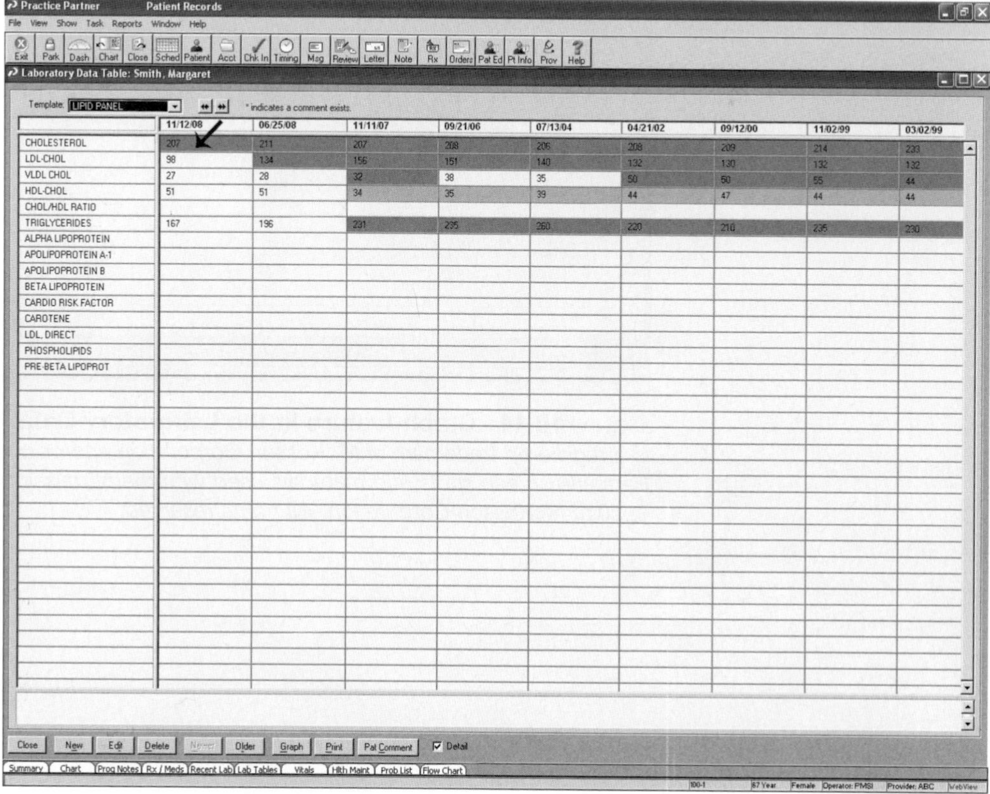

	11/12/08	06/25/08	11/11/07	09/21/06	07/13/04	04/21/02	09/12/00	11/02/99	03/02/99
CHOLESTEROL	207	211	207	208	206	208	209	214	233
LDL-CHOL	98	134	156	151	140	132	130	132	132
VLDL CHOL	27	28	32	38	35	50	50	55	44
HDL-CHOL	51	51	34	35	39	44	47	44	44
CHOL/HDL RATIO									
TRIGLYCERIDES	167	196	231	235	260	220	210	235	230
ALPHA LIPOPROTEIN									
APOLIPOPROTEIN A-1									
APOLIPOPROTEIN B									
BETA LIPOPROTEIN									
CARDIO RISK FACTOR									
CAROTENE									
LDL DIRECT									
PHOSPHOLIPIDS									
PRE-BETA LIPOPROT									

Figure **10-13** **Margaret Smith's cholesterol.** *Practice Partner® is a registered trademark of McKesson Corporation and/or one of its subsidiaries. Practice Partner® screen shots and materials used with the permission of McKesson Corporation. © 2010 McKesson Corporation. All rights reserved.*

From the Laboratory Data Table for Margaret Smith, the physician can also graph the results to see trends that have occurred over time for certain measures, such as glucose or cholesterol. For example, if Dr. Able wanted to see how Margaret's cholesterol levels trended over the last four visits, he would highlight the four entries for the time period 11/12/08 through 09/21/06 by placing the cursor in first block to be viewed, holding down the mouse button, and dragging the cursor over the blocks that contain the test results that he wanted included in the graph. Clicking the "Graph" button on the lower edge of the table displays the information as in **Figure 10-14**.

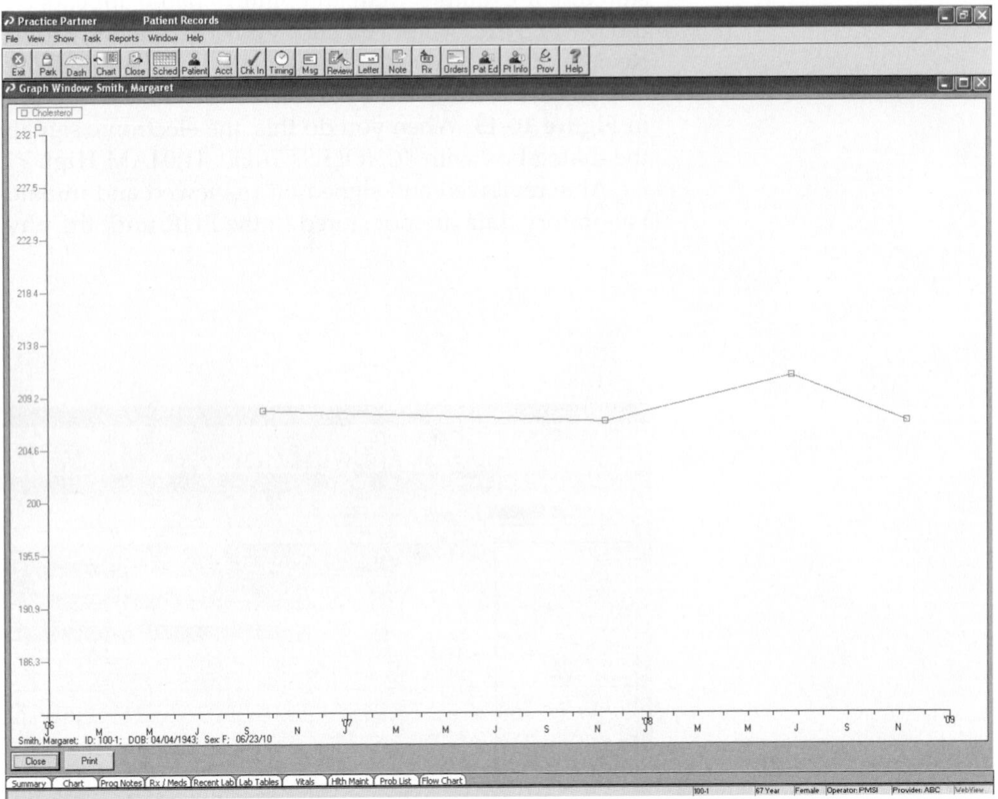

Figure **10-14 Graph feature in the Laboratory Data Table.** *Practice Partner® is a registered trademark of McKesson Corporation and/or one of its subsidiaries. Practice Partner® screen shots and materials used with the permission of McKesson Corporation. © 2010 McKesson Corporation. All rights reserved.*

Multiple elements can also be trended. For example, to display information as in **Figure 10-15**, highlight (drag the mouse cursor over text while pressing the mouse button) the first two elements (CHOLESTEROL and LDL-CHOL) for dates 11/12/08 through 09/21/06; then click the "Graph" button.

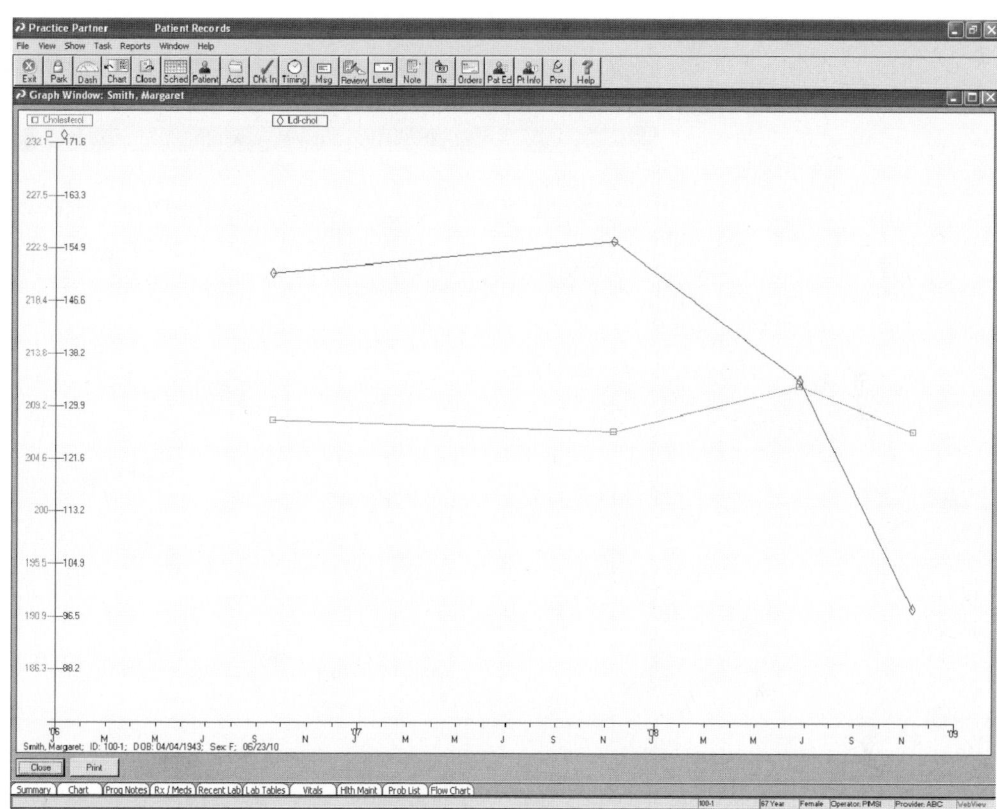

Figure **10-15** **Multiple elements in graph format.** *Practice Partner® is a registered trademark of McKesson Corporation and/or one of its subsidiaries. Practice Partner® screen shots and materials used with the permission of McKesson Corporation. © 2010 McKesson Corporation. All rights reserved.*

The visual trend data can also illustrate the test results over longer periods. For example, you could select to see all the cholesterol tests during the period of 2000 to 2008, as illustrated in **Figure 10-16**. This provides the physician with visual trending data that he may want to discuss with the patient.

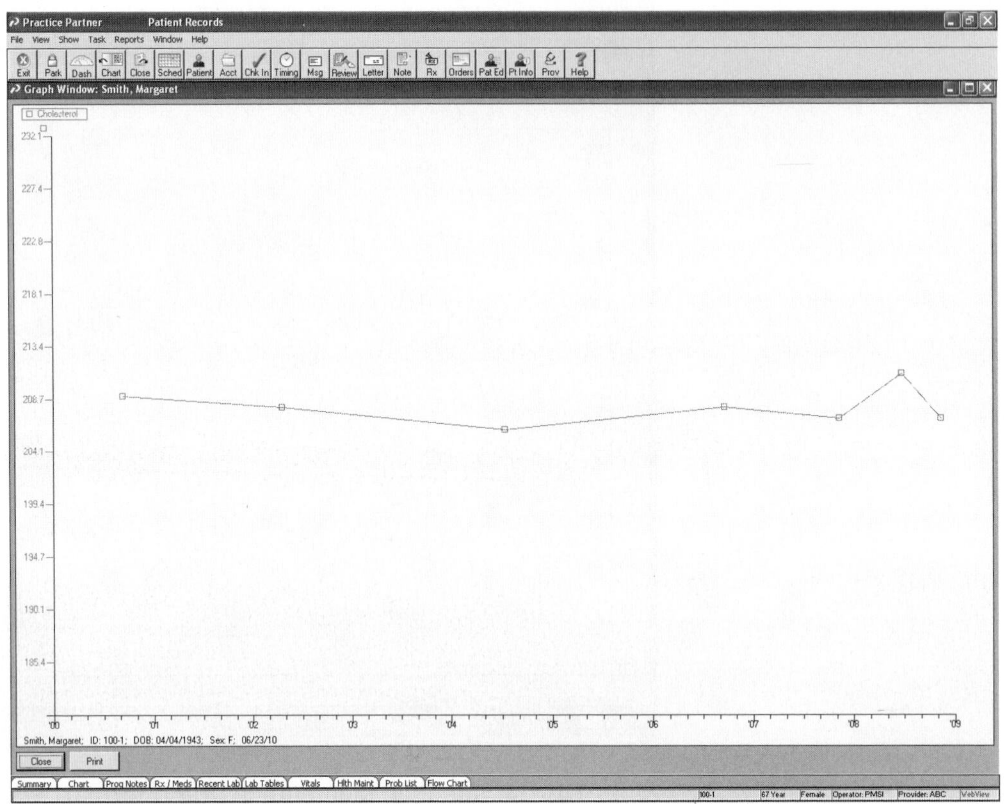

Figure **10-16** **Graphing over extended periods.** *Practice Partner® is a registered trademark of McKesson Corporation and/or one of its subsidiaries. Practice Partner® screen shots and materials used with the permission of McKesson Corporation. © 2010 McKesson Corporation. All rights reserved.*

Return to the Dashboard and open George Hall's Lab Review entry. From the Lab Table Review, the physician can review and sign the lab results. For example, click on the "Sign" button at the bottom of the Review screen as shown in **Figure 10-17**.

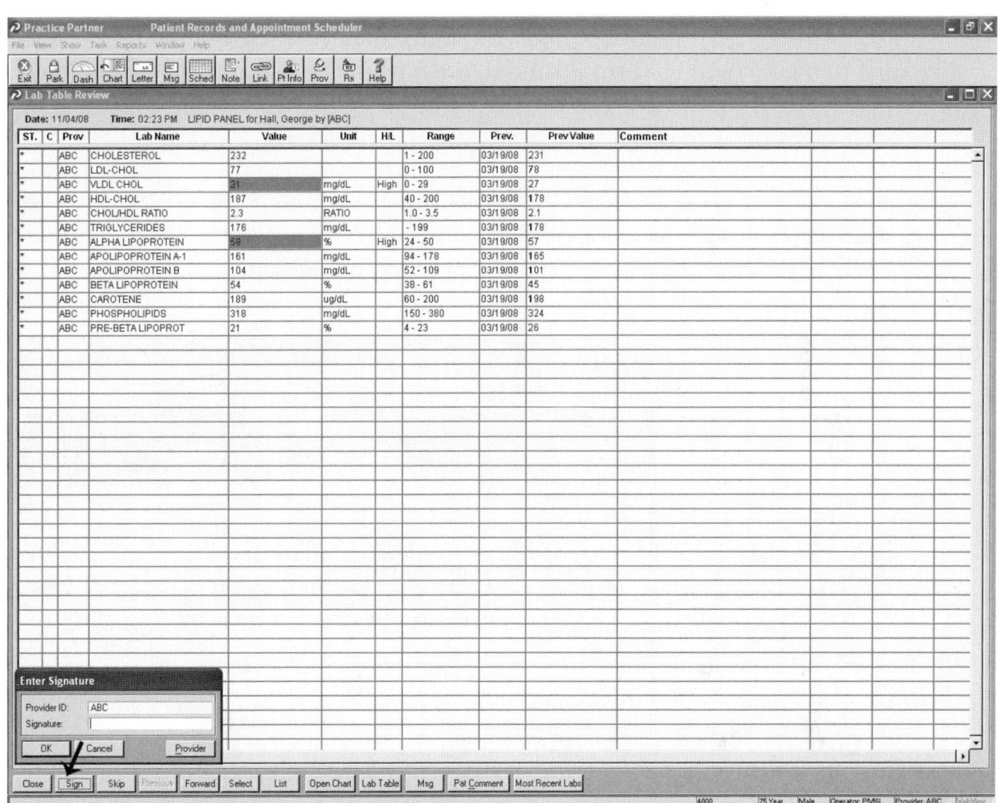

ST.	C	Prov	Lab Name	Value	Unit	H/L	Range	Prev.	Prev Value	Comment
*		ABC	CHOLESTEROL	232			1 - 200	03/19/08	231	
*		ABC	LDL-CHOL	77			0 - 100	03/19/08	78	
*		ABC	VLDL CHOL	31	mg/dL	High	0 - 29	03/19/08	27	
*		ABC	HDL-CHOL	187	mg/dL		40 - 200	03/19/08	178	
*		ABC	CHOL/HDL RATIO	2.3	RATIO		1.0 - 3.5	03/19/08	2.1	
*		ABC	TRIGLYCERIDES	176	mg/dL		- 199	03/19/08	178	
*		ABC	ALPHA LIPOPROTEIN	58	%	High	24 - 50	03/19/08	57	
*		ABC	APOLIPOPROTEIN A-1	161	mg/dL		94 - 178	03/19/08	165	
*		ABC	APOLIPOPROTEIN B	104	mg/dL		52 - 109	03/19/08	101	
*		ABC	BETA LIPOPROTEIN	54	%		38 - 61	03/19/08	45	
*		ABC	CAROTENE	189	ug/dL		60 - 200	03/19/08	198	
*		ABC	PHOSPHOLIPIDS	318	mg/dL		150 - 380	03/19/08	324	
*		ABC	PRE-BETA LIPOPROT	21	%		4 - 23	03/19/08	26	

Figure **10-17** **Physician signature area on Lab Table Review screen.** *Practice Partner® is a registered trademark of McKesson Corporation and/or one of its subsidiaries. Practice Partner® screen shots and materials used with the permission of McKesson Corporation. © 2010 McKesson Corporation. All rights reserved.*

DAY TEN TASK 10.4

Note that a Signature box appears. At this point, Dr. Able would enter his signature, which would remove George Hall's lab results from the Lab Review window and place them in his EHR. Cancel out of the Enter Signature box and return to the Dashboard.

From the Notes Review area of the Dashboard, scroll down to Richard Stein's EKG report from 04/07/2008 and open it by clicking on it. From the Review Provider Data screen, another patient's data can be accessed. For example, click on the "Older" button located on the right. This displays Julie Carter's note to review as shown in **Figure 10-18**. You can progress through all the messages on the review section of the Dashboard by clicking the "Newer" button to scroll through all the entries. You will notice that the progress notes you created for your patients, such as Karra Burthold, are now in the list of notes for review. Using this Older or Newer feature, the physician can quickly access the notes to be reviewed on the Dashboard.

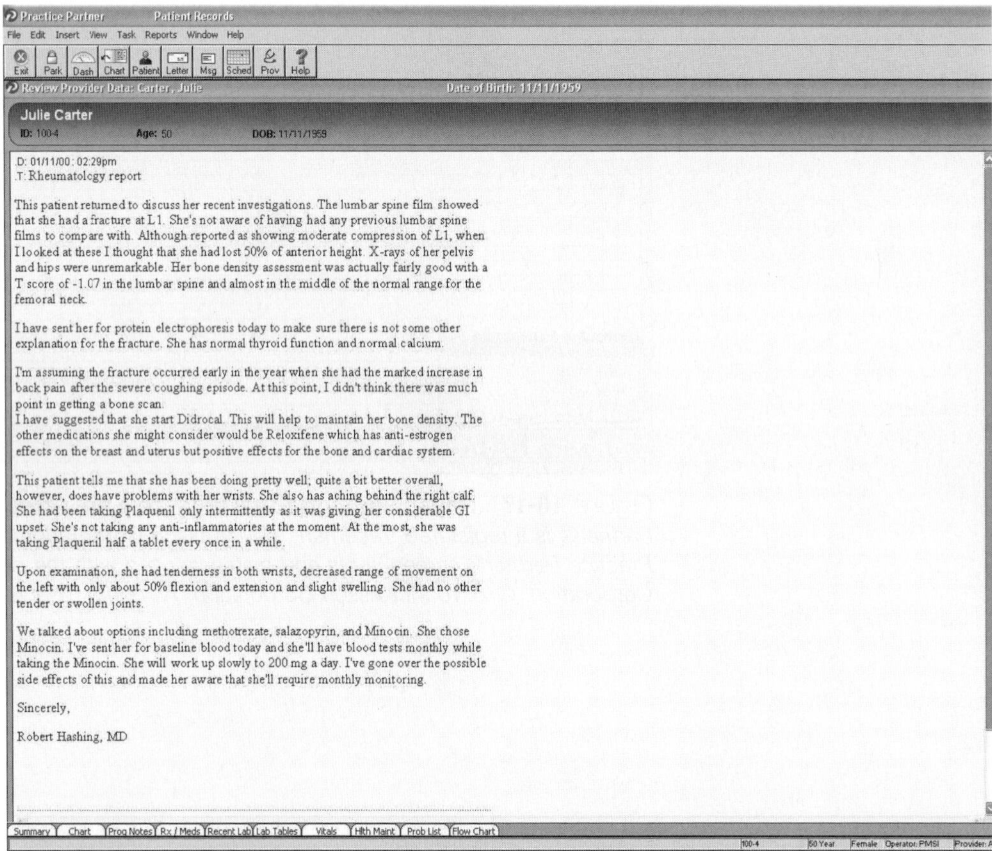

Figure **10-18** **Julie Carter's Report.** *Practice Partner® is a registered trademark of McKesson Corporation and/or one of its subsidiaries. Practice Partner® screen shots and materials used with the permission of McKesson Corporation. © 2010 McKesson Corporation. All rights reserved.*

From the Review Provider Data screen, the records can also be edited. For example, click on Julie Carter's rheumatology report and click on the "Edit" button on the right of the dialog box. When you do this, the note will open and you can now enter text into the report. Click "Cancel" and "Yes" to leave without saving changes.

The staff can also forward, fax, or print reports that need to be shared with other providers in the office by using the options to the right of the report. For example, if Dr. Able wanted to forward Julie Carter's rheumatology report to Abe Fromin, he would click "Forward" and select Abe Fromin from the "Provider Select" box and then enter his signature to forward the message.

***CONGRATULATIONS!* You did it, and it wasn't even that difficult, was it? It is like most new things; at first, new things seem harder than they actually turn out to be. You are going to be learning so many new things as you start your new health care career. Do not be concerned with the EHR software that you will encounter. You will find that it is user-friendly and will help you do your job in a more efficient and effective manner.**

This concludes your tasks for all 10 days. You did a great job!

Real difficulties can be overcome;
it is only the imaginary ones that are unconquerable.
—Theodore N. Vail

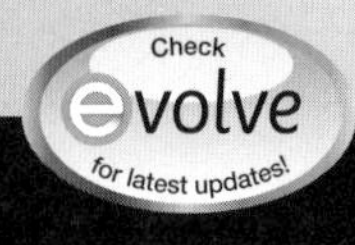
Check
evolve
for latest updates!

APPENDICES

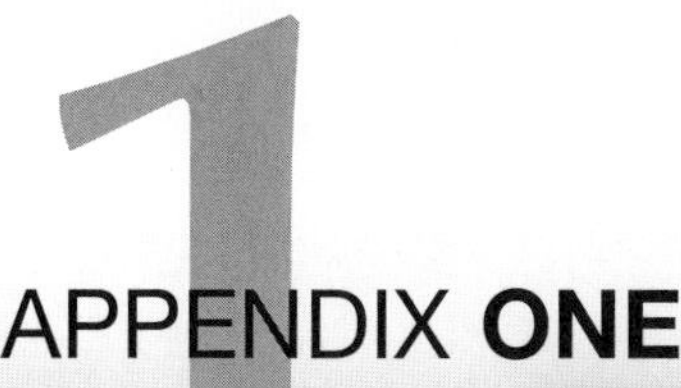

APPENDIX ONE

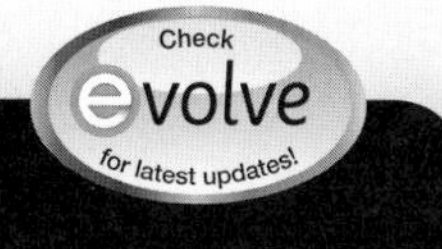
Check
evolve
for latest updates!

Welcome

Welcome to the South Padre Medical Center. You will find the Center to be a busy, friendly place to work where your skills, knowledge, and abilities will be appreciated and used. As in every office, there are standard procedures that we all follow to ensure that the office operates smoothly. The Policies and Procedures located in Appendix 2 will familiarize you with the operating procedures that are standard for all employees of the Center.

The employees of the Center are here to help you put your education and training into action by performing the tasks that you learned in your educational program. We have been involved in the internship process for more than a decade and see the internship experience as a vital part of your education. We want to help you be successful. You can expect that all employees will treat you as a professional member of the health care team. Mutual respect is absolutely necessary to ensure South Padre Medical Center has an environment conducive to superior patient care. On behalf of each member of the team, we are glad you are here and hope you find your experience with us rewarding.

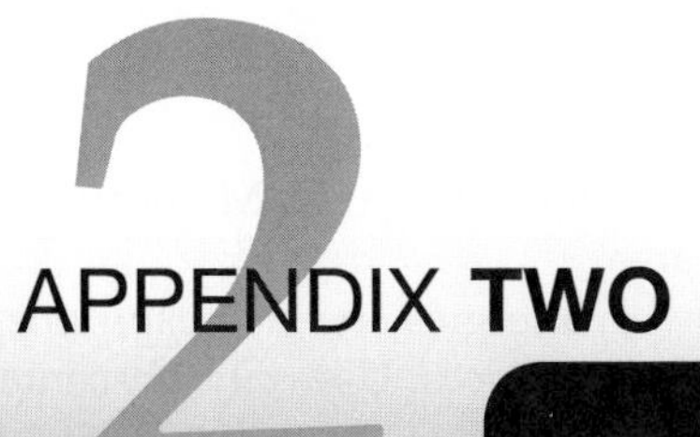

APPENDIX **TWO**

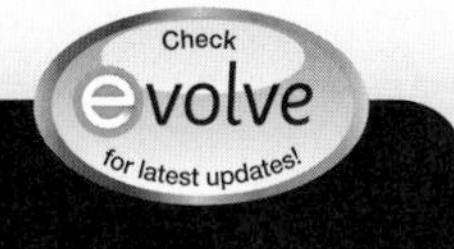

Policies and Procedures

A. Introduction

You are ready to begin your 2-week internship as a medical office assistant in the South Padre Medical Center, a medical office located in South Padre, Texas. The Center is a partnership of four physicians affiliated with Texas Health Corporation, a managed care corporation located in Houston, Texas. **Figure A2-1** displays the organizational structure of the Center and the affiliation with Texas Health Corporation.

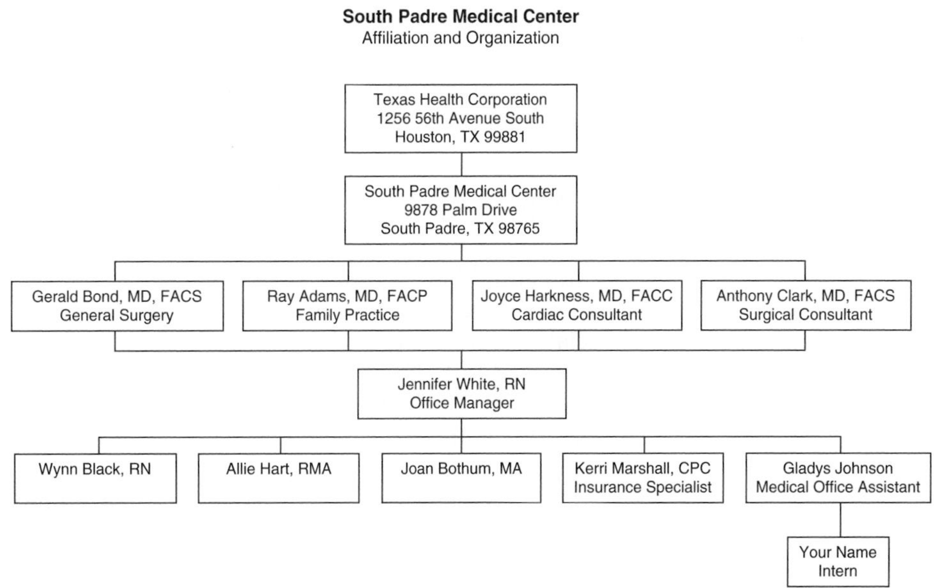

Figure **A2-1** **Affiliation and Organization of South Padre Medical Center.**

South Padre Medical Center is located at 9878 Palm Drive in South Padre in the South Padre Medical Complex. The one-story building houses several suites of professional offices. South Padre Medical Center is located in the middle of the building, just inside the front doors. The waiting room is the first area the patient enters. The front office area is separated from the patient waiting room by a registration desk.

There is a staff lounge located behind the lab area at the rear of the center. The lounge is used by all employees for breaks throughout the day. A picnic table is located outside the rear entrance and is also for employee use. There are lockers available in the lounge area, and all employees are required to place their personal items in a locker. Gladys Johnson, Medical Office Assistant, will assign you a locker and give you the combination to the lock located on the front of the locker. Personal items, such as purses and backpacks, are not allowed in the office area. Medically necessary items are, of course, allowed in the office area.

In consideration of our patients and employees with allergies and/or respiratory conditions, do not apply perfumes, colognes, or other fragrances. Use only unscented hairsprays, deodorants, and other personal care items.

Each of the physicians has a private office located a short distance from the seven patient examination rooms. When delivering mail or messages for the physicians, delivery is to be to the physician's private office. Never interrupt the physician in the patient examination rooms unless specifically told to do so by your supervisor.

A small lab is located in the Center and is used for a variety of laboratory procedures. Staff members collect specimens and some of the less complex analyses are conducted in the Center's laboratory by Center personnel. The Center has contracted Island Express Labs to do all the Center's outside specimen analysis. The more complex analyses are sent to Island Express Labs, an outside laboratory. Each evening, a messenger from Island Express Labs delivers the results of previous analyses and picks up the specimens that are being sent to Island Express Labs for analysis. Island Express Labs also returns results using the U.S. mail system.

Minor surgical procedures are sometimes conducted in the Center, but the physicians are on staff at Island Hospital, where they admit patients for more major surgeries on either an inpatient or outpatient basis.

The South Padre Medical Complex building also houses offices of an independent radiologist; psychiatrist; and an ear, nose, and throat (ENT) specialist. The physicians from the Center often refer patients to these physicians for consultation. You will be receiving patient information from each of these offices regarding patients that have been referred for services, and you will be sending patient information to these offices while performing your office tasks.

B. About Our Physicians

South Padre Medical Center was established to meet the health needs of South Padre residents in general surgery and family practice, with consultation affiliates specializing in cardiology and surgery.

- Dr. Gerald Bond, a general surgeon, and Dr. Ray Adams, a family practitioner, founded the Center 20 years ago to provide health care to private patients and patients participating in Texas Health Corporation, a managed care organization.
- Dr. Joyce Harkness, a cardiologist, and Dr. Anthony Clark, a surgeon, serve as consultants to the Center. Dr. Harkness and Dr. Clark are from San Antonio and commute 2 days a week to see patients in the Center and at the hospital.
- All four physicians are registered with Texas Health Corporation as preferred providers. All physicians also have staff privileges at the South Padre Island Hospital and the South Padre Island Nursing Home.

C. Your Internship Duties

Your education has prepared you for this internship as a medical office assistant. Your internship will require you to do a variety of front office tasks in the areas of written correspondence, records management, telephone messages, patient appointments, mail, transcription, insurance claim, travel arrangements, banking services, bookkeeping, payroll, and arranging for meetings. Jennifer White is the office manager and has assigned Gladys Johnson, medical office assistant, to provide your orientation, training, and supervision. You will also spend some time working for Kerri Marshall, who is the insurance specialist for the Center; however, Gladys will remain your supervisor throughout the duration of your internship.

D. Calendar and Work Hours

Your internship covers a 2-week period from April 7 to April 18, 2008.

April 2008						
S	M	T	W	T	F	S
		1	2	3	4	5
6	**7**	**8**	**9**	**10**	**11**	12
13	**14**	**15**	**16**	**17**	**18**	19
20	21	22	23	24	25	26
27	28	29	30			

Your work hours are from 7:45 AM to 4:45 PM each day. Gladys and you should arrive 15 minutes prior to the start of office hours to open the office and begin answering the telephones promptly at 8 AM. Kerri Marshall arrives at 8:15 AM and works until 5:15 PM and covers the reception desk from 4:45 PM until 5:15 PM. The nursing personnel cover the reception desk from 5:15 PM until closing.

All staff take an hour lunch break, except on Wednesdays when all staff take a half-hour lunch break while three of the physicians are seeing office patients. All staff take a 15-minutue break in the morning and afternoon at various times to ensure continuous coverage of all Center services. Kerri Marshall covers the reception area for Gladys Johnson and you when both of you are on breaks.

E. Confidentiality

Every employee is required to read and sign a confidentiality statement, **Figure A2-2.** Confidentiality is a critically important aspect of your position. The patients' names, addresses, telephone numbers, disorders, and financial information are all confidential information. Even the fact that the patient is a Center patient is confidential, as is *all* information about the patient. You will be allowed access to patient information on a need-to-know basis. You are not allowed to access patient information that you do not have a reason to access. Do not discuss patient information unless you need to do so to complete your assigned tasks. If you should need to discuss patient information, please do so quietly, being cautious that other patients do not overhear your discussions.

When you receive a request for release of information, you are to verify that the release documentation has the signature of the patient or, in the case of a minor or incompetent patient, the signature of the legal guardian. As an intern or a new employee, you are to ask your supervisor/trainer to verify the correctness of the release documentation before releasing any information.

All documentation containing patient information, of any kind, is to be kept from public view. This includes, but is not limited to, appointment schedules, patient

South Padre Medical Center
Confidentiality Agreement

All information regarding patients and their health care that is acquired during the course of employment at South Padre Medical Center shall be considered confidential.

Confidential information must never be disclosed for non-employment related purposes. Disclosure of confidential information outside of an employee's assigned duties will constitute unauthorized release of confidential information and can be grounds for dismissal.

By signing this document, I acknowledge that I understand this statement.

Employee name ______________________ Date ______________

Figure **A2-2** **Confidentiality statement.** *(Modified from Potter BP:* Medical office administration: a worktext, *ed 2, St. Louis, 2010, Saunders.)*

records, laboratory/pathology reports, surgery reports, insurance forms, financial information, and telephone logs. All patient medical documentation is to be kept on your desk in a location that will not allow others to view it.

The respect that you show for our patients by keeping their information confidential should also be extended to our physicians. You are a reflection of the Center in all you do and say, especially in what you say about the Center and the staff. Professionalism and respect for the privacy of the physicians and employees of the South Padre Medical Center is an expectation of all Center employees.

F. Telephone and Request for Inpatient Consultation Forms

The telephone is a vital business tool in the Center. When your responsibilities include this valuable task, answer the telephone with: "South Padre Medical Center, this is (your name)." You are to complete the following blocks of the Telephone Record **(Figure A2-3)** for each patient message (though not all messages will include all of the items of information listed here):

Left side

- **PRIORITY**—if patient/caller indicates an urgency, place a 3 in the box.
- **Patient**—patient's first and last name.
- **Age**—note if patient/caller indicates the age.
- **Caller**—if the caller is not the patient but is calling for the patient, indicate the relationship of the caller to the patient. For example, Jane Smith, mother of Carrie Smith.
- **Telephone**—the patient/caller's telephone number and area code if patient is calling from outside the local area code.
- **Referred to**—the physician or team member to whom you delivered the call.
- **Chart #**—if known.
- **Chart attached**—yes or no (for all tasks you will check "No" on all Chart Attached areas).

PRIORITY ☐

Telephone Record

Patient Age

Caller

Telephone

Referred to

Chart #

Chart Attached ☐ YES ☐ NO

Date / / Time Rec'd By

Message

Temp	Allergies

Response

PHY/RN Initials	Date / /	Time	Handled By

Figure **A2-3** **Telephone Record.**

- **Date**—for this simulation, each patient/caller will state the date of the telephone call (MM/DD/YY).
- **Time**—for this simulation, each patient/caller will state the time called. Be sure to use AM or PM with all times.
- **Rec'd by**—your first name.

Right side

- **Message**—as precise and short as you can make it.
- **Temp**—if patient/caller indicates temperature, record it.
- **Allergies**—if patient specifically states an allergy, record it; if not, leave blank.
- **Response**—note the day, date, and time you scheduled any tentative appointment. Use the MM/DD/YY format. For example 04/09/08.
- **PHY/RN Initials, Date, Time, Handled By**—located in lower right-hand corner of the form are ***not*** to be completed by you but rather the person who approves your response. For example, if the patient called on Saturday and requested an appointment for Monday, and you had an appropriate appointment time available, you would schedule the appointment and record the time of appointment in the "Response" section of the telephone record. Your supervisor would then review your suggested appointment time prior to the patient being contacted with the appointment time. Whoever calls the patient with the appointment time would complete this section of the Telephone Record.

The Telephone Records are printed four to a page.

REQUEST FOR INPATIENT CONSULTATION FORM

You are to complete the following items on the Request for Inpatient Consultation form **(Figure A2-4)**:

- **To**—check the physician from whom the consultation is requested.
- **ATTENDING**—record the name of the **requesting** physician.
- **TELEPHONE**—record the **requesting** physician's telephone number, if provided.
- **Request date and time**—complete with the date and time of the telephone call.
- **PATIENT**—the patient for whom the consultation is requested.
- **ADMIT DATE**—the date the patient was admitted to the hospital, also known as the admitting date or admission date. Provide this information if the requesting physician/caller indicates it (MM/DD/YY).
- **FACILITY**—the hospital or other inpatient facility that the patient was admitted to.

REQUEST FOR INPATIENT CONSULTATION

To: ❑ Gerald Bond, MD
❑ Ray Adams, MD
❑ Joyce Harkness, MD
❑ Anthony Clark, MD

ATTENDING: ____________
TELEPHONE: ____________
Request Date and Time: ____________

PATIENT: ____________ ADMIT DATE: ____________

FACILITY: ____________ FLOOR: ____________ ROOM: ____________

REASON FOR CONSULTATION: ____________

PLEASE COMPLETE BY: ____________ (DATE) RECEIVED BY: ____________

Figure **A2-4** **Request for Inpatient Consultation form.**

- **FLOOR**—the hospital floor number on which the patient is located.
- **ROOM**—the hospital room number in which the patient is located.
- **REASON FOR CONSULTATION**—record as stated by the requesting physician/caller.
- **PLEASE COMPLETE BY**—the date (MM/DD/YY) that the requesting physician has asked that the consultation be competed by.
- **RECEIVED BY**—your first name.

When a physician requests one of the Center physicians to provide a consultation at the hospital, place the consultation on the appointment schedule. For example, Dr. Thompson requests an inpatient consultation Monday afternoon by Dr. Bond. You would identify adequate time on the schedule, at either the requested time or a convenient time for the Center physician, and enter the information about the patient (i.e., name, room number, reason for consultation, requesting physician, and if the patient was a new or established patient) onto the schedule. Remember to schedule 15 minutes of travel time before the consultation.

G. Mail

The U.S. Postal Service delivers the mail each day between 9 AM and 10 AM. The front desk receptionist receives the mail and does the initial sorting. The mail should be sorted and handled as follows:

1. **Patients' laboratory or pathology results.**
   - Scan the results and write "rec'd" and the date (i.e., 04/08/08) received in the upper right-hand corner of each report as illustrated in **Figure A2-5.** Results that are positive are of the greatest priority.
   - Positive results are to be attached to the patient's medical record and placed on the top of the physician's incoming mail stack for immediate physician attention. If the physician is out of the office for more than a day, give the results and the medical record to the physician's nurse.
   - Negative results are to be placed in a file folder and placed in the physician's mail stack to be reviewed and initialed before the reports are filed into the medical records.

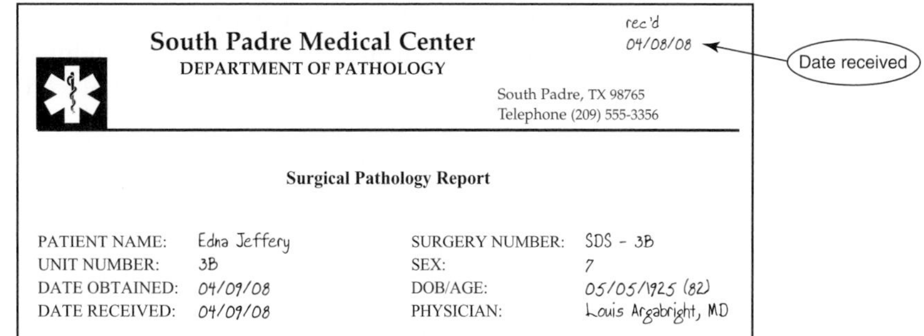

South Padre Medical Center
DEPARTMENT OF PATHOLOGY

rec'd
04/08/08

South Padre, TX 98765
Telephone (209) 555-3356

Surgical Pathology Report

PATIENT NAME:	Edna Jeffery	SURGERY NUMBER:	SDS - 3B
UNIT NUMBER:	3B	SEX:	?
DATE OBTAINED:	04/09/08	DOB/AGE:	05/05/1925 (82)
DATE RECEIVED:	04/09/08	PHYSICIAN:	Louis Argabright, MD

Figure **A2-5** **Date received.**

2. **Mail marked "Personal" or "Confidential."**
   - These items are not to be opened by you but placed on the mail stack as they were received with the date received (rec'd) on the front of the envelope in the lower left-hand corner as illustrated in **Figure A2-6.**

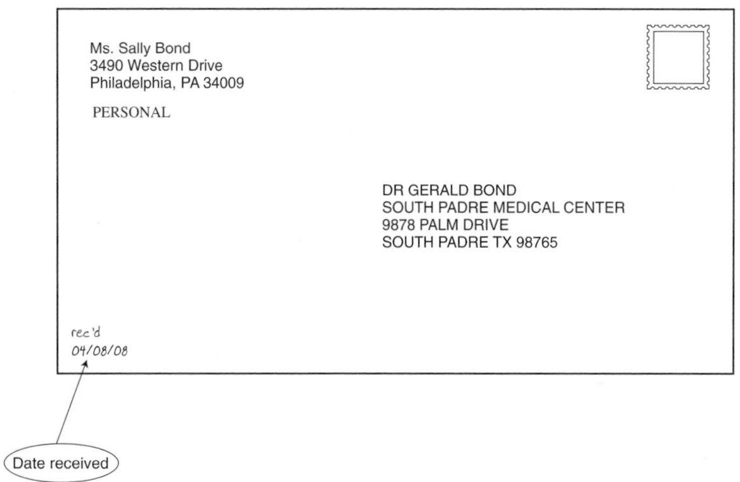

Ms. Sally Bond
3490 Western Drive
Philadelphia, PA 34009

PERSONAL

DR GERALD BOND
SOUTH PADRE MEDICAL CENTER
9878 PALM DRIVE
SOUTH PADRE TX 98765

rec'd
04/08/08

Figure **A2-6** **Personal or confidential mail.**

3. **Important letters, memos, documents.**
   - Open the mail and date stamp each item.
   - Review each item to ensure that it cannot be handled by another Center employee. When you are a new employee, you are to review these mail items with your supervisor/trainer until you are familiar with the office team and each employee's duties.

4. **Payments from patients or insurance companies.**
   - Sort the payments into two stacks—one for patient payments and the other for insurance company payments.
   - Payments are to be delivered to accounts receivable.
   - Place the envelope in which the payment was received behind each check or cash payment. Secure the envelope, payment, and any correspondence that accompanied the payment together with a paper clip. This step is especially important for payments that are made with cash and will ensure that all payments are credited to the correct accounts.

5. **Financial documents.**
   - Bank statements, invoices, statements, payroll forms, and state and federal tax information are to be dated and grouped together.

6. **Medical newsletters, journals, periodicals.**
   - These medical materials are to be delivered to the physician to whom they are addressed and are never to be placed in the patient waiting room.

7. **Reception room magazines and newspapers.**
   - *People, Good Housekeeping,* and other general reading magazines are to be placed in the waiting room.
   - Some physicians have personal magazine subscriptions sent to the office. These personal magazines are to be delivered to the physician, not placed in the waiting room. Dr. Bond's personal subscriptions are *RV World* and *Gold Prospector* magazines. Dr. Adams subscribes to *Money Monthly* and *Downhill Ski.*

8. **Advertisements.**
   - Delivered to Gladys.

9. **Other**
   - Stationery, business cards, check blanks, and other items from a printer are to be delivered to Gladys, who will review and approve the items for distribution or storage.

H. Delivery Service Items

A variety of delivery services deliver packages and letters to the Center each day (e.g., Federal Express, United Parcel Service, private delivery services). The times for these deliveries vary; however, deliveries are usually made before 4 PM each day. When a service delivers an item, you are to follow the same procedures as outlined for U.S. mail service. Many of the supplies for the Center are delivered by the delivery service method and you should notify the department to whom the package is addressed immediately by telephone when a department item has been received. Write the department name on the top of the item so as to facilitate pickup by department personnel. Set these items under the reception counter for pickup by the receiving department's personnel.

I. Office Hours and Physicians' Schedules

Office hours are from 8 AM to 6 PM Monday through Friday. Hours for each of the physicians are as follows:

Physician	Monday	Tuesday	Wednesday	Thursday	Friday
Dr. Gerald Bond	10-6	9-5	9-12	9-12	8-5
Dr. Ray Adams	9-6	9-6	10-5	9-12	9-5
Dr. Joyce Harkness			2-6	2-6	
Dr. Anthony Clark			2-6	2-6	

Note: You are not *to mark the following physician preferences on the appointment schedule at this time. You will be directed to mark the preferences in Task 1.1 when you begin working with the schedule. For now you are to only read about the preferences.*

J. Physicians' Lunch Hours

Lunch breaks for physicians are 1 hour in length and should be scheduled from noon to 1 PM for physicians on days when his/her office hours begin at 8 AM or 9 AM and from 1 PM to 2 PM when his/her office hours begin at 10 AM. When a physician's office hours are only scheduled from 9 AM to noon or 10 AM to noon, you do not schedule a lunch break. Drs. Harkness and Clark request a 1 PM to 2 PM lunch break on the 2 days they are scheduled in the office. Should a physician change his/her office hours, you will change the lunch break accordingly.

K. Surgery Schedules

If the physician is scheduled in the office before a surgery is scheduled at the hospital, you are to block off the hour before the first surgery is scheduled. On days with a surgery schedule, you are to mark off as "Unavailable" any time following the last possible time to schedule surgery if the surgery schedule is in the afternoon. For example, Dr. Bond wants to have surgeries scheduled beginning at 1 PM, with the last starting time for a surgery no later than 4 PM. You would mark off the time periods from 12 PM through 12:45 PM, and label the 12:45 to 1 PM block "Surgery," with an arrow pointing to the surgery block of time. Refer to **Figure A2-7** for an

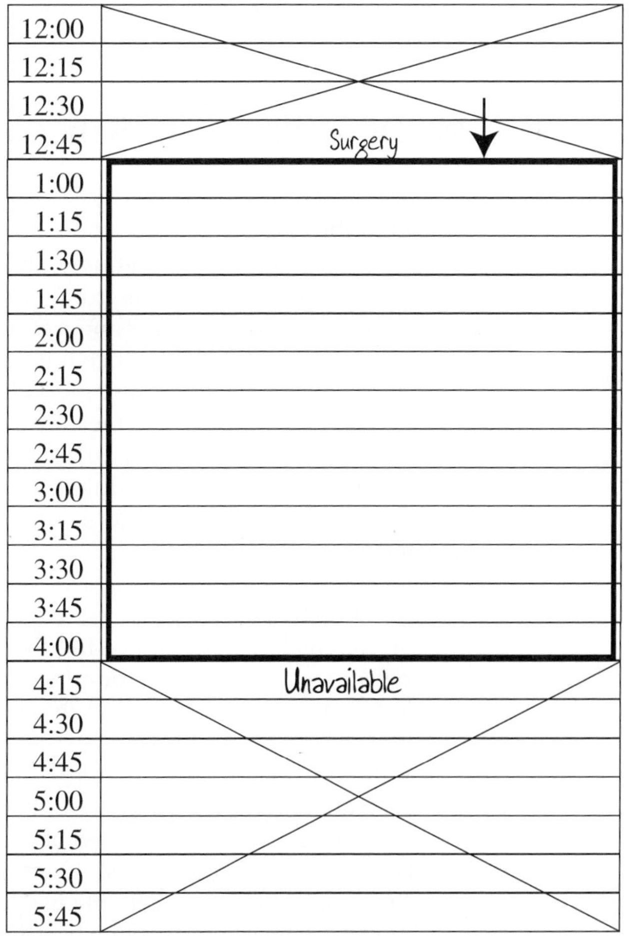

Figure **A2-7** **Surgery hours marked off on an appointment sheet.**

APPENDIX 2

illustration of marking off the surgery time. You outline the hours from 1 PM through 4 PM to set the surgery hours apart from the regular office scheduling time. You would also mark off the time blocks from 4:15 PM through 5:45 PM as "Unavailable" so no one schedules further surgeries or patients into this time for Dr. Bond. Dr. Harkness and Dr. Clark have morning surgery schedules followed by an hour of lunch, then begin seeing office patients at 2 PM on Wednesdays and Thursdays. See "M" for individual physician scheduling preferences.

L. Marking Off the End-of-Day Time Blocks

You are to mark off any time periods at the end of the day that the physician has indicated are not to be scheduled. For example, Dr. Bond wants to finish no later than 5 PM on Tuesdays; therefore, you would mark off the four 15-minute time blocks from 5 PM through 5:45 PM **(Figure A2-8)**.

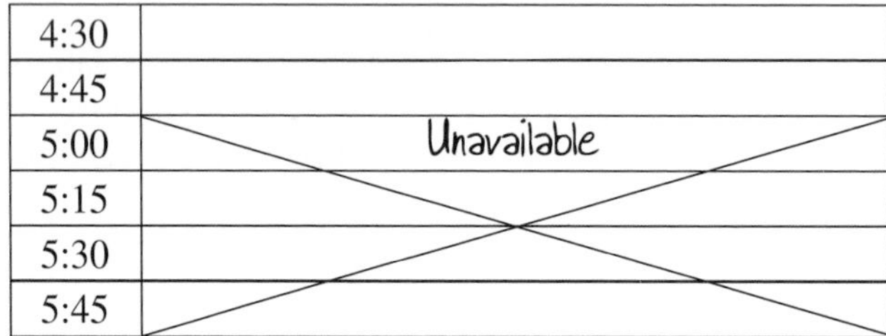

Figure **A2-8** **End-of-day time marked off on an appointment sheet.**

M. Other Physician Scheduling Preferences

DR. BOND

- Dr. Bond has a board meeting each Thursday from 7:30 AM to 8:45 AM and conducts inpatient rounds from 6 AM to 8:45 AM every Tuesday and Wednesday. He has requested a 15-minute travel time at the end of his rounds and board meeting to travel to the office but you do not need to write "travel" on the schedule, just block off the time as indicated.
- Dr. Bond has selected Wednesday and Thursday afternoons beginning at 1 PM as the preferred time for scheduling surgical procedures. He has requested that the last surgery never be scheduled later than a starting time of 4 PM. He has requested that an hour before surgery be marked off to provide desk, travel, and/or lunch time.

DR. ADAMS

- Dr. Adams has a board meeting the second Wednesday of each month from 8 AM to 9:45 AM and conducts rounds from 7 AM to 8:45 AM on Monday, Thursday, and Friday. He has requested that he have 15 minutes of travel time scheduled after the board meeting and rounds to travel to the office but you do not need to write "Travel" on the schedule, just block off the time because the physician is not leaving from the office or returning to the office.
- Dr. Adams also teaches a class at the local medical school from 1 PM to 3 PM each Thursday and has requested 30 minutes "Travel" be written on his schedule (as illustrated in **Figure A2-9**). He has lunch from noon to 1 PM but wants the "travel" note as a reminder. Dr. Adams does not return to the office after the class is finished. Mark off his time from 3 PM and after as "Unavailable."

12:30	Travel
12:45	
1:00	Medical School
1:15	
1:30	
1:45	
2:00	
2:15	
2:30	
2:45	
3:00	Unavailable
3:15	
3:30	
3:45	
4:00	
4:15	
4:30	
4:45	
5:00	
5:15	
5:30	
5:45	

Figure **A2-9** **Dr. Adams' schedule on Thursday.**

DR. HARKNESS AND DR. CLARK

- Drs. Harkness and Clark have selected 8 AM to 9 AM on Wednesday and Thursday for hospital rounds. They have requested that surgeries be scheduled from 9 AM and ending at or before 1 PM on Wednesdays and Thursdays. Mark off Monday, Tuesday, and Friday as "Unavailable."
- Both Dr. Harkness and Dr. Clark request patients be scheduled beginning at 2 PM on Wednesday and Thursday. Inpatient consultations are to be scheduled at the end of the day.

N. Appointment Scheduling Guidelines

For billing purposes, a **new patient** is defined as one who has not seen the physician or another physcian of the same specialty within the South Padre Medical Center within the past 3 years. An **established patient** is one who has seen any physician or another physician of the same specialty within the South Padre Medical Center within the past 3 years. Because the patient has seen a physician within the Center within 3 years means that the patient's medical record is available and only needs to be updated. Because updating requires less time than does development of a new patient record, physicians get paid more for a new patient office visit than they do for an established patient visit. But, for purposes of the schedule, if the patient has been seen in the Center by any of the Center physicians, he/she is considered an established patient because there is a medical record available for that patient.

When an established patient is scheduled for an appointment, "Est" is to be placed on the appointment schedule behind the patient's name. When a new patient is scheduled, "New" is placed behind the name on the appointment schedule. In this way, you will know which patients need their medical records retrieved from storage and which patients need new medical records assembled.

It is your responsibility to schedule patient appointments and to ensure that the correct information is recorded on the appointment schedule. The physicians have developed a list of the length of time you are to allow for the most common patient complaints. The following are the scheduling guidelines you will use when scheduling both new and established patients:

15 MINUTES

- Allergies
- Burns
- Cast recheck
- Conjunctivitis
- Cough
- Ear pain or infection
- Ear wash
- Elevated temperature
- Flu symptoms
- Pharyngitis
- Rash, hives
- Recheck flu
- Recheck Pap
- Sinus
- Sore throat
- URI
- UTI
- Wart treatment

30 MINUTES

- Abdominal pain
- Asthma
- Bronchitis
- Cast change
- Chest congestion
- Chest pain
- Confusion
- Depression
- Diabetic new problem
- Diabetic recheck
- Dizziness
- Eye injury
- Foreign body removal (location)
- Headache
- Infection
- Ingrown toenail
- Lesion removal (1)
- Menstrual problems
- Muscle strain
- OB check
- Pap
- Postoperative visit
- Preop physical
- Shortness of breath (SOB)
- Sprain or suspected fracture
- STD
- Varicocele recheck

45 MINUTES

- Breast pain
- Dog bite
- Lump
- Postoperative complication or pain
- Varicose veins

15 TO 60 MINUTES

- Pap included for female patients (over age 18)
- Physicals (px) and preoperatives (preop) (schedule by age)

Under 18	15 minutes
18–40	30 minutes
41–65	45 minutes
Over 65	60 minutes

CONSULTATION

Request for an inpatient consultation: Prefer an hour but can use 45 minutes. Note reason for consultation when placing inpatient consultation on schedule.

CARDIAC 1 HOUR

- New cardiac outpatient
- New inpatient consultation

SURGERY, ECHOCARDIOGRAM, AND MISCELLANEOUS 1 HOUR

- Lymphadenectomy
- Pacemaker
- Surgical echocardiogram

45 MINUTES

- Hearing check
- Hernia repair, periumbilical
- Lesion removal (2 or more)
- Outpatient echocardiogram
- Proctosigmoidoscopy (procto)

60 MINUTES

- Breast biopsy
- Initial (new) OB visit
- Kidney biopsy
- Liver biopsy
- Lymph biopsy
- Needle biopsy
- New surgical patient

90 MINUTES

- Diskectomy

If a patient requires an appointment for a complaint not listed, you are to use your judgment in making the appointment based on the similarity of the complaint to those on the scheduling guidelines.

O. Patient Lists

Prior to the physician's arrival for the day, a Patient List is prepared that displays all of the appointments for physicians for that day. **Figure A2-10** illustrates a previous

PATIENT LIST
for
Monday, March 31, 2008

Gerald Bond, MD

8:00-10:00	Unavailable
10:00-10:30	McCormick, Matthew, New, Preop physical
10:30-11:00	Norman, Patty, New, Ulcer
11:00-11:30	Stout, Henry, New, Hernia
11:30-12:00	Meuler, Darrin, New, Preop physical
12:00-12:30	O'Leary, Corwin, New, Abdominal pain
12:30-1:00	Garcia, Manuel, New, Upper GI pain
1:00-2:00	Lunch
2:00-2:45	SPH Consultation, Lopez, Jesus, Room 522, pancreatic CA, Ref: Dr. Orlando
2:45-	Open

Figure **A2-10** **Sample Patient List.**

Patient List prepared for Dr. Bond. Patient Lists are keyed onto blank paper. The Patient List has many purposes and is a necessary tool in the medical office:

- At the receptionist desk to mark off the patients as they arrive for their appointments and to ensure that the correct medical record is available for each patient.
- By the nursing staff to prepare the examination rooms and supplies needed for each patient's visit.
- By medical records personnel to pull from the filing shelves the records for the day's patients.
- By the physicians as their daily schedules.
- To check the daysheet of charges against the Patient List each day.

The Patient List is prepared the morning before the day represented on the list. The list is updated throughout the remainder of the day and the next morning before the first patient arrives. There are always changes to the schedule after the day begins, and it is the receptionist's responsibility to keep the master Patient List current throughout the day. At the end of the day the Patient Lists (one for each physician seeing patients in the office that day) are given to Gladys Johnson, who routes the updated lists to Kerri Marshall to ensure that all patients have been billed for services provided on that day. This extra step is a backup to the regular accounting system and a valuable reference in this busy office.

P. Patient Reception

When the patient arrives for his/her appointment, first cheerfully greet the patient. It is important to greet the patient quietly by name whenever possible. A simple greeting for an established patient could be: "Good morning, Mr. Wilson." (Don't forget to SMILE with your greeting.)

For an established patient, ask the patient to verify his/her address, telephone number, and insurance information as stated in the medical record, check the patient's name off the Patient List, and place the patient's medical record in the "Patients to Be Seen" inbox for the physician's nurse.

When a new patient arrives for his/her appointment, type a file folder label in capital letters with the last name, first name, middle initial. Secure the label to a file folder and place a blank Subsequent Findings form (see Figure 2-1) in the folder. Have the patient complete a Patient Information form (see Figure 2-2) and place the form in the folder. The newly created patient's medical record is then placed in the "Patients to Be Seen" inbox for the physician's nurse.

Ask the patient to be seated in the waiting area and assure him/her that the nurse will call his/her name when it is time to go into the examination room. For example, you could state, "Thank you, Mr. Wilson. Please be seated in the waiting room and the nurse will call you in about 5 minutes." If the appointments are running late, give the patient some idea of how long a wait to expect, with a brief explanation such as "The doctor is running a little behind today, so it will be about 15 minutes before the nurse will call you."

Q. Filing

There are two types of filing most commonly used in the medical setting—alphabetic and numeric. Numeric is often preferred because it provides anonymity to the patient. Numeric filing requires the use of an accession ledger that keeps track of each number that is assigned to a patient. The numbering system would begin with a higher number, such as 1000. The first patient assigned a number would be 1000 and the patient's name would be registered to that number by means of the accession ledger. Numbers are always assigned in consecutive order.

There are two commonly used numeric filing methods—consecutive and terminal digit filing. Consecutive number filing is when the charts are filed in order of the lowest to the highest number. For example, the following four file numbers are placed in consecutive order in a six-digit consecutive filing system:

004569
098122
560011
890103

Note that two zeros were added to 4569 and one zero to 98122 to maintain a six-digit consecutive filing system.

When using a terminal digit filing system, the numbers are separated into groups. For example, 890103 becomes 89 01 03. The 89 is the primary unit, 01 the secondary unit, and 03 the tertiary (third) unit. The 89 indicates that the record is filed in the "89" section of the medical records room, in the 01 section, with the record placed behind the "02" medical record. Using the terminal digit filing method, the file numbers used above would be filed as follows:

00	45	69
09	81	22
56	00	11
89	01	03

Color coding of the numbers in the filing system is often used to speed the filing process and reduce misfiles. For example, in an alphabetic filing system, the R would be orange and the I would be yellow. Ann Riggs's file would be have her name on the side of the file "RIGGS, ANN" and also along the side would be an orange R and a yellow I, as illustrated in **Figure A2-11.** Another example is the letter **S** in yellow and the letter **A** in grey, as in Monica Sartori's file in **Figure A2-12.** As an added feature, note that at the top edge of Ann Riggs's file is 2000 to indicate she became a patient in the year 2000. Monica Sartori's file has a 99 to indicate she became a patient in 1999.

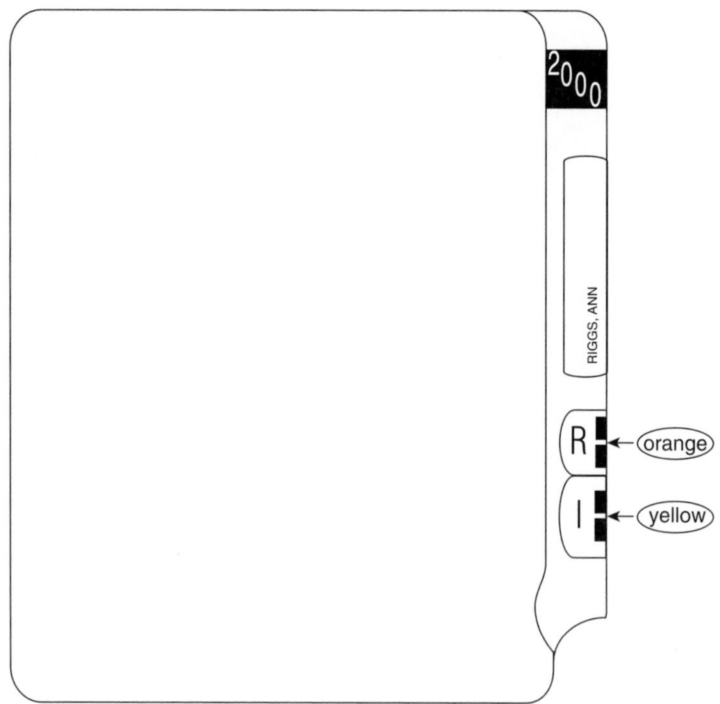

Figure **A2-11** **Example of color-coded file for Ann Riggs.**

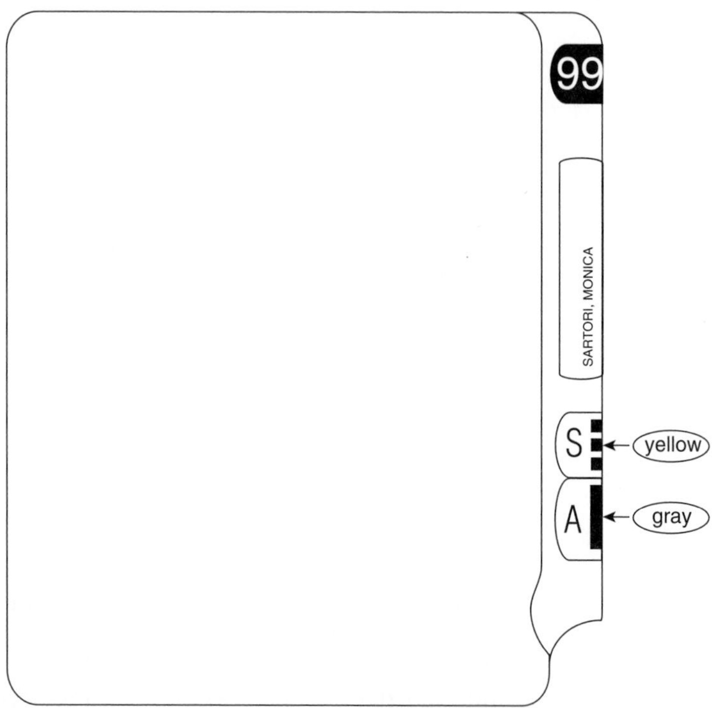

Figure **A2-12** **Example of color-coded file for Monica Sartori.**

Color coding is used in a numeric filing system by having each number or a group of numbers assigned a certain color. The colored numbers are preprinted and come in rolls similar to file folder labels. The medical records clerk then applies the colored labels for each number. The following is an example of a color-coding system for a numeric system and an alphabetic system:

Using this color-coding system, chart number 004569 would have two grey zeros, a red 4, tan 5, white 6, and a blue 9. If the alphabetic filing system used color coding for the first two letters of the last name, Paul Smith's name would have a yellow **S** and a purple **M** on the medical record. You can see that these color-coding methods would certainly speed filing. It is also much easier to locate misfiled records when the added feature of color coding is used.

Number	Letter	Color
0	A, K, U	Grey
1	B, L, V	Pink
2	C, M, W	Purple
3	D, N, X	Green
4	E, O, Y	Red
5	F, P, Z	Tan
6	G, Q	White
7	H, R	Orange
8	I, S	Yellow
9	J, T	Blue

R. Inventory Management

The Center's medical office assistant has established an inventory system that is used throughout the Center to inventory equipment and furniture in excess of $50. Items less than $50 are not inventoried using the inventory process; rather they are considered supplies. The inventory form contains the inventory number, product name, description, date purchased, and the room in which the item is located. Inventory checks are completed every 6 months in all rooms of the Center. Gladys assigns staff to various rooms in the Center, and those staff members are responsible for submitting a completed inventory form for the room(s) for which they are responsible. Gladys uses a computer program to manage the inventory and prints a copy of the items in each room and distributes the copies to the responsible employee. The employee is to determine that the equipment/furniture is in the assigned room and the inventory number is the same as is indicated on the equipment/furniture item. The inventory number is located on a tag that is glued to the back or underside of the item. When completing an inventory form, be certain the inventory number and the item are as listed on the form and then initial in the dated column (far right column). Your initials verify the item is located in the room indicated and that the inventory number is located on the item.

S. Referral

Figure A2-13 illustrates a Referral form that is used when one of the Center's physicians wants a patient to be seen and/or treated by a physician who is not a member of our staff. In the "From" area of the form, place an "X" on the line indicating the referring physician. On the "To" line indicate the name of the physician to whom the patient is being referred. Indicate the telephone number and address of the physician to whom the patient is being referred. On the "Patient" line indicate the name of the patient being referred and the patient's telephone number on the "Patient's Phone Number" line. The "Address" line is for the patient's home address—street, city, state, and zip code. Indicate the reason the patient is being referred on the "Reason for Referral" line. The "Appointment Date and Time" line is left blank until a member of the office staff calls the physician to whom the patient is being referred and obtains a time and date. You will not be doing this, so leave the Appointment Date and Time area blank. Last, place your initials and date on the "Referral Completed By" line to indicate when you completed the Referral form. Leave the "Arrangements Made By" line blank as this area will be used by the staff member who obtains the time and date for the referral appointment.

REFERRAL

FROM: Gerald Bond, MD _______
Ray Adams, MD _______
Joyce Harkness, MD _______
Anthony Clark, MD _______

TO: ____________________
TELEPHONE: ____________________
ADDRESS: ____________________
Requested Date and Time: ____________________

PATIENT: ____________________ PATIENT'S PHONE NUMBER: ____________________

ADDRESS: ____________________

REASON FOR REFERRAL: ____________________

____

____

APPOINTMENT DATE AND TIME: ____________________

REFERRAL COMPLETED BY: ____________________ (INITIAL AND DATE)

ARRANGEMENTS MADE BY: ____________________ (INITIAL AND DATE)

Figure **A2-13** **Example of a Referral form.**

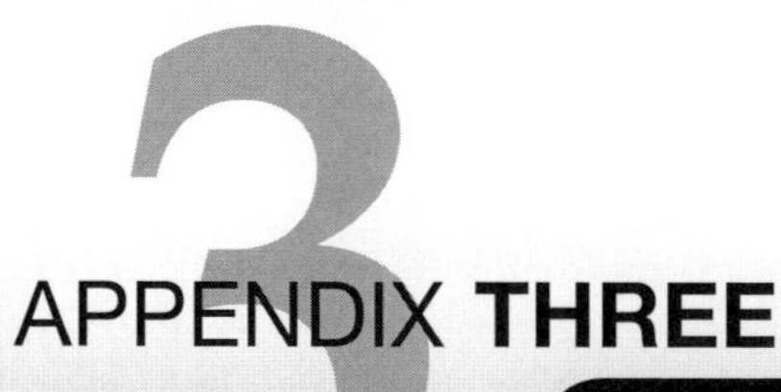

APPENDIX THREE

Third-Party Payer List and Directions

Check evolve for latest updates!

The CMS-1500 form is located in the Forms Library on the companion Evolve site and in the Supplies section of this text. The CMS-1500 is the universal insurance form used to submit charges to third-party payers or insurance companies. Some third-party payers have their own forms and require submission on those forms for claims made on behalf of patients covered by their insurance. Blocks 1 through 13 on the CMS-1500 contain patient information and blocks 14 through 33 contain provider information. Table 1 indicates the information that is to be placed in each block for the patient and provider information.

Assume that all patients have signed a previous authorization to submit insurance and receive payment directly from the payer. The insurance personnel enter "SOF" on the signature lines to indicate that the facility has the patient's signature on file.

The Center's Federal identification number is **00789200**.

By regulation, Medicare health care providers must obtain National Provider Identification (NPI) numbers. On the CMS-1500 (08/05), the referring provider's NPI is entered in 17b and the rendering provider's NPI is entered in 24J. The facility NPI is entered in 33a. The Center and each physician have an NPI number:

South Padre Medical Center	8866905213
Gerald Bond, MD	4682943911
Ray Adams, MD	7824443110
Anthory Clark, MD	8291458624
Joyce Harkness, MD	6894597377

Referring physicians' NPI numbers are:

Thomas Thompson, MD	1100986210
Bert Bethos, MD	3120981144
Clarence McDonald, MD	5925442862
Theodore Blackburn, MD	7739745986

The CMS-1500 is to be completed in capital letters with no punctuation. The following directions for completing the CMS-1500 are excerpts from the Medicare Claims Processing Manual, Chapter 26, Completing and Processing, 10.2, revised 02-24-06:

1500

HEALTH INSURANCE CLAIM FORM

APPROVED BY NATIONAL UNIFORM CLAIM COMMITTEE 08/05

PICA | PICA

CARRIER

1. MEDICARE (Medicare #) | MEDICAID (Medicaid #) | TRICARE CHAMPUS (Sponsor's SSN) | CHAMPVA (Member ID#) | GROUP HEALTH PLAN (SSN or ID) | FECA BLK LUNG (SSN) | OTHER (ID)

1a. INSURED'S I.D. NUMBER (For Program in Item 1)

PATIENT AND INSURED INFORMATION

2. PATIENT'S NAME (Last Name, First Name, Middle Initial)

3. PATIENT'S BIRTH DATE MM DD YY SEX M F

4. INSURED'S NAME (Last Name, First Name, Middle Initial)

5. PATIENT'S ADDRESS (No., Street)

6. PATIENT RELATIONSHIP TO INSURED Self Spouse Child Other

7. INSURED'S ADDRESS (No., Street)

CITY STATE

8. PATIENT STATUS Single Married Other

CITY STATE

ZIP CODE TELEPHONE (Include Area Code) ( )

Employed Full-Time Student Part-Time Student

ZIP CODE TELEPHONE (Include Area Code) ( )

9. OTHER INSURED'S NAME (Last Name, First Name, Middle Initial)

10. IS PATIENT'S CONDITION RELATED TO:

11. INSURED'S POLICY GROUP OR FECA NUMBER

a. OTHER INSURED'S POLICY OR GROUP NUMBER

a. EMPLOYMENT? (Current or Previous) YES NO

a. INSURED'S DATE OF BIRTH MM DD YY SEX M F

b. OTHER INSURED'S DATE OF BIRTH MM DD YY SEX M F

b. AUTO ACCIDENT? YES NO PLACE (State)

b. EMPLOYER'S NAME OR SCHOOL NAME

c. EMPLOYER'S NAME OR SCHOOL NAME

c. OTHER ACCIDENT? YES NO

c. INSURANCE PLAN NAME OR PROGRAM NAME

d. INSURANCE PLAN NAME OR PROGRAM NAME

10d. RESERVED FOR LOCAL USE

d. IS THERE ANOTHER HEALTH BENEFIT PLAN? YES NO ***If yes***, return to and complete item 9 a-d.

READ BACK OF FORM BEFORE COMPLETING & SIGNING THIS FORM.

12. PATIENT'S OR AUTHORIZED PERSON'S SIGNATURE I authorize the release of any medical or other information necessary to process this claim. I also request payment of government benefits either to myself or to the party who accepts assignment below.

SIGNED ______ DATE ______

13. INSURED'S OR AUTHORIZED PERSON'S SIGNATURE I authorize payment of medical benefits to the undersigned physician or supplier for services described below.

SIGNED ______

PHYSICIAN OR SUPPLIER INFORMATION

14. DATE OF CURRENT: MM DD YY ILLNESS (First symptom) OR INJURY (Accident) OR PREGNANCY(LMP)

15. IF PATIENT HAS HAD SAME OR SIMILAR ILLNESS. GIVE FIRST DATE MM DD YY

16. DATES PATIENT UNABLE TO WORK IN CURRENT OCCUPATION MM DD YY FROM TO MM DD YY

17. NAME OF REFERRING PROVIDER OR OTHER SOURCE

17a.

17b. NPI

18. HOSPITALIZATION DATES RELATED TO CURRENT SERVICES MM DD YY FROM TO MM DD YY

19. RESERVED FOR LOCAL USE

20. OUTSIDE LAB? YES NO $ CHARGES

21. DIAGNOSIS OR NATURE OF ILLNESS OR INJURY (Relate Items 1, 2, 3 or 4 to Item 24E by Line)

1. ___ . ___ 3. ___ . ___

2. ___ . ___ 4. ___ . ___

22. MEDICAID RESUBMISSION CODE ORIGINAL REF. NO.

23. PRIOR AUTHORIZATION NUMBER

24. A. DATE(S) OF SERVICE From MM DD YY To MM DD YY	B. PLACE OF SERVICE	C. EMG	D. PROCEDURES, SERVICES, OR SUPPLIES (Explain Unusual Circumstances) CPT/HCPCS MODIFIER	E. DIAGNOSIS POINTER	F. $ CHARGES	G. DAYS OR UNITS	H. EPSDT Family Plan	I. ID. QUAL.	J. RENDERING PROVIDER ID. #
1								NPI	
2								NPI	
3								NPI	
4								NPI	
5								NPI	
6								NPI	

25. FEDERAL TAX I.D. NUMBER SSN EIN

26. PATIENT'S ACCOUNT NO.

27. ACCEPT ASSIGNMENT? (For govt. claims, see back) YES NO

28. TOTAL CHARGE $

29. AMOUNT PAID $

30. BALANCE DUE $

31. SIGNATURE OF PHYSICIAN OR SUPPLIER INCLUDING DEGREES OR CREDENTIALS (I certify that the statements on the reverse apply to this bill and are made a part thereof.)

SIGNED DATE

32. SERVICE FACILITY LOCATION INFORMATION

a. b.

33. BILLING PROVIDER INFO & PH # ( )

a. b.

NUCC Instruction Manual available at: www.nucc.org PLEASE PRINT OR TYPE APPROVED OMB-0938-0999 FORM CMS-1500 (08-05)

Figure **A3-1** **Items shaded are to be left blank when patient has basic Medicare coverage.**

1500

HEALTH INSURANCE CLAIM FORM

APPROVED BY NATIONAL UNIFORM CLAIM COMMITTEE 08/05

PICA | PICA | CARRIER

1. MEDICARE (Medicare #) MEDICAID (Medicaid #) TRICARE CHAMPUS (Sponsor's SSN) CHAMPVA (Member ID#) GROUP HEALTH PLAN (SSN or ID) FECA BLK LUNG (SSN) OTHER (ID)		1a. INSURED'S I.D. NUMBER (For Program in Item 1)
2. PATIENT'S NAME (Last Name, First Name, Middle Initial)	3. PATIENT'S BIRTH DATE MM DD YY SEX M F	4. INSURED'S NAME (Last Name, First Name, Middle Initial)
5. PATIENT'S ADDRESS (No., Street)	6. PATIENT RELATIONSHIP TO INSURED Self Spouse Child Other	7. INSURED'S ADDRESS (No., Street)
CITY STATE	8. PATIENT STATUS Single Married Other	CITY STATE
ZIP CODE TELEPHONE (Include Area Code) ( )	Employed Full-Time Student Part-Time Student	ZIP CODE TELEPHONE (Include Area Code) ( )
9. OTHER INSURED'S NAME (Last Name, First Name, Middle Initial)	10. IS PATIENT'S CONDITION RELATED TO:	11. INSURED'S POLICY GROUP OR FECA NUMBER
a. OTHER INSURED'S POLICY OR GROUP NUMBER	a. EMPLOYMENT? (Current or Previous) YES NO	a. INSURED'S DATE OF BIRTH MM DD YY SEX M F
b. OTHER INSURED'S DATE OF BIRTH MM DD YY SEX M F	b. AUTO ACCIDENT? YES NO PLACE (State)	b. EMPLOYER'S NAME OR SCHOOL NAME
c. EMPLOYER'S NAME OR SCHOOL NAME	c. OTHER ACCIDENT? YES NO	c. INSURANCE PLAN NAME OR PROGRAM NAME
d. INSURANCE PLAN NAME OR PROGRAM NAME	10d. RESERVED FOR LOCAL USE	d. IS THERE ANOTHER HEALTH BENEFIT PLAN? YES NO *If yes*, return to and complete item 9 a-d.

PATIENT AND INSURED INFORMATION

READ BACK OF FORM BEFORE COMPLETING & SIGNING THIS FORM.

12. PATIENT'S OR AUTHORIZED PERSON'S SIGNATURE I authorize the release of any medical or other information necessary to process this claim. I also request payment of government benefits either to myself or to the party who accepts assignment below.

SIGNED ______ DATE ______

13. INSURED'S OR AUTHORIZED PERSON'S SIGNATURE I authorize payment of medical benefits to the undersigned physician or supplier for services described below.

SIGNED ______

14. DATE OF CURRENT: MM DD YY ◀ ILLNESS (First symptom) OR INJURY (Accident) OR PREGNANCY(LMP)	15. IF PATIENT HAS HAD SAME OR SIMILAR ILLNESS. GIVE FIRST DATE MM DD YY	16. DATES PATIENT UNABLE TO WORK IN CURRENT OCCUPATION FROM MM DD YY TO MM DD YY
17. NAME OF REFERRING PROVIDER OR OTHER SOURCE	17a. / 17b. NPI	18. HOSPITALIZATION DATES RELATED TO CURRENT SERVICES FROM MM DD YY TO MM DD YY
19. RESERVED FOR LOCAL USE		20. OUTSIDE LAB? YES NO $ CHARGES
21. DIAGNOSIS OR NATURE OF ILLNESS OR INJURY (Relate Items 1, 2, 3 or 4 to Item 24E by Line) 1. ___ . ___ 3. ___ . ___ 2. ___ . ___ 4. ___ . ___		22. MEDICAID RESUBMISSION CODE ORIGINAL REF. NO.
		23. PRIOR AUTHORIZATION NUMBER

	24. A. DATE(S) OF SERVICE From MM DD YY To MM DD YY	B. PLACE OF SERVICE	C. EMG	D. PROCEDURES, SERVICES, OR SUPPLIES (Explain Unusual Circumstances) CPT/HCPCS MODIFIER	E. DIAGNOSIS POINTER	F. $ CHARGES	G. DAYS OR UNITS	H. EPSDT Family Plan	I. ID. QUAL.	J. RENDERING PROVIDER ID. #
1									NPI	
2									NPI	
3									NPI	
4									NPI	
5									NPI	
6									NPI	

25. FEDERAL TAX I.D. NUMBER SSN EIN	26. PATIENT'S ACCOUNT NO.	27. ACCEPT ASSIGNMENT? (For govt. claims, see back) YES NO	28. TOTAL CHARGE $	29. AMOUNT PAID $	30. BALANCE DUE $
31. SIGNATURE OF PHYSICIAN OR SUPPLIER INCLUDING DEGREES OR CREDENTIALS (I certify that the statements on the reverse apply to this bill and are made a part thereof.) SIGNED DATE	32. SERVICE FACILITY LOCATION INFORMATION a. b.		33. BILLING PROVIDER INFO & PH # ( ) a. b.		

PHYSICIAN OR SUPPLIER INFORMATION

NUCC Instruction Manual available at: www.nucc.org PLEASE PRINT OR TYPE APPROVED OMB-0938-0999 FORM CMS-1500 (08-05)

Figure **A3-2** **Items shaded are to be left blank when private insurance is the primary and only coverage.**

1500

HEALTH INSURANCE CLAIM FORM

APPROVED BY NATIONAL UNIFORM CLAIM COMMITTEE 08/05

PICA | PICA

CARRIER

PATIENT AND INSURED INFORMATION

1. MEDICARE (Medicare #) | MEDICAID (Medicaid #) | TRICARE CHAMPUS (Sponsor's SSN) | CHAMPVA (Member ID#) | GROUP HEALTH PLAN (SSN or ID) | FECA BLK LUNG (SSN) | OTHER (ID)

1a. INSURED'S I.D. NUMBER (For Program in Item 1)

2. PATIENT'S NAME (Last Name, First Name, Middle Initial)

3. PATIENT'S BIRTH DATE MM DD YY — SEX M F

4. INSURED'S NAME (Last Name, First Name, Middle Initial)

5. PATIENT'S ADDRESS (No., Street)

6. PATIENT RELATIONSHIP TO INSURED — Self, Spouse, Child, Other

7. INSURED'S ADDRESS (No., Street)

CITY — STATE

8. PATIENT STATUS — Single, Married, Other

CITY — STATE

ZIP CODE — TELEPHONE (Include Area Code) ( )

Employed, Full-Time Student, Part-Time Student

ZIP CODE — TELEPHONE (Include Area Code) ( )

9. OTHER INSURED'S NAME (Last Name, First Name, Middle Initial)

10. IS PATIENT'S CONDITION RELATED TO:

11. INSURED'S POLICY GROUP OR FECA NUMBER

a. OTHER INSURED'S POLICY OR GROUP NUMBER

a. EMPLOYMENT? (Current or Previous) YES NO

a. INSURED'S DATE OF BIRTH MM DD YY — SEX M F

b. OTHER INSURED'S DATE OF BIRTH MM DD YY — SEX M F

b. AUTO ACCIDENT? YES NO — PLACE (State)

b. EMPLOYER'S NAME OR SCHOOL NAME

c. EMPLOYER'S NAME OR SCHOOL NAME

c. OTHER ACCIDENT? YES NO

c. INSURANCE PLAN NAME OR PROGRAM NAME

d. INSURANCE PLAN NAME OR PROGRAM NAME

10d. RESERVED FOR LOCAL USE

d. IS THERE ANOTHER HEALTH BENEFIT PLAN? YES NO *If yes*, return to and complete item 9 a-d.

READ BACK OF FORM BEFORE COMPLETING & SIGNING THIS FORM.

12. PATIENT'S OR AUTHORIZED PERSON'S SIGNATURE I authorize the release of any medical or other information necessary to process this claim. I also request payment of government benefits either to myself or to the party who accepts assignment below.

SIGNED ______ DATE ______

13. INSURED'S OR AUTHORIZED PERSON'S SIGNATURE I authorize payment of medical benefits to the undersigned physician or supplier for services described below.

SIGNED ______

PHYSICIAN OR SUPPLIER INFORMATION

14. DATE OF CURRENT: MM DD YY — ILLNESS (First symptom) OR INJURY (Accident) OR PREGNANCY(LMP)

15. IF PATIENT HAS HAD SAME OR SIMILAR ILLNESS. GIVE FIRST DATE MM DD YY

16. DATES PATIENT UNABLE TO WORK IN CURRENT OCCUPATION FROM MM DD YY TO MM DD YY

17. NAME OF REFERRING PROVIDER OR OTHER SOURCE — 17a. — 17b. NPI

18. HOSPITALIZATION DATES RELATED TO CURRENT SERVICES FROM MM DD YY TO MM DD YY

19. RESERVED FOR LOCAL USE

20. OUTSIDE LAB? YES NO — $ CHARGES

21. DIAGNOSIS OR NATURE OF ILLNESS OR INJURY (Relate Items 1, 2, 3 or 4 to Item 24E by Line)

1. ___ . ___ 3. ___ . ___

2. ___ . ___ 4. ___ . ___

22. MEDICAID RESUBMISSION CODE — ORIGINAL REF. NO.

23. PRIOR AUTHORIZATION NUMBER

24. A. DATE(S) OF SERVICE From MM DD YY To MM DD YY	B. PLACE OF SERVICE	C. EMG	D. PROCEDURES, SERVICES, OR SUPPLIES (Explain Unusual Circumstances) CPT/HCPCS MODIFIER	E. DIAGNOSIS POINTER	F. $ CHARGES	G. DAYS OR UNITS	H. EPSDT Family Plan	I. ID. QUAL.	J. RENDERING PROVIDER ID. #
1								NPI	
2								NPI	
3								NPI	
4								NPI	
5								NPI	
6								NPI	

25. FEDERAL TAX I.D. NUMBER SSN EIN

26. PATIENT'S ACCOUNT NO.

27. ACCEPT ASSIGNMENT? (For govt. claims, see back) YES NO

28. TOTAL CHARGE $

29. AMOUNT PAID $

30. BALANCE DUE $

31. SIGNATURE OF PHYSICIAN OR SUPPLIER INCLUDING DEGREES OR CREDENTIALS (I certify that the statements on the reverse apply to this bill and are made a part thereof.)

SIGNED ______ DATE ______

32. SERVICE FACILITY LOCATION INFORMATION — a. — b.

33. BILLING PROVIDER INFO & PH # ( ) — a. — b.

NUCC Instruction Manual available at: www.nucc.org — PLEASE PRINT OR TYPE — APPROVED OMB-0938-0999 FORM CMS-1500 (08-05)

Figure **A3-3** **Items shaded are to be left blank when another insurance is the primary and Medicare is the secondary.**

1500

HEALTH INSURANCE CLAIM FORM

APPROVED BY NATIONAL UNIFORM CLAIM COMMITTEE 08/05

PICA — PICA

CARRIER

1. MEDICARE (Medicare #) — MEDICAID (Medicaid #) — TRICARE CHAMPUS (Sponsor's SSN) — CHAMPVA (Member ID#) — GROUP HEALTH PLAN (SSN or ID) — FECA BLK LUNG (SSN) — OTHER (ID)

1a. INSURED'S I.D. NUMBER (For Program in Item 1)

2. PATIENT'S NAME (Last Name, First Name, Middle Initial)

3. PATIENT'S BIRTH DATE MM | DD | YY — SEX M F

4. INSURED'S NAME (Last Name, First Name, Middle Initial)

5. PATIENT'S ADDRESS (No., Street)

6. PATIENT RELATIONSHIP TO INSURED — Self Spouse Child Other

7. INSURED'S ADDRESS (No., Street)

CITY — STATE

8. PATIENT STATUS — Single Married Other

CITY — STATE

ZIP CODE — TELEPHONE (Include Area Code) ( )

Employed — Full-Time Student — Part-Time Student

ZIP CODE — TELEPHONE (Include Area Code) ( )

9. OTHER INSURED'S NAME (Last Name, First Name, Middle Initial)

10. IS PATIENT'S CONDITION RELATED TO:

11. INSURED'S POLICY GROUP OR FECA NUMBER

a. OTHER INSURED'S POLICY OR GROUP NUMBER

a. EMPLOYMENT? (Current or Previous) — YES NO

a. INSURED'S DATE OF BIRTH MM | DD | YY — SEX M F

b. OTHER INSURED'S DATE OF BIRTH MM | DD | YY — SEX M F

b. AUTO ACCIDENT? — YES NO — PLACE (State)

b. EMPLOYER'S NAME OR SCHOOL NAME

c. EMPLOYER'S NAME OR SCHOOL NAME

c. OTHER ACCIDENT? — YES NO

c. INSURANCE PLAN NAME OR PROGRAM NAME

d. INSURANCE PLAN NAME OR PROGRAM NAME

10d. RESERVED FOR LOCAL USE

d. IS THERE ANOTHER HEALTH BENEFIT PLAN? — YES NO — *If yes*, return to and complete item 9 a-d.

READ BACK OF FORM BEFORE COMPLETING & SIGNING THIS FORM.

12. PATIENT'S OR AUTHORIZED PERSON'S SIGNATURE I authorize the release of any medical or other information necessary to process this claim. I also request payment of government benefits either to myself or to the party who accepts assignment below.

SIGNED ____________ DATE ____________

13. INSURED'S OR AUTHORIZED PERSON'S SIGNATURE I authorize payment of medical benefits to the undersigned physician or supplier for services described below.

SIGNED ____________

PATIENT AND INSURED INFORMATION

14. DATE OF CURRENT: MM | DD | YY — ILLNESS (First symptom) OR INJURY (Accident) OR PREGNANCY(LMP)

15. IF PATIENT HAS HAD SAME OR SIMILAR ILLNESS. GIVE FIRST DATE MM | DD | YY

16. DATES PATIENT UNABLE TO WORK IN CURRENT OCCUPATION — FROM MM | DD | YY — TO MM | DD | YY

17. NAME OF REFERRING PROVIDER OR OTHER SOURCE — 17a. — 17b. NPI

18. HOSPITALIZATION DATES RELATED TO CURRENT SERVICES — FROM MM | DD | YY — TO MM | DD | YY

19. RESERVED FOR LOCAL USE

20. OUTSIDE LAB? YES NO — $ CHARGES

21. DIAGNOSIS OR NATURE OF ILLNESS OR INJURY (Relate Items 1, 2, 3 or 4 to Item 24E by Line)

1. ___ . ___   3. ___ . ___

2. ___ . ___   4. ___ . ___

22. MEDICAID RESUBMISSION CODE — ORIGINAL REF. NO.

23. PRIOR AUTHORIZATION NUMBER

24. A. DATE(S) OF SERVICE From MM DD YY	To MM DD YY	B. PLACE OF SERVICE	C. EMG	D. PROCEDURES, SERVICES, OR SUPPLIES (Explain Unusual Circumstances) CPT/HCPCS | MODIFIER	E. DIAGNOSIS POINTER	F. $ CHARGES	G. DAYS OR UNITS	H. EPSDT Family Plan	I. ID. QUAL.	J. RENDERING PROVIDER ID. #
1									NPI	
2									NPI	
3									NPI	
4									NPI	
5									NPI	
6									NPI	

PHYSICIAN OR SUPPLIER INFORMATION

25. FEDERAL TAX I.D. NUMBER — SSN EIN

26. PATIENT'S ACCOUNT NO.

27. ACCEPT ASSIGNMENT? (For govt. claims, see back) YES NO

28. TOTAL CHARGE $

29. AMOUNT PAID $

30. BALANCE DUE $

31. SIGNATURE OF PHYSICIAN OR SUPPLIER INCLUDING DEGREES OR CREDENTIALS (I certify that the statements on the reverse apply to this bill and are made a part thereof.)

SIGNED ____________ DATE ____________

32. SERVICE FACILITY LOCATION INFORMATION — a. — b.

33. BILLING PROVIDER INFO & PH # ( ) — a. — b.

NUCC Instruction Manual available at: www.nucc.org — PLEASE PRINT OR TYPE — APPROVED OMB-0938-0999 FORM CMS-1500 (08-05)

Figure **A3-4** **Items shaded are to be left blank when Medicaid is the only coverage.**

APPENDIX 3

Item 1	Check the appropriate box for the patient's insurance.
Item 1a	Enter insured's identification number.
Item 2	Enter the patient's last name, first name, and middle initial, if any, as shown on the patient's Medicare card.
Item 3	Enter the patient's 8-digit birth date (MM/DD/CCYY) and sex.
Item 4	If there is insurance primary to Medicare, from any source, list the name of the insured here. When the insured and the patient are the same, enter the word SAME. If Medicare is primary, leave blank.
Item 5	Enter the patient's mailing address and telephone number. On the first line enter the street address; the second line, the city and state; the third line, the zip code and phone number.
Item 6	Check the appropriate box for patient's relationship to insured when item 4 is completed.
Item 7	Enter the insured's address and telephone number. When the address is the same as the patient's, enter the word SAME. Complete this item only when items 4, 6, and 11 are completed.
Item 8	Check the appropriate box for the patient's marital status and whether employed or a student.
Item 9a through 9d	Leave blank unless covered by Medigap.
Items 10a through 10c	Check "YES" or "NO" to indicate whether employment, auto liability, or other accident involvement applies to one or more of the services described in item 24.
Item 10d	Use this item exclusively for Medicaid (MCD) information. If the patient is entitled to Medicaid, enter the patient's Medicaid number preceded by MCD.
Item 11	By completing this item, the physician/supplier acknowledges having made a good faith effort to determine whether Medicare is the primary or secondary payer. If there is insurance primary to Medicare, enter the insured's policy or group number and proceed to items 11a, 11c. Items 4, 6, and 7 must also be completed. Enter the appropriate information in item 11c if insurance primary to Medicare is indicated in item 11. If there is no insurance primary to Medicare, enter the word "NONE" and proceed to item 12.
Item 11a	Enter the insured's 8-digit birth date (MM/DD/CCYY) and sex if different from item 3.
Item 11b	Enter employer's name, if applicable.
Item 11c	Enter the 9-digit PAYERID number of the primary insurer. If no PAYERID number exists, then enter the **complete** primary payer's program or plan name. If the primary payer's EOB does not contain the claims processing address, record the primary payer's claims processing address directly on the EOB. This is required if there is insurance primary to Medicare that is indicated in item 11.
Item 11d	Leave blank. Not required by Medicare.
Item 12	The patient or authorized representative must sign and enter either a 6-digit date (MM/DD/YY), 8-digit date (MM/DD/CCYY), or an alpha-numeric date (e.g., January 1, 1998) unless the signature is on file. In lieu of signing the claim, the patient may sign a statement to be retained in the provider, physician, or supplier file in accordance with Chapter 1, "General Billing Requirements." This can be "Signature on File" (SOF) and/or a computer-generated signature. The patient's signature authorizes release of medical information necessary to process the claim. It also authorizes payment of benefits to the provider of service or supplier when the provider of service or supplier accepts assignment on the claim.

Item 13	The signature in this item authorizes payment of benefits to the participating physician or supplier. This can be "Signature on File" signature and/or a computer-generated signature.
Item 14	Enter either an 8-digit (MM/DD/CCYY) or 6-digit (MM/DD/YY) date of current illness, injury, or pregnancy.
Item 15	Leave blank. Not required by Medicare.
Item 16	If the patient is employed and is unable to work in his/her current occupation, enter an 8-digit (MM/DD/CCYY) or 6-digit (MM/DD/YY) date when patient is unable to work.
Item 17	Enter the name of the referring or ordering physician if the service or item was ordered or referred by a physician.
Item 17a	Enter the NPI of the referring/ordering physician listed in item 17. This field is required when a service was ordered or referred by a physician.
Item 18	Enter either an 8-digit (MM/DD/CCYY) or a 6-digit (MM/DD/YY) date when a medical service is furnished as a result of, or subsequent to, a related hospitalization.
Item 19	Leave blank. Reserved for local use.
Item 20	Leave blank. Reserved for local use.
Item 21	Enter the patient's diagnosis/condition.
Item 22	Leave blank. Not required by Medicare.
Item 23	Enter any prior authorization number for procedures requiring prior approval.
Item 24A	Enter a 6-digit or 8-digit (MM/DD/CCYY) date for each procedure, service, or supply. When "from" and "to" dates are shown for a series of identical services, enter the number of days or units in column G.
Item 24B	Enter the appropriate place of service code(s) from the list provided *(partial list):* *11 Office* *12 Home* *21 Inpatient hospital* *22 Outpatient hospital* *23 ED hospital*
Item 24C	Medicare providers are not required to complete this item.
Item 24D	Enter the CPT/HCPCS codes for the procedures, services, or supplies. When applicable, show modifiers with the code.
Item 24E	Enter the diagnosis code reference number as shown in item 21 to relate the date of service and the procedures performed to the primary diagnosis.
Item 24F	Enter the charge for each listed service.
Item 24G	Enter the number of days or units. This field is most commonly used for multiple visits, units of supplies, anesthesia minutes, or oxygen volume. If only one service is performed, the numeral 1 must be entered.
Item 24H	Leave blank. Not required by Medicare.
Item 24I	Leave blank. Not required by Medicare.
Item 24J	Leave blank. Not required by Medicare.
Item 24K	Enter the NPI of the performing provider of service/supplier if the provider is a member of a group practice.

Item 25	Enter the provider of service or supplier Federal Tax ID (Employer Identification Number) or Social Security Number. ***The Federal tax identification number for the South Padre Medical Center is 00789200.***
Item 26	Enter the patient's account number assigned by the provider's of service.
Item 27	Check the appropriate block to indicate whether the provider of service accepts assignment of Medicare benefits.
Item 28	Enter total charges for the services.
Item 29	Enter the total amount the patient paid on the covered services only.
Item 30	Leave blank. Not required by Medicare.
Item 31	Enter the signature of provider of service or supplier, or his/her representative, and either the 6-digit date (MM/DD/YY), 8-digit date (MM/DD/CCYY), or alpha-numeric date (e.g., January 1, 1998) the form was signed.
Item 32	Enter the name and address, and ZIP code of the facility if the services were furnished in a hospital, clinic, laboratory, or facility other than the patient's home or physician's office. Effective for claims received on or after April 1, 2004, the name, address, and zip code of the service location for all services other than those furnished in place of service home—12.
Item 33	Enter the provider of service/supplier's billing name, address, zip code, and telephone number. This is a required field. Enter the group NPI, for the performing provider of service/supplier who is a member of a group practice.

TABLE **1: CMS-1500 (08/05) Medicare Claims**

Item Number	Patient Information
	Left printer alignment block
	Right printer alignment block
1	Medicare
1	Medicaid
1	Tricare Champus
1	Champva
1	Group Health Plan
1	FECA Blk Lung
1	Other
1a	Insured's ID Number
2	Patient's Name (Last, First, MI)
3	Patient's Birth Date (Month)
3	Patient's Birth Date (Day)
3	Patient's Birth (Year)
3	Sex-Male
3	Sex-Female
4	Insured Name (Last, First, MI)
5	Patient's Address
6	Patient Relationship to Insured (Self)
6	Patient Relationship to Insured (Spouse)
6	Patient Relationship to Insured (Child)
6	Patient Relationship to Insured (Other)
7	Insured's Address
5	Patient's City
5	Patient's State
8	Patient Status (Single)
8	Patient Status (Other)
7	Insured's City7
7	Insured's State
5	Patient's Zip Code
5	Patient's Area Code
5	Patient's Phone Number
8	Patient Status (Employed)
8	Patient Status (Full Time Student)
8	Patient Status (Part Time Student)

Continued

APPENDIX 3

TABLE **1: cont'd**

Item Number	Patient Information
7	Insured's Zip Code
7	Insured's Area Code
7	Insured's Phone Number
9	Other Insured's Name (Last, First, MI)
11	Insured's Policy, Group or FECA Number
9a	Other Insured's Policy or Group Number
10a	Condition Related (Employment C/P, Yes)
10a	Condition Related (Employment C/P, No)
11a	Insured's Date of Birth (Month)
11a	Insured's Date of Birth (Day)
11a	Insured's Date of Birth (Year)
11a	Sex-Male
11a	Sex-Female
9b	Other Insured's Date of Birth (Month)
9b	Other Insured's Date of Birth (Day)
9b	Other Insured's Date of Birth (Year)
9b	Sex-Male
9b	Sex-Female
10b	Condition Related To: (Auto Accident-Yes)
10b	Condition Related To: (Auto Accident-No)
10b	Condition Related To: (Auto Accident-State)
11b	Insured's Employer's Name or School Name
9c	Other Insured's Employer's Name or School Name
10c	Other Accident (Yes)
10c	Other Accident (No)
11c	Insured's Insurance Plan or PayerID
9d	Other Insured's Insurance Plan Name or PayerID
10d	(Reserved for Local Use)
11d	Another Benefit Health Plan (Yes)
11d	Another Benefit Health Plan (No)
12	Left Blank for Patient's Signature & Date
13	Left Blank for Insured's Signature
14	Date of Current Illness, Injury, Pregnancy (Month)
14	Date of Current Illness, Injury, Pregnancy (Day)
14	Date of Current Illness, Injury, Pregnancy—(Year)

TABLE **1: cont'd**

Item Number	Patient Information
15	First Date Has Had Same or Similar Illness (Month)
15	First Date Has Had Same or Similar Illness (Day)
15	First Date Has Had Same or Similar Illness—(Year)
16	Dates Patient Unable to Work (From Month)
16	Dates Patient Unable to Work (From Day)
16	Dates Patient Unable to Work (From Year)
16	Dates Patient Unable to Work (To Month)
16	Dates Patient Unable to Work (To Day)
16	Dates Patient Unable to Work (To Year)
17a	Legacy Qualifier/Provider Number of Referring Physician
17	Name of Referring Physician or Other Source
17b	NPI Number of Referring Physician
18	Hospitalization Related Current Svcs (From Month)
18	Hospitalization Related Current Svcs (From Day)
18	Hospitalization Related Current Svcs (From Year)
18	Hospitalization Related Current Svcs (To Month)
18	Hospitalization Related Current Svcs (To Day)
18	Hospitalization Related Current Svcs (To Year)
19	Reserved for Local Use
19	Reserved for Local Use
20	Outside Lab (Yes)
20	Outside Lab (No)
20	$ Charges
21.1	Diagnosis or Nature of Illness or Injury (Code)
21.3	Diagnosis or Nature of Illness or Injury (Code)
22	Medicaid Resubmission Code
22.2	Original Reference Number
21.2	Diagnosis or Nature of Illness or Injury (Code)
21.4	Diagnosis or Nature of Illness or Injury (Code)
23	Prior Authorization Number
24	Line Detail Narrative
24.1i	Legacy Qualifier Rendering Provider
24.1j	Legacy Provider Number Rendering Provider
24.1a	Date(s) of Service—(From Month)
24.1a	Date(s) of Service—(From Day)

Continued

TABLE **1: cont'd**

Item Number	Patient Information
24.1a	Date(s) of Service—(From Year)
24.1a	Date(s) of Service—(To Month)
24.1a	Date(s) of Service—(To Day)
24.1a	Date(s) of Service—(To Year)
24.1b	Place of Service
24.1c	EMG
24.1d	Procedures, Svcs or Supplies (CPT/HCPCS)
24.1d	Procedures, Svcs or Supplies (Modifier 1)
24.1d	Procedures, Svcs or Supplies (Modifier 2)
24.1d	Procedures, Svcs or Supplies (Modifier 3)
24.1d	Procedures, Svcs or Supplies (Modifier 4)
24.1e	Diagnosis Pointer
24.1f	$ Charges
24.1g	Days or Units
24.1h	EPSDT Family Plan
24.1i	Legacy Qualifier Rendering Provider (Leave Bank)
24.1j	Legacy Provider Number Rendering Provider
24	Line Detail Narrative
24.2i	Legacy Qualifier Rendering Provider
24.2j	Legacy Provider Number Rendering Provider
24.2a	Date(s) of Service—(From Month)
24.2a	Date(s) of Service—(From Day)
24.2a	Date(s) of Service—(From Year)
24.2a	Date(s) of Service—(To Month)
24.2a	Date(s) of Service—(To Day)
24.2a	Date(s) of Service—(To Year)
24.2b	Place of Service
24.2c	EMG
24.2d	Procedures, Svcs or Supplies (CPT/HCPCS)
24.2d	Procedures, Svcs or Supplies (Modifier 1)
24.2d	Procedures, Svcs or Supplies (Modifier 2)
24.2d	Procedures, Svcs or Supplies (Modifier 3)
24.2d	Procedures, Svcs or Supplies (Modifier 4)
24.2e	Diagnosis Pointer
24.2f	$ Charges

TABLE **1: cont'd**

Item Number	Patient Information
24.2g	Days or Units
24.2h	EPSDT Family Plan
24.2i	Legacy Qualifier Rendering Provider (Leave Blank)
24.2j	Legacy Provider Number Rendering Provider
24	Line Detail Narrative
24.3i	Legacy Qualifier Rendering Provider
24.3j	Legacy Provider Number Rendering Provider
24.3a	Date(s) of Service—(From Month)
24.3a	Date(s) of Service—(From Day)
24.3a	Date(s) of Service—(From Year)
24.3a	Date(s) of Service—(To Month)
24.3a	Date(s) of Service—(To Day)
24.3a	Date(s) of Service—(To Year)
24.3b	Place of Service
24.3c	EMG
24.3d	Procedures, Svcs or Supplies (CPT/HCPCS)
24.3d	Procedures, Svcs or Supplies (Modifier 1)
24.3d	Procedures, Svcs or Supplies (Modifier 2)
24.3d	Procedures, Svcs or Supplies (Modifier 3)
24.3d	Procedures, Svcs or Supplies (Modifier 4)
24.3e	Diagnosis Pointer
24.3f	$ Charges
24.3g	Days or Units
24.3h	EPSDT Family Plan
24.3i	Legacy Qualifier Rendering Provider (Leave Blank)
24.3j	Legacy Provider Number Rendering Provider
24	Line Detail Narrative
24.4i	Legacy Qualifier Rendering Provider
24.4j	Legacy Provider Number Rendering Provider
24.4a	Date(s) of Service—(From Month)
24.4a	Date(s) of Service—(From Day)
24.4a	Date(s) of Service—(From Year)
24.4a	Date(s) of Service—(To Month)
24.4a	Date(s) of Service—(To Day)
24.4a	Date(s) of Service—(To Year)

Continued

TABLE **1: cont'd**

Item Number	Patient Information
24.4b	Place of Service
24.4c	EMG
24.4d	Procedures, Svcs or Supplies (CPT/HCPCS)
24.4d	Procedures, Svcs or Supplies (Modifier 1)
24.4d	Procedures, Svcs or Supplies (Modifier 2)
24.4d	Procedures, Svcs or Supplies (Modifier 3)
24.4d	Procedures, Svcs or Supplies (Modifier 4)
24.4e	Diagnosis Pointer
24.4f	$ Charges
24.4g	Days or Units
24.4h	EPSDT Family Plan
24.4i	Legacy Qualifier Rendering Provider (Leave Blank)
24.4j	Legacy Provider Number Rendering Provider
24	Line Detail Narrative
24.5i	Legacy Qualifier Rendering Provider
24.5j	Legacy Provider Number Rendering Provider
24.5a	Date(s) of Service—(From Month)
24.5a	Date(s) of Service—(From Day)
24.5a	Date(s) of Service—(From Year)
24.5a	Date(s) of Service—(To Month)
24.5a	Date(s) of Service—(To Day)
24.5a	Date(s) of Service—(To Year)
24.5b	Place of Service
24.5c	EMG
24.5d	Procedures, Svcs or Supplies (CPT/HCPCS)
24.5d	Procedures, Svcs or Supplies (Modifier 1)
24.5d	Procedures, Svcs or Supplies (Modifier 2)
24.5d	Procedures, Svcs or Supplies (Modifier 3)
24.5d	Procedures, Svcs or Supplies (Modifier 4)
24.5e	Diagnosis Pointer
24.5f	$ Charges
24.5g	Days or Units
24.5h	EPSDT Family Plan
24.5i	Legacy Qualifier Rendering Provider (Leave Blank)
24.5j	Legacy Provider Number Rendering Provider

TABLE **1: cont'd**

Item Number	Patient Information
24	Line Detail Narrative
24.6i	Legacy Qualifier Rendering Provider
24.6j	Legacy Provider Number Rendering Provider
24.6a	Date(s) of Service—(From Month)
24.6a	Date(s) of Service—(From Day)
24.6a	Date(s) of Service—(From Year)
24.6a	Date(s) of Service—(To Month)
24.6a	Date(s) of Service—(To Day)
24.6a	Date(s) of Service—(To Year)
24.6b	Place of Service
24.6c	EMG
24.6d	Procedures, Svcs or Supplies (CPT/HCPCS)
24.6d	Procedures, Svcs or Supplies (Modifier 1)
24.6d	Procedures, Svcs or Supplies (Modifier 2)
24.6d	Procedures, Svcs or Supplies (Modifier 3)
24.6d	Procedures, Svcs or Supplies (Modifier 4)
24.6e	Diagnosis Pointer
24.6f	$ Charges
24.6g	Days or Units
24.6h	EPSDT Family Plan
24.6i	Legacy Qualifier Rendering Provider (Leave Blank)
24.6j	Legacy Provider Number Rendering Provider
25	Federal Tax ID Number
25	Federal Tax ID Number (SSN)
25	Federal Tax ID Number (EIN)
26	Patient's Account Number
27	Accept Assignment (Yes)
27	Accept Assignment (No)
28	Total Charge
29	Amount Paid
30	Balance Due
33	Billing Provider Phone Number Area Code
33	Billing Provider Phone Number
32	Name of Facility Where Svcs Rendered
33	Physician/Supplier Billing Name

Continued

TABLE **1: cont'd**

Item Number	Patient Information
32	Address of Facility Where Svcs Rendered
33	Physician/Supplier Address
31	Left Blank for Signature Physician/Supplier
32	City, State and Zip Code of Facility
33	City, State and Zip Code of Billing Provider
32a	Facility NPI Number
32b	Facility Qualifier and Legacy Number
33a	Billing Provider NPI Number
33b	Billing Provider Qualifier and Legacy Number

Modified from Department of Health and Human Services (DHHS), Centers for Medicare and Medicaid Services (CMS): CMS manual system: Pub 100-04 Medicare claims processing *(Transmittal 899), March 31, 2006, Change Request 4293.*

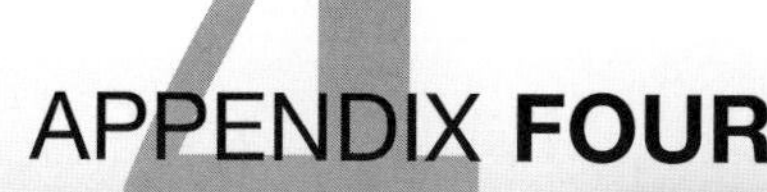

APPENDIX FOUR

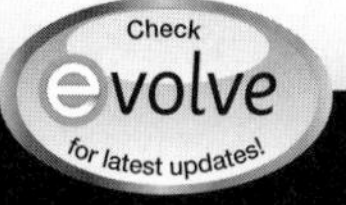

Forms Library

APPENDIX 4

South Padre Medical Center
9878 Palm Drive
SOUTH PADRE, TX 98765

FIRST NATIONAL BANK
100 FIRST STREET
SOUTH PADRE, TX 98765

98-95
1251

NO 999

PAY ______________________________ DOLLARS

DATE	CHECK NO.	AMOUNT	

TO THE
ORDER OF ______________________________

⑆0⑈0123⑆ ⑈4567⑉8901⑈ ⑆1234567890⑆

1500

HEALTH INSURANCE CLAIM FORM

APPROVED BY NATIONAL UNIFORM CLAIM COMMITTEE 08/05

PICA | PICA

CARRIER

1. MEDICARE (Medicare #) | MEDICAID (Medicaid #) | TRICARE CHAMPUS (Sponsor's SSN) | CHAMPVA (Member ID#) | GROUP HEALTH PLAN (SSN or ID) | FECA BLK LUNG (SSN) | OTHER (ID)

1a. INSURED'S I.D. NUMBER (For Program in Item 1)

2. PATIENT'S NAME (Last Name, First Name, Middle Initial)

3. PATIENT'S BIRTH DATE MM | DD | YY — SEX M F

4. INSURED'S NAME (Last Name, First Name, Middle Initial)

5. PATIENT'S ADDRESS (No., Street)

6. PATIENT RELATIONSHIP TO INSURED — Self Spouse Child Other

7. INSURED'S ADDRESS (No., Street)

CITY — STATE

8. PATIENT STATUS — Single Married Other

CITY — STATE

ZIP CODE — TELEPHONE (Include Area Code) ( )

Employed — Full-Time Student — Part-Time Student

ZIP CODE — TELEPHONE (Include Area Code) ( )

9. OTHER INSURED'S NAME (Last Name, First Name, Middle Initial)

10. IS PATIENT'S CONDITION RELATED TO:

11. INSURED'S POLICY GROUP OR FECA NUMBER

a. OTHER INSURED'S POLICY OR GROUP NUMBER

a. EMPLOYMENT? (Current or Previous) YES NO

a. INSURED'S DATE OF BIRTH MM | DD | YY — SEX M F

b. OTHER INSURED'S DATE OF BIRTH MM | DD | YY — SEX M F

b. AUTO ACCIDENT? YES NO — PLACE (State)

b. EMPLOYER'S NAME OR SCHOOL NAME

c. EMPLOYER'S NAME OR SCHOOL NAME

c. OTHER ACCIDENT? YES NO

c. INSURANCE PLAN NAME OR PROGRAM NAME

d. INSURANCE PLAN NAME OR PROGRAM NAME

10d. RESERVED FOR LOCAL USE

d. IS THERE ANOTHER HEALTH BENEFIT PLAN? YES NO *If yes*, return to and complete item 9 a-d.

READ BACK OF FORM BEFORE COMPLETING & SIGNING THIS FORM.

12. PATIENT'S OR AUTHORIZED PERSON'S SIGNATURE I authorize the release of any medical or other information necessary to process this claim. I also request payment of government benefits either to myself or to the party who accepts assignment below.

SIGNED ____ DATE ____

13. INSURED'S OR AUTHORIZED PERSON'S SIGNATURE I authorize payment of medical benefits to the undersigned physician or supplier for services described below.

SIGNED ____

PATIENT AND INSURED INFORMATION

14. DATE OF CURRENT: MM | DD | YY — ILLNESS (First symptom) OR INJURY (Accident) OR PREGNANCY(LMP)

15. IF PATIENT HAS HAD SAME OR SIMILAR ILLNESS. GIVE FIRST DATE MM | DD | YY

16. DATES PATIENT UNABLE TO WORK IN CURRENT OCCUPATION MM | DD | YY FROM — TO

17. NAME OF REFERRING PROVIDER OR OTHER SOURCE — 17a. — 17b. NPI

18. HOSPITALIZATION DATES RELATED TO CURRENT SERVICES MM | DD | YY FROM — TO

19. RESERVED FOR LOCAL USE

20. OUTSIDE LAB? YES NO — $ CHARGES

21. DIAGNOSIS OR NATURE OF ILLNESS OR INJURY (Relate Items 1, 2, 3 or 4 to Item 24E by Line)

1. ___ . ___ 3. ___ . ___

2. ___ . ___ 4. ___ . ___

22. MEDICAID RESUBMISSION CODE — ORIGINAL REF. NO.

23. PRIOR AUTHORIZATION NUMBER

24. A. DATE(S) OF SERVICE From MM DD YY To MM DD YY	B. PLACE OF SERVICE	C. EMG	D. PROCEDURES, SERVICES, OR SUPPLIES (Explain Unusual Circumstances) CPT/HCPCS MODIFIER	E. DIAGNOSIS POINTER	F. $ CHARGES	G. DAYS OR UNITS	H. EPSDT Family Plan	I. ID. QUAL.	J. RENDERING PROVIDER ID. #
1								NPI	
2								NPI	
3								NPI	
4								NPI	
5								NPI	
6								NPI	

25. FEDERAL TAX I.D. NUMBER SSN EIN

26. PATIENT'S ACCOUNT NO.

27. ACCEPT ASSIGNMENT? (For govt. claims, see back) YES NO

28. TOTAL CHARGE $

29. AMOUNT PAID $

30. BALANCE DUE $

31. SIGNATURE OF PHYSICIAN OR SUPPLIER INCLUDING DEGREES OR CREDENTIALS (I certify that the statements on the reverse apply to this bill and are made a part thereof.)

SIGNED DATE

32. SERVICE FACILITY LOCATION INFORMATION — a. b.

33. BILLING PROVIDER INFO & PH # ( ) — a. b.

PHYSICIAN OR SUPPLIER INFORMATION

NUCC Instruction Manual available at: www.nucc.org — PLEASE PRINT OR TYPE — APPROVED OMB-0938-0999 FORM CMS-1500 (08-05)

CONTINUATION

DEPOSIT TICKET

SOUTH PADRE MEDICAL CENTER
9878 PALM DRIVE
SOUTH PADRE, TX 98765

FIRST NATIONAL BANK
100 FIRST STREET
SOUTH PADRE, TX 98765

DATE ______________________

DEPOSITS MAY NOT BE AVAILABLE FOR IMMEDIATE WITHDRAWAL

	DOLLARS	CENTS
CURRENCY		
COIN		
CHECKS LIST EACH SEPARATELY		
1 2		
3 4		
5 6		
7 8		
9 10		
11 12		
13 14		
15 16		
17 18		
19 20		
21 22		
23 24		
25 26		
27 28		
TOTAL FROM OTHER SIDE OR ATTACHED LIST		
PLEASE RE-ENTER TOTAL HERE — TOTAL		

000100100 2005

$

Checks and other items are received for deposit subject to the provisions of the Uniform Commercial Code or any applicable collection agreement.

Gerald Bond, MD
Ray Adams, MD
Joyce Harkness, MD
Anthony Clark, MD

South Padre Medical Center

9878 Palm Drive
South Padre, TX 98765
Telephone (209) 555-3356

HISTORY AND PHYSICAL EXAMINATION

APPENDIX 4

South Padre Medical Center

Interoffice Memo

JOURNAL OF DAILY CHARGES & PAYMENTS

	DATE	PROFESSIONAL SERVICE	FEE	PAYMENT	ADJUST-MENT	NEW BALANCE	OLD BALANCE	PATIENT'S NAME	
1									1
2									2
3									3
4									4
5									5
6									6
7									7
8									8
9									9
10									10
11									11
12									12
13									13
14									14
15									15
16									16
17									17
18									18
19									19
20									20
21									21
22									22
23									23
24									24
25									25
26									26
27									27
28									28
29									29
30									30
31								**TOTALS THIS PAGE**	31
32								**TOTAL PREVIOUS PAGE**	32
33								**TOTALS MONTH TO DATE**	33
			COLUMN A	COLUMN B	COLUMN C	COLUMN D	COLUMN E		

MEMO ______________________

DAILY - FROM LINE 31

ARITHMETIC POSTING PROOF	
Column E	$
Plus Column A	
Sub-Total	
Minus Column B	
Sub-Total	
Minus Column C	
Equals Column D	

MONTH - FROM LINE 31

ACCOUNTS RECEIVABLE PROOF	
Accts. Receivable Previous Day	$
Plus Column A	
Sub-Total	
Minus Column B	
Sub-Total	
Minus Column C	
Accts. receivable End of Day	

YEAR TO DATE - FROM LINE 33

ACCOUNTS RECEIVABLE PROOF	
Accts. Receivable beginning of Month	$
Plus Column A MONTH TO DATE	
Sub-Total C	
Minus Column B MONTH TO DATE	
Sub-Total	
Minus Column C MONTH TO DATE	
Accts. receivable End of Day MONTH TO DATE	

APPENDIX 4

Gerald Bond, MD
Ray Adams, MD
Joyce Harkness, MD
Anthony Clark, MD

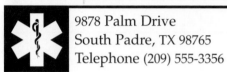

South Padre Medical Center

9878 Palm Drive
South Padre, TX 98765
Telephone (209) 555-3356

Gerald Bond, MD
Ray Adams, MD
Joyce Harkness, MD
Anthony Clark, MD

South Padre Medical Center

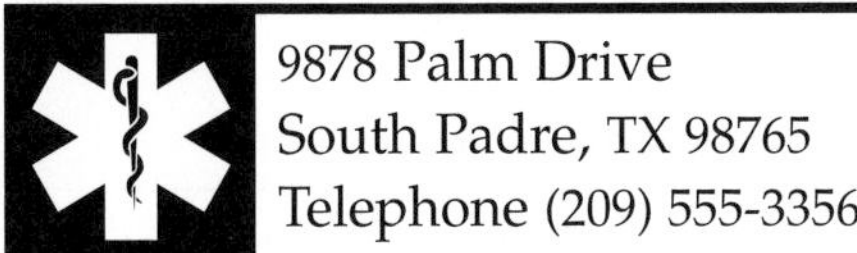

9878 Palm Drive
South Padre, TX 98765
Telephone (209) 555-3356

PATIENT INFORMATION

Please Print

Today's Date ____________________

Last Name ____________________ First Name ____________________ Initial ______

Date of Birth ____________________ Age __________ Sex __________ SS# ______-_____-______

Home Address Street ____________________ City ____________________

State ____________________ Zip__________ Home Phone (______)____________________

Occupation ____________________ Employer ____________________

Employer Address Street ____________________ City____________________

State ____________________ Zip __________ Work Phone (______)____________________

Are you currently a student? Yes No Name of School ____________________

Spouse's Name ____________________ Marital Status M S D W SEP

Spouse's SS# ______-_____-________ Spouse's Employer ____________________

In case of emergency, notify ____________________ Relationship____________________

Home Phone (____) ____________________ Work Phone (____) ____________________

If you are a minor: Parent's Name ____________________SS# ______-_____-______

Street ____________________ City ______________ State ______ Zip__________

Home Phone (____) ____________________ Work Phone (____) ____________________

Reason for Visit ____________________

Work related injury? Yes No Date of injury____________________

Automobile accident? Yes No Date of injury____________________

Other injury? Yes No Date of injury____________________

Insurance (Primary) Company Name: ____________________

Street ____________________ City ______________ State ______ Zip__________

Subscriber's Name ____________________

Relationship to Subscriber: ____________________

Policy #____________________ Group #____________________

Insurance (Secondary) Company Name: ____________________

Street ____________________ City ______________ State ______ Zip__________

Subscriber's Name ____________________

Relationship to Subscriber: ____________________

Policy #____________________ Group #____________________

Assignment of Benefits:

I directly assign all medical/surgical benefits, including major medical benefits and Medicare, to South Padre Medical Center. I understand that this authorization for assignment remains in effect until I revoke it in writing. A photocopy of this assignment will be considered as valid as this original assignment. I further understand that I am responsible for my indebtedness no matter what charges the insurance pays for.

Insured or Guardian's Signature ____________________ Date ______________

SOUTH PADRE MEDICAL CENTER
PETTY CASH JOURNAL

Beginning Balance:

DATE	STAFF	PURPOSE	AMOUNT	BALANCE

PRIORITY ☐

Telephone Record

Patient Age

Caller

Telephone

Referred to

Chart #

Chart Attached ☐ YES ☐ NO

Date / / Time Rec'd By

Message

Temp | Allergies

Response

PHY/RN Initials | Date / / | Time | Handled By

PRIORITY ☐

Telephone Record

Patient Age

Caller

Telephone

Referred to

Chart #

Chart Attached ☐ YES ☐ NO

Date / / Time Rec'd By

Message

Temp | Allergies

Response

PHY/RN Initials | Date / / | Time | Handled By

PRIORITY ☐

Telephone Record

Patient Age

Caller

Telephone

Referred to

Chart #

Chart Attached ☐ YES ☐ NO

Date / / Time Rec'd By

Message

Temp | Allergies

Response

PHY/RN Initials | Date / / | Time | Handled By

PRIORITY ☐

Telephone Record

Patient Age

Caller

Telephone

Referred to

Chart #

Chart Attached ☐ YES ☐ NO

Date / / Time Rec'd By

Message

Temp | Allergies

Response

PHY/RN Initials | Date / / | Time | Handled By

APPENDIX 4

REFERRAL

FROM: Gerald Bond, MD ________
Ray Adams, MD ________
Joyce Harkness, MD ________
Anthony Clark, MD ________

TO: ________________________________

TELEPHONE: ________________________
ADDRESS: __________________________

Requested Date and Time: ______________

PATIENT: ______________________ PATIENT'S PHONE NUMBER: ____________________

ADDRESS: ____

REASON FOR REFERRAL: ____

____

____

APPOINTMENT DATE AND TIME: ____

REFERRAL COMPLETED BY: ______________ ARRANGEMENTS MADE BY: ______________
(INITIAL AND DATE) (INITIAL AND DATE)

REQUEST FOR INPATIENT CONSULTATION

To:
- ❑ Gerald Bond, MD
- ❑ Ray Adams, MD
- ❑ Joyce Harkness, MD
- ❑ Anthony Clark, MD

ATTENDING: ______________________

TELEPHONE: ______________________

Request Date and Time: ______________________

PATIENT: ______________________ ADMIT DATE: ______________________

FACILITY: ______________________ FLOOR: ____________ ROOM: ____________

REASON FOR CONSULTATION: ____

____

____

____

PLEASE COMPLETE BY: ______________________ RECEIVED BY: ______________________
(DATE)

APPENDIX 4

REQUEST FOR PREAUTHORIZATION FOR SURGERY

Surgeon: Gerald Bond, MD
(circle one) Ray Adams, MD
Joyce Harkness, MD
Anthony Clark, MD

PATIENT NAME: ______________________ FACILITY: ______________________

DATE OF BIRTH: ______________________ ADMIT DATE: ______________________

ACCOUNT #: ______________________ SURGERY DATE: ______________________

INSURANCE: ______________________ POLICY#: ______________________

PROCEDURE: ____

DIAGNOSIS: ____

AUTHORIZATION: ______________________

COMPLETED BY: ______________________

DATE COMPLETED: ______________________

SOUTH PADRE MEDICAL CENTER
9878 Palm Drive
South Padre, TX 98765

Gerald Bond, MD
Ray Adams, MD
Joyce Harkness, MD
Anthony Clark, MD

Affiliated with:
Texas Health Corporation
1256 56th Avenue South
Houston, TX 99881

STATEMENT TO:

TEAR OFF AND RETURN UPPER PORTION WITH PAYMENT

Balance Forward

DATE	PROFESSIONAL SERVICE	FEE		PAYMENT		ADJUST-MENT		NEW BALANCE	

APPENDIX 4

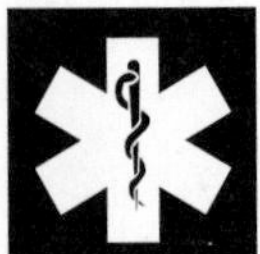

South Padre Medical Center

Patient's Name ______________________ Age _____ Sex _____ Marital Status S M W D

Address ______________________ Insurance ______________________

Telephone ______________________ Referred ______________________

Date	Subsequent Findings

South Padre Medical Center

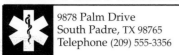

9878 Palm Drive
South Padre, TX 98765
Telephone (209) 555-3356

Gerald Bond, MD
Ray Adams, MD
Joyce Harkness, MD
Anthony Clark, MD

PATIENT'S LAST NAME	FIRST	ACCOUNT #	BIRTHDATE	SEX	TODAY'S DATE
			/ /	☐ MALE ☐ FEMALE	/ /

INSURANCE COMPANY	SUBSCRIBER	GROUP/PLAN #	SUB. #	TIME

ASSIGNMENT: I hereby assign my insurance benefits to be paid directly to the undersigned physician. I am financially responsible for non-covered services.
SIGNED: (Patient,
Or parent, if Minor)____________________ DATE: / /

RELEASE: I hereby authorize the physician to release to my insurance carriers any information required to process this claim.

SIGNED: (Patient,
Or Parent, if Minor) ____________________ DATE: / /

√	DESCRIPTION	CPT	Diag.	FEE	√	DESCRIPTION	CPT	Diag.	FEE	√	DESCRIPTION	CPT	Diag.	FEE
	OFFICE VISIT					**IMMUNIZATIONS/INJECTIONS**					**PROCEDURES**			
	NEW PATIENT					Admin of Vaccine 1	90471				Inhalation treatment	94640		
	Problem Focused					Admin of Vac 2+	90472				Demo/eval treatment	94664		
	Exp Problem Focused	99202				TB Tine, skin	86486				Vital Capacity	94150		
	Detailed	99203				Pneumococcal	90732				Spirometry	94010		
	Comp/ Mod MDM	99204				Medicare code	G0009				EKG w/interpretation	93000		
	Comp/ High MDM	99205				Influenza <3	90657				I&D abscess	10060		
	ESTABLISHED PATEINT					Influenza 3 and >	90658				Remove skin tag <15	11200		
	Minimal/Nurse Visit	99211				Medicare code	G0008				EXCISION BENIGN LESIONS (inc. margins)			
	Problem Focused	99212				Varicella	90716				Trunk, arms, legs			
	Exp Problem Forcused	99213				DPT	90701				0.5 cm or less	11400		
	Detailed	99214				DT children	90702				0.6 to 1.0 cm	11401		
	Comprehensive	99215				Td adult	90718				1.1 to 2.0 cm	11402		
	CONSULTATION					DtaP	90700				2.1 to 3.0 cm	11403		
	Problem Focused	99241				IPV	90713				Scalp, neck, hand, ft			
	Exp Problem Focused	99242				Rubella	90706				0.5 cm or less	11420		
	Detailed	99243				MMR	90707				0.6 to 1.0 cm	11421		
	Comp/ Mod MDM	99244				Hep B Child	90744				1.1 to 2.0 cm	11422		
	Comp/High MDM	99245				Hep B Adult	90746				2.1 to 3.0 cm	11423		
	Requesting Provider ________________					IM Administration	96372				Face, ears, eyelids, lip			
						Compazine	J0780				0.5 cm or less	11440		
	Post-op Exam	99024		0.00		Demerol	J2175				0.6 to 1.0 cm	11441		
	PREVENTIVE MEDICINE					Depo-Provera	J1055				1.1 to 2.0 cm	11442		
	NEW PATIENT					Dexamethasone	J1100				2.1 to 3.0 cm	11443		
	Infant – 1 yr	99381				Solumedrol	J1720				EXCISION MALIGNANT LESIONS (inc. margins)			
	1 yr – 4 yr	99382				Antigen admin 1	95115				Trunk, arms, legs			
	5 yr – 11 yr	99383				Antigen admin 2+	95117				0.5 cm or less	11600		
	12 yr – 17 yr	99384				**LABORATORY**					0.6 to 1.0 cm	11601		
	18 yr – 39 yr	99385				Blood collect Vein	36415				1.1 to 2.0 cm	11602		
	40 yr – 64 yr	99386				Capillary	36416				2.1 to 3.0 cm	11603		
	65 yr and over	99387				Hemoglobin	85018				Scalp, neck, hand, ft			
	ESTABLISHED PATIENT					Glucose, reagent	82948				0.5 cm or less	11620		
	Infant – 1 yr	99391				Pregnancy, Serum	84702				0.6 to 1.0 cm	11621		
	1 yr – 4 yr	99392				Pregnancy, Urine	81025				1.1 to 2.0 cm	11622		
	5 yr – 11 yr	99393				Health panel	80050				2.1 to 3.0 cm	11623		
	12 yr – 17 yr	99394				B Met Pan Cal ion	80047				Face, ears, eyelids, lip			
	18 yr – 39 yr	99395				B Met Pan Cal tot	80048				0.5 cm or less	11640		
	40 yr – 64 yr	99396				C Metabolic panel	80053				0.6 to 1.0 cm	11641		
	65 yr and over	99397				Ob panel	80055				1.1 to 2.0 cm	11642		
	SUPPLIES					Lipid panel	80061				2.1 to 3.0 cm	11643		
	Take home burn kit	99070				UA Auto w/o micro	81003				***Awaiting path report***	☐ ***Yes***		☐ ***No***
	Take home wound kit	99070				UA dip stck	81000				Wart destruction < 14	17110		
	Miscellaneous					Strep test	87880				Cerumen removal	69210		
						Hemoccult	82270				Endometrial biopsy	58100		
	MODIFIERS					Lab Handling	99000							

√	MODIFIERS	
	Significant/Sep EM provided with other service	-25
	Unrelated EM in post op period	-24
	Repeat procedure, same physician, same day	-76

30 DAYS	60 DAYS	90 DAYS

DIAGNOSIS:

1) ______________________

2) ______________________

3) ______________________

4) ______________________

RETURN APPOINTMENT:
(days) (wks) (mos) (PRN)

NEXT APPOINTMENT:
M - T - W - TH - F - S

DATE / / TIME

Provider's Signature:

TODAY'S TOTAL	
PREVIOUS BALANCE	
AMOUNT REC'D TODAY REC'D BY ________	
BALANCE DUE	

APPENDIX 4

South Padre Medical Center

SURGICAL REQUEST AND INFORMATION

This portion is to be completed by requesting surgeon.

Surgeon: ❑ Gerald Bond, MD
❑ Ray Adams, MD
❑ Joyce Harkness, MD
❑ Anthony Clark, MD

Schedule: ❑ URGENT ❑ IMMEDIATE ❑ PATIENT CONVENIENCE

Date Requested: ______________________ Time Requested: ______________________

Patient Name: ______________________

Procedure: ______________________

Procedure Code(s): ______________________

Diagnosis(es): ______________________

Diagnosis(es) Code(s): ______________________

Estimated Surgery Time: ______________________

Surgical Assistant Requested: ______________________

Additional Information: ______________________

This portion is to be completed by scheduling personnel.

Surgery Date: ______________________ Time: ______________________
Day Date

Authorization Obtained: ❑ YES ❑ NO ❑ REQUESTED

If authorization has been requested and response is pending, list date and contact information from the initial request.

Requested From: ______________________ Date: ______________________
(Carrier and person)

Telephone: ______________________ Ext: ____________

Completed By: ______________________

Date Completed: ______________________

South Padre Medical Center

Patient Health History

Today's Date: ______________________

Name: ______________________ Date of Birth: ______________

Marital Status: S M D W

Reason for today's visit: ______________________

Nutrition and Activity

Diet (check one): ❑ Good ❑ Poor

Level of Physical Activity (check one):

❑ Very Active ❑ Active ❑ Sedentary ❑ Inactive

Medical History (Please list any you currently have or have had in the past)

Allergies: ______________________

Significant illnesses or conditions: ______________________

____

Current medications: ______________________

Hospitalizations or Surgery: ______________________

Injuries requiring medical treatment: ______________________

Family History

Have any members of your family had any of the following (check one):

❑ Asthma ❑ Diabetes ❑ Bleeding Disorder

❑ Glaucoma ❑ Heart Disease ❑ Drug/Alcohol Addiction

❑ Hypertension ❑ Mental Illness ❑ Strokes

❑ Cancer (list) ______________ ❑ Other (list) ______________

Family relationship for any of the above condition(s) checked: ______________________

____

Social History

Occupation: ______________________

Are you sexually active? ❑ Yes ❑ No

Have you ever had a sexually transmitted infection (STI)? ❑ Yes ❑ No

If yes, please list the STI type(s) and treatment(s) used ______________________

Do you consume alcohol? ❑ Yes ❑ No

Do you smoke? ❑ Yes ❑ No

If yes, average weekly consumption and drink of choice ______________________

If yes, check all that apply: ❑ Cigarettes ❑ Pipe tobacco ❑ Cigars

Do you chew tobacco? ❑ Yes ❑ No

How much tobacco do you consume on average per day? ______________________

How long have you used tobacco? ______________________

Do you or have you used illegal substance(s)? ❑ Yes ❑ No

If yes, please list ______________________

APPENDIX 4

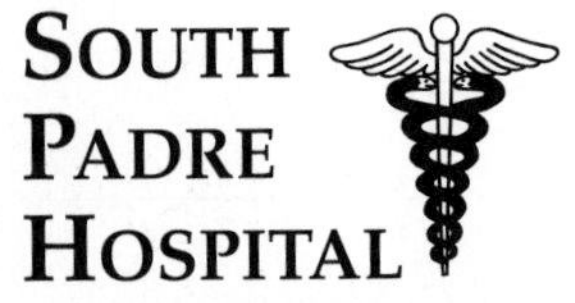

980 Lagona Drive • South Padre, TX 98765 • Telephone (209) 555-4289

OPERATIVE REPORT

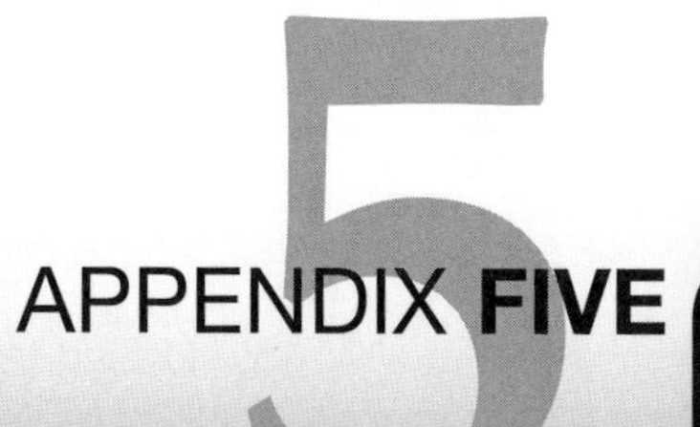

APPENDIX **FIVE**

Other Physician, Business, Third-Party Payer Directory

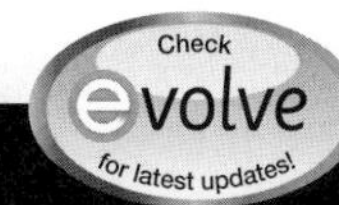
Check
evolve
for latest updates!

Physicians

Dr. John Andrews
Louis Argabright, MD
Bert Bethos, MD
    (209) 555-8231
Dr. Blackburn
Dr. Evans
Dr. Green
Dr. Greggory
Dr. McDonald
    (209) 555-8292
Dr. Morgan
Dr. Peters
Dr. Smith, Fort Worth
Morton Samson, MD
    1256 56th Avenue South
    Houston, TX 99881
    (956) 934-6120
Thomas Thompson, MD
    (209) 555-0090

Business Information

First National Bank
South Padre, TX 98765
100 First Street

South Padre Medical Center
9878 Palm Drive
South Padre, TX 98765
(209) 555-3356

South Padre Hospital
980 Lagona Drive
South Padre, TX 98765
(209) 555-4289

South Padre Surgery Center
(209) 555-8247

Texas Health Corporation
1256 56th Avenue South
Houston, TX 99881

Texas Health Corporation
884 Worthington Rd
San Antonio, TX 99784

Third-Party Payers

BC/BS of Texas
1514 West Road
Houston, TX 99881

Delta of New York
8119 Tower
New York, NY 59800

Medicare/Medicaid
402 Main Street
South Padre, TX 98765

Primer Mutual
897 Wayland Rd
Boston, MA 82643

Primer West
4200 Douglas St
San Diego, CA 98110

Prudential
86410 Worldum Avenue
St. Louis, MO 88488

South Padre Insurance Company
2702 Oak Line Drive
South Padre, TX 98765

Traveler's Insurance
42110 West Road
Houston, TX 99881

Workers' Compensation Claims
10 State Highway
Houston, TX 99881

SUPPLIES

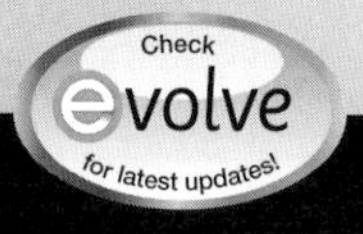
Check
evolve
for latest updates!

Equipment Maintenance and Desk Security

INTERN: ______________________________

INTERNSHIP DATES: April 7-April 18, 2008

SUPERVISOR: Gladys Johnson

DATE	MAINTAINED EQUIPMENT	SECURED DESK
April 7		
April 8		
April 9		
April 10		
April 11		
April 14		
April 15		
April 16		
April 17		
April 18		

Gerald Bond, MD
Ray Adams, MD
Joyce Harkness, MD
Anthony Clark, MD

South Padre Medical Center

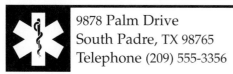

9878 Palm Drive
South Padre, TX 98765
Telephone (209) 555-3356

HISTORY AND PHYSICAL EXAMINATION

PATIENT: Gloria Hydorn
DATE: Thursday, April 3, 2008
PHYSICIAN: Ray Adams, MD

This 68-year-old female presents to the office today requesting a complete physical examination. She has recently moved to our area and states she would like to establish with a family practitioner. She has a history of coronary artery disease, status post coronary artery bypass x 3 in 1978. She has been doing well. Gravid 3, para 3, postmenopausal x 20 years. History is also significant for hypertension, controlled by diet. Otherwise no complaints.

Past Medical History: Remarkable for conditions stated above.

Operations:
1. Hysterectomy with bladder repair, 1973
2. Bilateral blepharoplasty
3. D&C x 4

Allergies: None.

Medications: Digoxin in 0.25 mg, Lasix 40 mg p.o.q.d. Estrogen.

Tobacco: Does not smoke. Alcohol: Occasional.

Social History: Homemaker, mother of three. Husband recently deceased.

Family History: Mother deceased from heart disease. Father has had multiple strokes. Two brothers, one with polio. Three children, health is good. One sister, died of breast cancer at age 35.

Review of systems: Denies nausea, vomiting, headaches, dysuria, incontinence; dyspnea. Occasional bouts of atrial fibrillation, always converts spontaneously.

Hydorn, Gloria
2

HEENT: Wears glasses. Otherwise negative.

Respiratory: Negative.

Cardiovascular: Negative except as discussed above.

GI/GU: Postmenopausal, on estrogen.

Endocrine: No diabetes or thyroid problems.

Musculoskeletal: Some arthritis, both hands.

Psychiatric: Negative.

Physical examination: Reveals a very pleasant elderly female, in no distress.

Vitals: Blood pressure is 140/84; pulse 90 and regular, right arm sitting position. 150/90 left arm sitting position.

Weight: 115 pounds.

Skin: No skin lesions are present.

Nodes: No lymphadenopathy.

ENT: Negative.

Chest: Clear to auscultation.

Cardiac: Reveals a regular rhythm. I did not hear any murmurs or gallops.

Breast exam: Right side free from lumps or masses. Small lump noted in left breast upon examination which is painless, without discharge, without retraction.

Assessment and plan:

1. History of coronary artery disease, status post coronary artery bypass. No complaints at present, no abnormal findings. Continue medications as previously prescribed.
2. Breast mass on examination. Suggest mammography. If positive, consultation will be requested from surgery.
3. Postmenopausal, continue on estrogen therapy.

SUPPLIES TASK 1.4

Gerald Bond, MD
Ray Adams, MD
Joyce Harkness, MD
Anthony Clark, MD

South Padre Medical Center

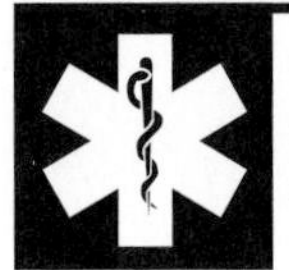

9878 Palm Drive
South Padre, TX 98765
Telephone (209) 555-3356

HISTORY AND PHYSICAL EXAMINATION

CONTINUATION

PATIENT: Gloria Hydorn

DATE: Friday, April 4, 2008

Patient has bilateral diagnostic mammography that shows normal finding on the right, but dense, suspicious area on the left. Suggestion by radiologist is further clinical study. Referred to Dr. Gerald Bond for evaluation of left breast lump.

Ray Adams, MD

CONTINUATION

FILING

Colors for Alphabetic Filing Method

1. Carrie Anderson ________ , ________
2. Karra Burthold ________ , ________
3. Aggy Carlisle ________ , ________
4. Kathy Forest ________ , ________
5. Adam Hoverson ________ , ________

Patient names from the Accession Ledger for a six-place filing system

Name	Number	Order	First Two Colors
1. Tony Mayer	345692	___	________ , ________
2. Mathew Owens	560122	___	________ , ________
3. Dalmer Garcia	789211	___	________ , ________
4. Missy Butler	34099	___	________ , ________
5. Kathy Sue Thompson	5678	___	________ , ________
6. Louise Carabin	58900	___	________ , ________
7. Hilton Smart	009091	___	________ , ________
8. Ellisa Talbot	762900	___	________ , ________
9. Joan Woods	980001	___	________ , ________
10. Maureen Loopstoe	509821	___	________ , ________

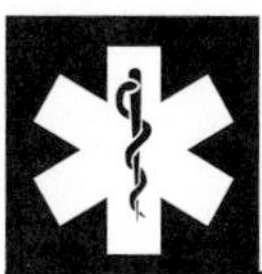

South Padre Medical Center

Patient's Name ______________________ Age _____ Sex ______ Marital Status S M W D

Address ______________________ Insurance ______________________

Telephone ______________________ Referred ______________________

Date	Subsequent Findings

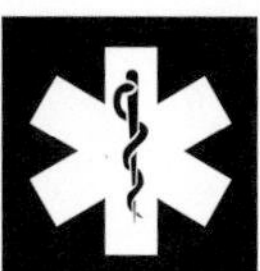

South Padre Medical Center

Patient's Name ______________________________ Age _____ Sex ______ Marital Status S M W D

Address ______________________________ Insurance ______________________________

Telephone ______________________ Referred ______________________________

Date	Subsequent Findings

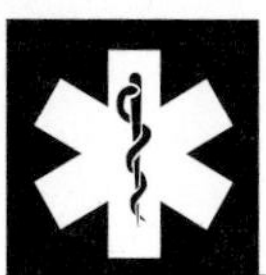

South Padre Medical Center

Patient's Name ______________________ Age _____ Sex ______ Marital Status S M W D

Address ______________________ Insurance ______________________

Telephone ______________________ Referred ______________________

Date	Subsequent Findings

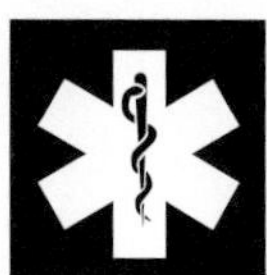

South Padre Medical Center

Patient's Name ______________________________ Age _____ Sex ______ Marital Status S M W D

Address ______________________________ Insurance ______________________________

Telephone ______________________ Referred ______________________________

Date	Subsequent Findings

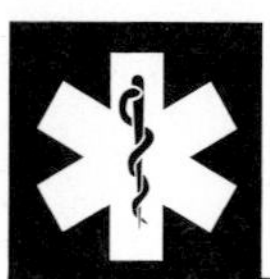

South Padre Medical Center

Patient's Name ______________________________ Age _____ Sex ______ Marital Status S M W D

Address ______________________________ Insurance ______________________________

Telephone ____________________ Referred ______________________________

Date	Subsequent Findings

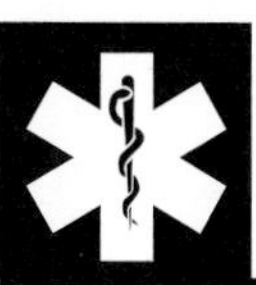

South Padre Medical Center

Patient's Name ____________________ Age _____ Sex _____ Marital Status S M W D

Address ____________________ Insurance ____________________

Telephone ____________________ Referred ____________________

Date	Subsequent Findings

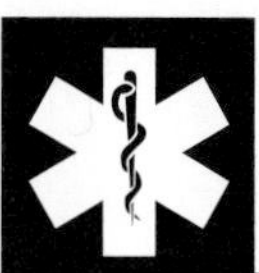

South Padre Medical Center

Patient's Name ______________________________ Age _____ Sex ______ Marital Status S M W D

Address ______________________________ Insurance ______________________________

Telephone ____________________ Referred ______________________________

Date	Subsequent Findings

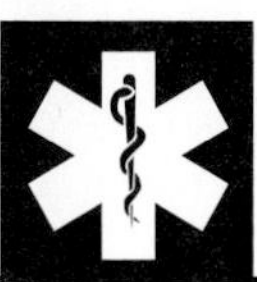

South Padre Medical Center

Patient's Name ______________________ Age _____ Sex ______ Marital Status S M W D

Address ______________________ Insurance ______________________

Telephone ______________________ Referred ______________________

Date	Subsequent Findings

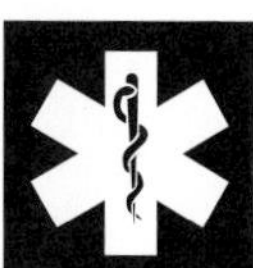

South Padre Medical Center

Patient's Name ______________________________ Age _____ Sex ______ Marital Status S M W D

Address ______________________________ Insurance ______________________________

Telephone ______________________ Referred ______________________________

Date	Subsequent Findings

RAYMOND EDWARDS

PROBLEM: RECHECK EARS

SUBJECTIVE: THE PATIENT RETURNS TO THE CLINIC 04/04/08. HE STILL HAS THE SENSATION OF STUFFINESS AND PLUGGED FEELING IN HIS EARS. HE HAS HAD TWO COURSES OF ANTIBIOTICS NOW WITHOUT ANY REAL RELIEF. HE HAD PREVIOUS PE TUBES A NUMBER OF YEARS AGO FOR RECURRENT EAR PROBLEMS. HE DOES NOT APPEAR TO HAVE ANY OBVIOUS HEARING DEFICIT, ALTHOUGH HE SOMETIMES HAS AN ECHO IN HIS EARS. HE HAS BEEN TRYING TYLENOL AND SUDAFED. THE ANTIBIOTIC DID NOT SEEM TO HELP AT ALL. HE HAS NO ALLERGIES TO MEDICINES.

PHYSICAL EXAM: HIS TMS DO NOT APPEAR RED OR DULL. THEY DO HAVE THE TYMPANOSCLEROSIS. I DO NOT DETECT AN OBVIOUS EFFUSION, BUT THE AREA OF TYMPANOSCLEROSIS IS PROMINENT ENOUGH THAT I DO NOT THINK I COULD SEE AN EFFUSION IF IT WAS PRESENT.

ASSESSMENT: TYMPANOSCLEROSIS.

PLAN: WE ARE GOING TO CHECK A TYPANOGRAM AND AUDIOGRAM AND HAVE HIM BE RECHECKED BY EAR, NOSE AND THROAT TO SEE IF THERE IS ANYTHING ELSE THAT HE NEEDS.

GERALD BOND, MD

SUPPLIES TASK 3.4

Gerald Bond, MD
Ray Adams, MD
Joyce Harkness, MD
Anthony Clark, MD

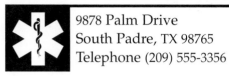

South Padre Medical Center

9878 Palm Drive
South Padre, TX 98765
Telephone (209) 555-3356

Gerald Bond, MD
Ray Adams, MD
Joyce Harkness, MD
Anthony Clark, MD

South Padre Medical Center

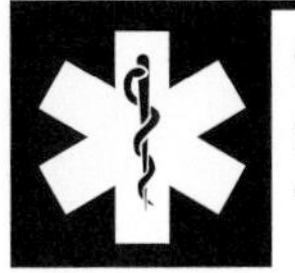

9878 Palm Drive
South Padre, TX 98765
Telephone (209) 555-3356

INCOMING MAIL FORM
THURSDAY, APRIL 10

1. Letter to Dr. Bond from Dr. Andrews
2. BC/BS of TX (payments)
3. Good Housekeeping magazine (Dr. Harkness's office)
4. Completed job applications from Job Service of TX
5. Letter from the Medicare Appeals Division
6. Pathology results State of Texas Pathology, Attn: Dr. Adams
7. Texas Health (payments)
8. People Magazine (Dr. Adams' office)
9. X-ray pouches for Dr. Clark
10. Blank IRS/W-4 forms
11. Envelope containing CMS-1500 forms, attn: Kerri Marshall
12. Personal marked letter to Dr. Harkness
13. 3 boxes of check blanks/South Padre Medical Center
14. *South Padre Living* (2 copies, magazine)
15. 1 box from South Padre Printing Company containing letterhead stationery
16. BC/BS of TX Appeals Division
17. Gold Prospector magazine (Dr. Gerald Bond)
18. 4 boxes of business cards, one for each Dr. in the clinic
19. Request for surgical consultation for Dr. Clark
20. Medicare (reimbursement)

MAIL SORTING

Dr. Bond

Dr. Harkness

Dr. Adams

Dr. Clark

Gladys

Accounts receivable

Insurance

Human Resources

Waiting Room

South Padre Medical Center

Gerald Bond, MD
Ray Adams, MD
Joyce Harkness, MD
Anthony Clark, MD

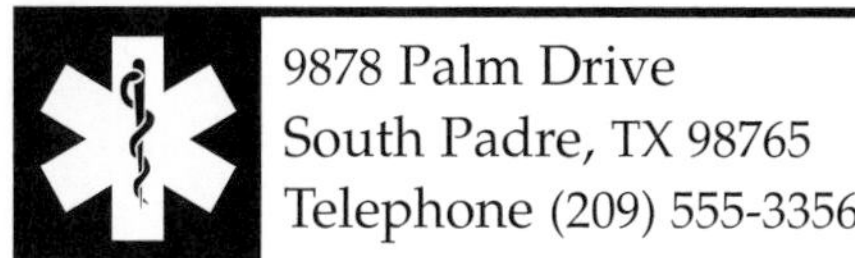

9878 Palm Drive
South Padre, TX 98765
Telephone (209) 555-3356

PATIENT INFORMATION

Please Print

Today's Date ____________________

Last Name ____________________ First Name ____________________ Initial ______

Date of Birth ____________________ Age __________ Sex __________ SS# ______-_____-______

Home Address Street ____________________ City ____________________

State ____________________ Zip__________ Home Phone (______)____________________

Occupation ____________________ Employer ____________________

Employer Address Street ____________________ City____________________

State ____________________ Zip __________ Work Phone (______)____________________

Are you currently a student? Yes No Name of School ____________________

Spouse's Name ____________________ Marital Status M S D W SEP

Spouse's SS# ______-_____-________ Spouse's Employer ____________________

In case of emergency, notify ____________________ Relationship____________________

Home Phone (____) ____________________ Work Phone (____) ____________________

If you are a minor: Parent's Name ____________________SS# ______-_____-______

Street ____________________ City ____________________ State ______ Zip__________

Home Phone (____) ____________________ Work Phone (____) ____________________

Reason for Visit ____________________

Work related injury? Yes No Date of injury____________________

Automobile accident? Yes No Date of injury____________________

Other injury? Yes No Date of injury____________________

Insurance (Primary) Company Name: ____________________

Street ____________________ City ____________________ State ______ Zip__________

Subscriber's Name ____________________

Relationship to Subscriber: ____________________

Policy #____________________ Group #____________________

Insurance (Secondary) Company Name: ____________________

Street ____________________ City ____________________ State ______ Zip__________

Subscriber's Name ____________________

Relationship to Subscriber: ____________________

Policy #____________________ Group #____________________

Assignment of Benefits:

I directly assign all medical/surgical benefits, including major medical benefits and Medicare, to South Padre Medical Center. I understand that this authorization for assignment remains in effect until I revoke it in writing. A photocopy of this assignment will be considered as valid as this original assignment. I further understand that I am responsible for my indebtedness no matter what charges the insurance pays for.

Insured or Guardian's Signature ____________________ Date ____________________

Gerald Bond, MD
Ray Adams, MD
Joyce Harkness, MD
Anthony Clark, MD

South Padre Medical Center

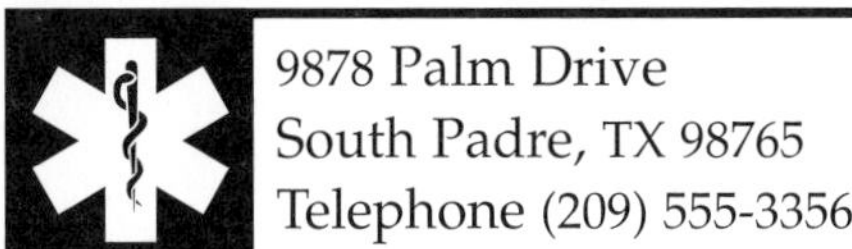

9878 Palm Drive
South Padre, TX 98765
Telephone (209) 555-3356

PATIENT INFORMATION

Please Print

Today's Date ____________________

Last Name ____________________ First Name ____________________ Initial ______

Date of Birth ____________________ Age ____________ Sex ____________ SS# ______-_____-______

Home Address Street ____________________ City ____________________

State ____________________ Zip__________ Home Phone (_____)________________

Occupation ____________________ Employer ____________________

Employer Address Street ____________________ City____________________

State ____________________ Zip ____________ Work Phone (_____)________________

Are you currently a student? Yes No Name of School ____________________

Spouse's Name ____________________ Marital Status M S D W SEP

Spouse's SS# ______-_____-________ Spouse's Employer ____________________

In case of emergency, notify ____________________ Relationship____________________

Home Phone (____) ________________ Work Phone (____) ________________

If you are a minor: Parent's Name ____________________SS# ______-_____-______

Street ____________________ City ____________ State ______ Zip__________

Home Phone (____) ________________ Work Phone (____) ________________

Reason for Visit ____________________

Work related injury? Yes No Date of injury____________________

Automobile accident? Yes No Date of injury____________________

Other injury? Yes No Date of injury____________________

Insurance (Primary) Company Name: ____________________

Street ____________________ City ____________ State ______ Zip__________

Subscriber's Name ____________________

Relationship to Subscriber: ____________________

Policy #____________________ Group #____________________

Insurance (Secondary) Company Name: ____________________

Street ____________________ City ____________ State ______ Zip__________

Subscriber's Name ____________________

Relationship to Subscriber: ____________________

Policy #____________________ Group #____________________

Assignment of Benefits:

I directly assign all medical/surgical benefits, including major medical benefits and Medicare, to South Padre Medical Center. I understand that this authorization for assignment remains in effect until I revoke it in writing. A photocopy of this assignment will be considered as valid as this original assignment. I further understand that I am responsible for my indebtedness no matter what charges the insurance pays for.

Insured or Guardian's Signature ____________________ Date ________________

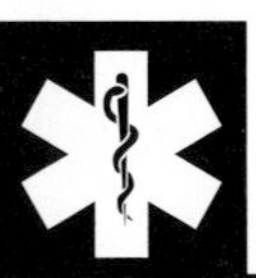

South Padre Medical Center

Patient's Name ____________________________________ Age _____ Sex ______ Marital Status S M W D

Address ____________________________________ Insurance ____________________________________

Telephone ____________________________ Referred ____________________________________

Date	Subsequent Findings

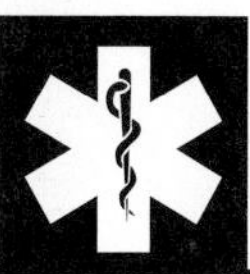

South Padre Medical Center

Patient's Name ______________________________ Age _____ Sex ______ Marital Status S M W D

Address ______________________________ Insurance ______________________________

Telephone ____________________ Referred ______________________________

Date	Subsequent Findings

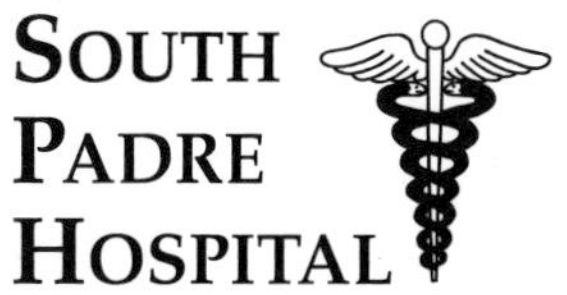

980 Lagona Drive • South Padre, TX 98765 • Telephone (209) 555-4289

OPERATIVE REPORT

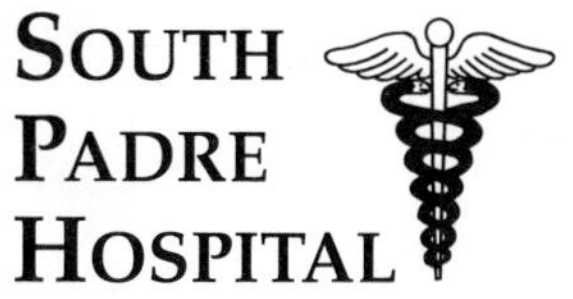

980 Lagona Drive • South Padre, TX 98765 • Telephone (209) 555-4289

OPERATIVE REPORT

South Padre Medical Center

Interoffice Memo

South Padre Medical Center

Interoffice Memo

SUPPLIES TASK 6.2

South Padre Medical Center

Interoffice Memo

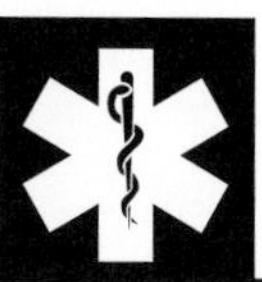

South Padre Medical Center

Interoffice Memo

South Padre Medical Center

Interoffice Memo

SUPPLIES TASK 6.2

Gerald Bond, MD
Ray Adams, MD
Joyce Harkness, MD
Anthony Clark, MD

South Padre Medical Center

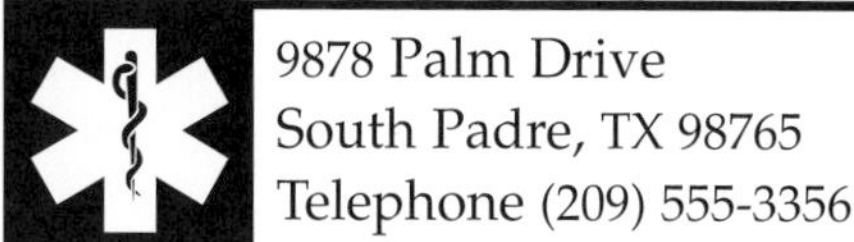

9878 Palm Drive
South Padre, TX 98765
Telephone (209) 555-3356

PATIENT INFORMATION

Please Print

Today's Date ____________________

Last Name ____________________ First Name ____________________ Initial ______

Date of Birth ____________________ Age __________ Sex __________ SS# ______-_____-______

Home Address Street ____________________ City ____________________

State ____________________ Zip__________ Home Phone (______)____________________

Occupation ____________________ Employer ____________________

Employer Address Street ____________________ City____________________

State ____________________ Zip __________ Work Phone (______)____________________

Are you currently a student? Yes No Name of School ____________________

Spouse's Name ____________________ Marital Status M S D W SEP

Spouse's SS# ______-_____-________ Spouse's Employer ____________________

In case of emergency, notify ____________________ Relationship____________________

Home Phone (____) ____________________ Work Phone (____) ____________________

If you are a minor: Parent's Name____________________SS# _______-_____-_______

Street ____________________ City ____________________ State ______ Zip__________

Home Phone (____) ____________________ Work Phone (____) ____________________

Reason for Visit ____________________

Work related injury? Yes No Date of injury____________________

Automobile accident? Yes No Date of injury____________________

Other injury? Yes No Date of injury____________________

Insurance (Primary) Company Name: ____________________

Street ____________________ City ____________________ State ______ Zip__________

Subscriber's Name ____________________

Relationship to Subscriber: ____________________

Policy #____________________ Group #____________________

Insurance (Secondary) Company Name: ____________________

Street ____________________ City ____________________ State ______ Zip__________

Subscriber's Name ____________________

Relationship to Subscriber: ____________________

Policy #____________________ Group #____________________

Assignment of Benefits:

I directly assign all medical/surgical benefits, including major medical benefits and Medicare, to South Padre Medical Center. I understand that this authorization for assignment remains in effect until I revoke it in writing. A photocopy of this assignment will be considered as valid as this original assignment. I further understand that I am responsible for my indebtedness no matter what charges the insurance pays for.

Insured or Guardian's Signature ____________________ Date ____________________

Gerald Bond, MD
Ray Adams, MD
Joyce Harkness, MD
Anthony Clark, MD

South Padre Medical Center

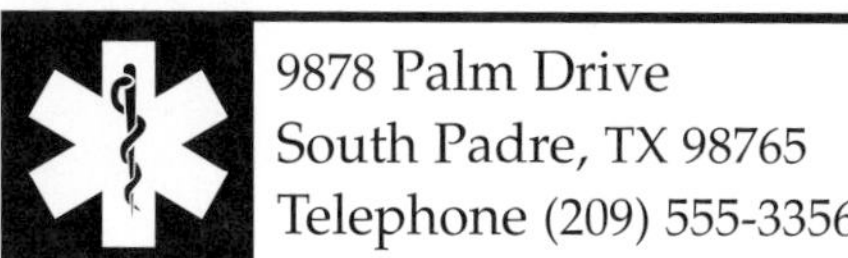

9878 Palm Drive
South Padre, TX 98765
Telephone (209) 555-3356

PATIENT INFORMATION

Please Print

Today's Date ____________________

Last Name ________________________________ First Name ________________________ Initial ______

Date of Birth ______________________ Age ____________ Sex ___________ SS# ______-_____-______

Home Address Street ____ City ________________________

State ____________________ Zip____________ Home Phone (______)____________________

Occupation ________________________________ Employer ____

Employer Address Street ____________________________________ City________________________

State ____________________ Zip ____________ Work Phone (______)____________________

Are you currently a student? Yes No Name of School ______________________________________

Spouse's Name ______________________________________ Marital Status M S D W SEP

Spouse's SS# ______-_____-________ Spouse's Employer ____

In case of emergency, notify __________________________________ Relationship_____________________

Home Phone (____) ____________________ Work Phone (____) ____________________

If you are a minor: Parent's Name ____SS# ______-_____-______

Street __________________________ City ______________ State ______ Zip__________

Home Phone (____) ____________________ Work Phone (____) ____________________

Reason for Visit ____

Work related injury? Yes No Date of injury__________________________

Automobile accident? Yes No Date of injury__________________________

Other injury? Yes No Date of injury__________________________

Insurance (Primary) Company Name: ____

Street __________________________ City ______________ State ______ Zip__________

Subscriber's Name ____

Relationship to Subscriber: ____

Policy #________________________________ Group #_________________________

Insurance (Secondary) Company Name: ____

Street __________________________ City ______________ State ______ Zip__________

Subscriber's Name ____

Relationship to Subscriber: ____

Policy #________________________________ Group #_________________________

Assignment of Benefits:

I directly assign all medical/surgical benefits, including major medical benefits and Medicare, to South Padre Medical Center. I understand that this authorization for assignment remains in effect until I revoke it in writing. A photocopy of this assignment will be considered as valid as this original assignment. I further understand that I am responsible for my indebtedness no matter what charges the insurance pays for.

Insured or Guardian's Signature ____ Date ________________

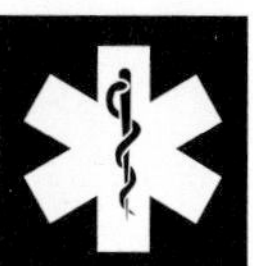

South Padre Medical Center

Patient's Name ______________________________ Age _____ Sex ______ Marital Status S M W D

Address ______________________________ Insurance ______________________________

Telephone ____________________ Referred ______________________________

Date	Subsequent Findings

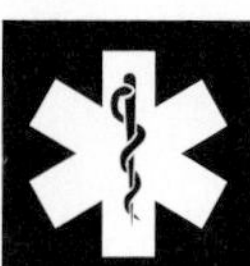

South Padre Medical Center

Patient's Name ______________________ Age _____ Sex ______ Marital Status S M W D

Address ______________________ Insurance ______________________

Telephone ______________________ Referred ______________________

Date	Subsequent Findings

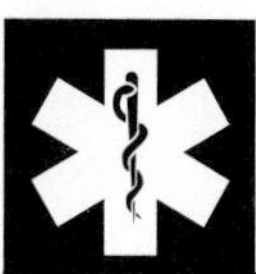

South Padre Medical Center

Patient's Name ______________________ Age _____ Sex ______ Marital Status S M W D

Address ______________________ Insurance ______________________

Telephone ______________________ Referred ______________________

Date	Subsequent Findings

REQUEST FOR PREAUTHORIZATION FOR SURGERY

Surgeon: Gerald Bond, MD
(circle one) Ray Adams, MD
Joyce Harkness, MD
Anthony Clark, MD

PATIENT NAME: ______________________________ FACILITY: ______________________________

DATE OF BIRTH: ______________________________ ADMIT DATE: ______________________________

ACCOUNT #: ______________________________ SURGERY DATE: ______________________________

INSURANCE: ______________________________ POLICY#: ______________________________

PROCEDURE: ____

DIAGNOSIS: ____

AUTHORIZATION: ______________________________

COMPLETED BY: ______________________________

DATE COMPLETED: ______________________________

REQUEST FOR PREAUTHORIZATION FOR SURGERY

Surgeon: Gerald Bond, MD
(circle one) Ray Adams, MD
Joyce Harkness, MD
Anthony Clark, MD

PATIENT NAME: ______________________ FACILITY: ______________________

DATE OF BIRTH: ______________________ ADMIT DATE: ______________________

ACCOUNT #: ______________________ SURGERY DATE: ______________________

INSURANCE: ______________________ POLICY#: ______________________

PROCEDURE: ____

DIAGNOSIS: ____

AUTHORIZATION: ______________________

COMPLETED BY: ______________________

DATE COMPLETED: ______________________

REQUEST FOR PREAUTHORIZATION FOR SURGERY

Surgeon: Gerald Bond, MD
(circle one) Ray Adams, MD
Joyce Harkness, MD
Anthony Clark, MD

PATIENT NAME: ______________________ FACILITY: ______________________

DATE OF BIRTH: ______________________ ADMIT DATE: ______________________

ACCOUNT #: ______________________ SURGERY DATE: ______________________

INSURANCE: ______________________ POLICY#: ______________________

PROCEDURE: ____

DIAGNOSIS: ____

AUTHORIZATION: ______________________

COMPLETED BY: ______________________

DATE COMPLETED: ______________________

REQUEST FOR PREAUTHORIZATION FOR SURGERY

Surgeon: Gerald Bond, MD
(circle one) Ray Adams, MD
Joyce Harkness, MD
Anthony Clark, MD

PATIENT NAME: ______________________ FACILITY: ______________________

DATE OF BIRTH: ______________________ ADMIT DATE: ______________________

ACCOUNT #: ______________________ SURGERY DATE: ______________________

INSURANCE: ______________________ POLICY#: ______________________

PROCEDURE: ____

DIAGNOSIS: ____

AUTHORIZATION: ______________________

COMPLETED BY: ______________________

DATE COMPLETED: ______________________

SUPPLIES TASK 7.6

REQUEST FOR PREAUTHORIZATION FOR SURGERY

Surgeon: Gerald Bond, MD
(circle one) Ray Adams, MD
Joyce Harkness, MD
Anthony Clark, MD

PATIENT NAME: ____________________ FACILITY: ____________________

DATE OF BIRTH: ____________________ ADMIT DATE: ____________________

ACCOUNT #: ____________________ SURGERY DATE: ____________________

INSURANCE: ____________________ POLICY#: ____________________

PROCEDURE: ____

DIAGNOSIS: ____

AUTHORIZATION: ____________________

COMPLETED BY: ____________________

DATE COMPLETED: ____________________

SUPPLIES TASK 7.6

REQUEST FOR PREAUTHORIZATION FOR SURGERY

Surgeon: Gerald Bond, MD
(circle one) Ray Adams, MD
Joyce Harkness, MD
Anthony Clark, MD

PATIENT NAME: ______________________ FACILITY: ______________________

DATE OF BIRTH: ______________________ ADMIT DATE: ______________________

ACCOUNT #: ______________________ SURGERY DATE: ______________________

INSURANCE: ______________________ POLICY#: ______________________

PROCEDURE: ____

DIAGNOSIS: ____

AUTHORIZATION: ______________________

COMPLETED BY: ______________________

DATE COMPLETED: ______________________

SUPPLIES TASK 7.6

South Padre Medical Center

SURGICAL REQUEST AND INFORMATION

This portion is to be completed by requesting surgeon.

Surgeon: ☒ Gerald Bond, MD
❑ Ray Adams, MD
❑ Joyce Harkness, MD
❑ Anthony Clark, MD

Schedule: ❑ URGENT ☒ IMMEDIATE ❑ PATIENT CONVENIENCE

Date Requested: 04-15-08 Time Requested: 8:10 AM

Patient Name: KLINT, SAM J. ACCOUNT #: 00000-0012

Procedure: BIOPSY OF KIDNEY

Procedure Code(s): 50200

Diagnosis(es): RENAL FAILURE

Diagnosis(es) Code(s): 586

Estimated Surgery Time: 1 HOUR OUTPATIENT

Surgical Assistant Requested: ——

Additional Information: ——

This portion is to be completed by scheduling personnel.

Surgery Date: ____________ Time: ____________
Day Date

Authorization Obtained: ❑ YES ❑ NO ❑ REQUESTED

If authorization has been requested and response is pending, list date and contact information from the initial request.

Requested From: ____________ Date: ____________
(Carrier and person)

Telephone: ____________ Ext: ____________

Completed By: ____________

Date Completed: ____________

SUPPLIES TASK 7.6

South Padre Medical Center

SURGICAL REQUEST AND INFORMATION

This portion is to be completed by requesting surgeon.

Surgeon: ❑ Gerald Bond, MD
❑ Ray Adams, MD
❑ Joyce Harkness, MD
☒ Anthony Clark, MD

Schedule: ❑ URGENT ☒ IMMEDIATE ❑ PATIENT CONVENIENCE

Date Requested: 04-15-08 Time Requested: 10:28 am

Patient Name: Adams, Tony W. account #: 00000-0223

Procedure: Biopsy of Lymph Node, Excisional

Procedure Code(s): 38510

Diagnosis(es): Lymphadenopathy

Diagnosis(es) Code(s): 785.6

Estimated Surgery Time: 1 hour Inpatient

Surgical Assistant Requested: Tony Andrews

Additional Information: —

This portion is to be completed by scheduling personnel.

Surgery Date: ______________________ Time: ______________________
Day Date

Authorization Obtained: ❑ YES ❑ NO ❑ REQUESTED

If authorization has been requested and response is pending, list date and contact information from the initial request.

Requested From: ______________________ Date: ______________
(Carrier and person)

Telephone: ______________________ Ext: __________

Completed By: ______________________

Date Completed: ______________________

SUPPLIES TASK 7.6

South Padre Medical Center

SURGICAL REQUEST AND INFORMATION

This portion is to be completed by requesting surgeon.

Surgeon: ☒ Gerald Bond, MD
❑ Ray Adams, MD
❑ Joyce Harkness, MD
❑ Anthony Clark, MD

Schedule: ❑ URGENT ☒ IMMEDIATE ❑ PATIENT CONVENIENCE

Date Requested: 04-15-08 Time Requested: 8:45 AM

Patient Name: HARKLAND, EMMY L. ACCOUNT #: 00000-0110

Procedure: BREAST BIOPSY

Procedure Code(s): 19101

Diagnosis(es): BREAST MASS

Diagnosis(es) Code(s): 239.3

Estimated Surgery Time: 1 HOUR OUTPATIENT

Surgical Assistant Requested: ______

Additional Information: ______

This portion is to be completed by scheduling personnel.

Surgery Date: ______ Time: ______
Day Date

Authorization Obtained: ❑ YES ❑ NO ❑ REQUESTED

If authorization has been requested and response is pending, list date and contact information from the initial request.

Requested From: ______ Date: ______
(Carrier and person)

Telephone: ______ Ext: ______

Completed By: ______

Date Completed: ______

SUPPLIES TASK 7.6

South Padre Medical Center

SURGICAL REQUEST AND INFORMATION

This portion is to be completed by requesting surgeon.

Surgeon: ☒ Gerald Bond, MD
❑ Ray Adams, MD
❑ Joyce Harkness, MD
❑ Anthony Clark, MD

Schedule: ❑ URGENT ☒ IMMEDIATE ❑ PATIENT CONVENIENCE

Date Requested: 04-15-08 Time Requested: 9:05 AM

Patient Name: BATES, MICHELLE L. ACCOUNT #: 00000-0069

Procedure: NEEDLE BIOPSY RT BREAST

Procedure Code(s): 19102

Diagnosis(es): BREAST NEOPLASM

Diagnosis(es) Code(s): 239.3

Estimated Surgery Time: 1 HOUR OUTPATIENT

Surgical Assistant Requested: —

Additional Information: —

This portion is to be completed by scheduling personnel.

Surgery Date: ______________________ Time: ______________________
Day Date

Authorization Obtained: ❑ YES ❑ NO ❑ REQUESTED

If authorization has been requested and response is pending, list date and contact information from the initial request.

Requested From: ______________________ Date: ______________________
(Carrier and person)

Telephone: ______________________ Ext: ______________________

Completed By: ______________________

Date Completed: ______________________

SUPPLIES TASK 7.6

South Padre Medical Center

SURGICAL REQUEST AND INFORMATION

This portion is to be completed by requesting surgeon.

Surgeon:
- ❑ Gerald Bond, MD
- ❑ Ray Adams, MD
- ☒ Joyce Harkness, MD
- ❑ Anthony Clark, MD

Schedule: ❑ URGENT ☒ IMMEDIATE ❑ PATIENT CONVENIENCE

Date Requested: 04-15-08 Time Requested: 10:40 am

Patient Name: Anderson, Charlie M. account #: 00000-0009

Procedure: Echocardiogram

Procedure Code(s): 93318

Diagnosis(es): Atrial Fibrillation

Diagnosis(es) Code(s): 427.31

Estimated Surgery Time: 45 minutes outpatient

Surgical Assistant Requested: —

Additional Information: —

This portion is to be completed by scheduling personnel.

Surgery Date: ______________________ Time: ______________________
Day Date

Authorization Obtained: ❑ YES ❑ NO ❑ REQUESTED

If authorization has been requested and response is pending, list date and contact information from the initial request.

Requested From: ______________________ Date: ______________________
(Carrier and person)

Telephone: ______________________ Ext: ______________

Completed By: ______________________

Date Completed: ______________________

SUPPLIES TASK 7.6

South Padre Medical Center

SURGICAL REQUEST AND INFORMATION

This portion is to be completed by requesting surgeon.

Surgeon:
- ☐ Gerald Bond, MD
- ☐ Ray Adams, MD
- ☐ Joyce Harkness, MD
- ☒ Anthony Clark, MD

Schedule: ☐ URGENT ☒ IMMEDIATE ☐ PATIENT CONVENIENCE

Date Requested: 04/15/08 Time Requested: 10:45 am

Patient Name: Wood, Tina J. account #: 00000-2123

Procedure: Cervical Diskectomy (2 disc, anterior)

Procedure Code(s): 63075, 63076

Diagnosis(es): Herniated disc C5-7

Diagnosis(es) Code(s): 722.0

Estimated Surgery Time: 1.5 hours Inpatient

Surgical Assistant Requested: Peggy Johnson

Additional Information: —

This portion is to be completed by scheduling personnel.

Surgery Date: ______________________ Time: ______________________
Day Date

Authorization Obtained: ☐ YES ☐ NO ☐ REQUESTED

If authorization has been requested and response is pending, list date and contact information from the initial request.

Requested From: ______________________ Date: ______________
(Carrier and person)

Telephone: ______________________ Ext: __________

Completed By: ______________________

Date Completed: ______________________

SUPPLIES TASK 7.6

Gerald Bond, MD
Ray Adams, MD
Joyce Harkness, MD
Anthony Clark, MD

South Padre Medical Center

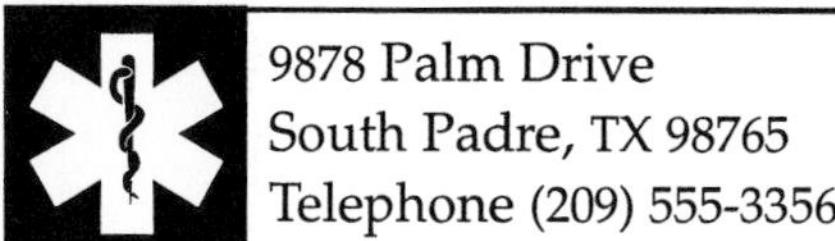

9878 Palm Drive
South Padre, TX 98765
Telephone (209) 555-3356

PATIENT INFORMATION

Please Print

Today's Date 04/15/08

Last Name Klint First Name Sam Initial J

Date of Birth 02/11/46 Age 62 Sex M SS# 504-11-4545

Home Address Street 5403 Fairview Dr. City South Padre

State TX Zip 98765 Home Phone (209) 555-0990

Occupation None - disabled Employer N/A

Employer Address Street ______ City ______

State ______ Zip ______ Work Phone (____) ______

Are you currently a student? Yes (No) Name of School ______

Spouse's Name Faye Klint Marital Status (M) S D W SEP

Spouse's SS# ___-___-___ Spouse's Employer ______

In case of emergency, notify ______ Relationship ______

Home Phone (____) ______ Work Phone (____) ______

If you are a minor: Parent's Name ______ SS# ___-___-___

Street ______ City ______ State ______ Zip ______

Home Phone (____) ______ Work Phone (____) ______

Reason for Visit Renal failure

Work related injury? Yes (No) Date of injury ______

Automobile accident? Yes (No) Date of injury ______

Other injury? Yes (No) Date of injury ______

Insurance (Primary) Company Name: BC/BS of Texas

Street 1514 West Road City Houston State TX Zip 99881

Subscriber's Name Self

Relationship to Subscriber: ______

Policy # MKL2211 Group # A1280

Insurance (Secondary) Company Name: ______

Street ______ City ______ State ______ Zip ______

Subscriber's Name ______

Relationship to Subscriber: ______

Policy # ______ Group # ______

Assignment of Benefits:

I directly assign all medical/surgical benefits, including major medical benefits and Medicare, to South Padre Medical Center. I understand that this authorization for assignment remains in effect until I revoke it in writing. A photocopy of this assignment will be considered as valid as this original assignment. I further understand that I am responsible for my indebtedness no matter what charges the insurance pays for.

Insured or Guardian's Signature ______ Date ______

SUPPLIES TASK 7.6

Gerald Bond, MD
Ray Adams, MD
Joyce Harkness, MD
Anthony Clark, MD

South Padre Medical Center

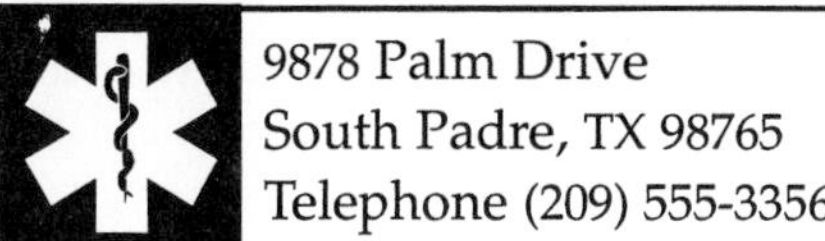

9878 Palm Drive
South Padre, TX 98765
Telephone (209) 555-3356

PATIENT INFORMATION

Please Print

Today's Date 04/15/08

Last Name Harkland First Name Emmy Initial L

Date of Birth 04/06/42 Age 66 Sex F SS# 009-99-0099

Home Address Street 1818 Oak Street City South Padre

State TX Zip 98765 Home Phone (209) 555-5209

Occupation Retired Employer N/A

Employer Address Street ____ City ____

State ____ Zip ____ Work Phone (____) ____

Are you currently a student? Yes (No) Name of School ____

Spouse's Name — Marital Status M S D (W) SEP

Spouse's SS# ___-___-___ Spouse's Employer ____

In case of emergency, notify ____ Relationship ____

Home Phone (____) ____ Work Phone (____) ____

If you are a minor: Parent's Name ____ SS# ___-___-___

Street ____ City ____ State ____ Zip ____

Home Phone (____) ____ Work Phone (____) ____

Reason for Visit Lump in breast

Work related injury? Yes (No) Date of injury ____

Automobile accident? Yes (No) Date of injury ____

Other injury? Yes (No) Date of injury ____

Insurance (Primary) Company Name: Medicare

Street 402 Main Street City South Padre State TX Zip 98765

Subscriber's Name ____

Relationship to Subscriber: Emmy Harkland

Policy # 00990099A Group # ____

Insurance (Secondary) Company Name: ____

Street ____ City ____ State ____ Zip ____

Subscriber's Name ____

Relationship to Subscriber: ____

Policy # ____ Group # ____

Assignment of Benefits:

I directly assign all medical/surgical benefits, including major medical benefits and Medicare, to South Padre Medical Center. I understand that this authorization for assignment remains in effect until I revoke it in writing. A photocopy of this assignment will be considered as valid as this original assignment. I further understand that I am responsible for my indebtedness no matter what charges the insurance pays for.

Insured or Guardian's Signature ____ Date ____

SUPPLIES TASK 7.6

Gerald Bond, MD
Ray Adams, MD
Joyce Harkness, MD
Anthony Clark, MD

South Padre Medical Center

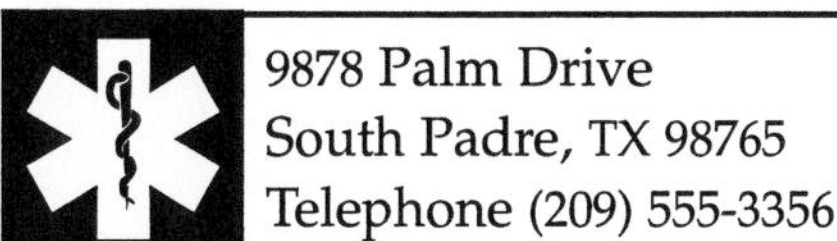

9878 Palm Drive
South Padre, TX 98765
Telephone (209) 555-3356

PATIENT INFORMATION

Please Print

Today's Date 04/15/08

Last Name Bates First Name Michelle Initial L

Date of Birth 11/09/61 Age 46 Sex F SS# 502-66-0066

Home Address Street 2204 2nd Ave City South Padre

State TX Zip 98765 Home Phone (209) 555-9737

Occupation Nurse Employer South Padre Nursing Home

Employer Address Street ______ City ______

State ______ Zip ______ Work Phone (____) ______

Are you currently a student? Yes (No) Name of School ______

Spouse's Name Dean Marital Status (M) S D W SEP

Spouse's SS# 180-52-9987 Spouse's Employer B&L Incorporated

In case of emergency, notify Dean Relationship Spouse

Home Phone (209) 555-9737 Work Phone (209) 555-1827

If you are a minor: Parent's Name ______ SS# ____-____-____

Street ______ City ______ State ______ Zip ______

Home Phone (____) ______ Work Phone (____) ______

Reason for Visit Breast mass

Work related injury? Yes (No) Date of injury ______

Automobile accident? Yes (No) Date of injury ______

Other injury? Yes (No) Date of injury ______

Insurance (Primary) Company Name: South Padre Insurance

Street 2702 Oak Line Dr. City South Padre State TX Zip 98765

Subscriber's Name Michelle Bates

Relationship to Subscriber: Self

Policy # KMK9236 Group # ______

Insurance (Secondary) Company Name: ______

Street ______ City ______ State ______ Zip ______

Subscriber's Name ______

Relationship to Subscriber: ______

Policy # ______ Group # ______

Assignment of Benefits:

I directly assign all medical/surgical benefits, including major medical benefits and Medicare, to South Padre Medical Center. I understand that this authorization for assignment remains in effect until I revoke it in writing. A photocopy of this assignment will be considered as valid as this original assignment. I further understand that I am responsible for my indebtedness no matter what charges the insurance pays for.

Insured or Guardian's Signature ______ Date ______

Gerald Bond, MD
Ray Adams, MD
Joyce Harkness, MD
Anthony Clark, MD

South Padre Medical Center

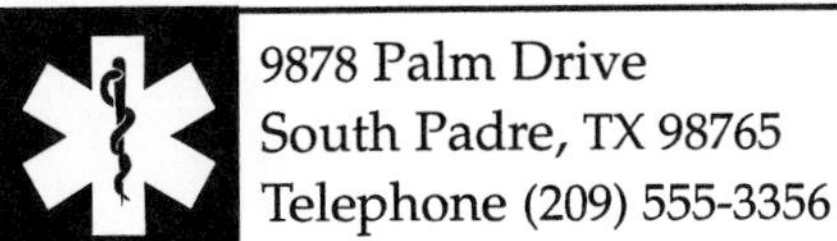

9878 Palm Drive
South Padre, TX 98765
Telephone (209) 555-3356

PATIENT INFORMATION

Please Print

Today's Date 04/15/08

Last Name Adams First Name Tony Initial W

Date of Birth 05/22/48 Age 59 Sex M SS# 509-81-8382

Home Address Street 1616 Todd Ave City South Padre

State TX Zip 98765 Home Phone (209) 555-1114

Occupation Lawyer Employer Adams Law Firm

Employer Address Street ______ City ______

State ______ Zip ______ Work Phone (____) ______

Are you currently a student? Yes (No) Name of School ______

Spouse's Name ______ Marital Status M S (D) W SEP

Spouse's SS# ___-___-___ Spouse's Employer ______

In case of emergency, notify ______ Relationship ______

Home Phone (____) ______ Work Phone (____) ______.

If you are a minor: Parent's Name ______ SS# ___-___-___

Street ______ City ______ State ______ Zip ______

Home Phone (____) ______ Work Phone (____) ______

Reason for Visit Excision Lymph Node/Neck

Work related injury? Yes (No) Date of injury ______

Automobile accident? Yes (No) Date of injury ______

Other injury? Yes (No) Date of injury ______

Insurance (Primary) Company Name: Texas Health

Street 1256 56th Ave S. City Houston State TX Zip 99881

Subscriber's Name ______

Relationship to Subscriber: Self

Policy # XCV4568 Group # ______

Insurance (Secondary) Company Name: ______

Street ______ City ______ State ______ Zip ______

Subscriber's Name ______

Relationship to Subscriber: ______

Policy # ______ Group # ______

Assignment of Benefits:

I directly assign all medical/surgical benefits, including major medical benefits and Medicare, to South Padre Medical Center. I understand that this authorization for assignment remains in effect until I revoke it in writing. A photocopy of this assignment will be considered as valid as this original assignment. I further understand that I am responsible for my indebtedness no matter what charges the insurance pays for.

Insured or Guardian's Signature ______ Date ______

SUPPLIES TASK 7.6

Assignment of Benefits

Gerald Bond, MD
Ray Adams, MD
Joyce Harkness, MD
Anthony Clark, MD

South Padre Medical Center

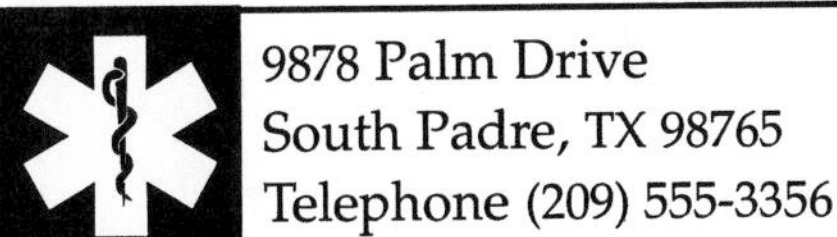

9878 Palm Drive
South Padre, TX 98765
Telephone (209) 555-3356

PATIENT INFORMATION

Please Print

Today's Date 04|15|08

Last Name Anderson First Name Charlie Initial M

Date of Birth 04/23/31 Age 76 Sex M SS# 011 - 22 - 3210

Home Address Street 919 36th Ave South City South Padre

State TX Zip 98765 Home Phone (209) 555 - 8838

Occupation Retired Employer N/A

Employer Address Street ______ City ______

State ______ Zip ______ Work Phone (____) ______

Are you currently a student? Yes (No) Name of School ______

Spouse's Name ______ Marital Status M S D (W) SEP

Spouse's SS# ___-___-___ Spouse's Employer ______

In case of emergency, notify ______ Relationship ______

Home Phone (____) ______ Work Phone (____) ______

If you are a minor: Parent's Name ______ SS# ___-___-___

Street ______ City ______ State ______ Zip ______

Home Phone (____) ______ Work Phone (____) ______

Reason for Visit Echocardiogram

Work related injury? Yes (No) Date of injury ______

Automobile accident? Yes (No) Date of injury ______

Other injury? Yes (No) Date of injury ______

Insurance (Primary) Company Name: Medicare

Street 402 Main Street City South Padre State TX Zip 98765

Subscriber's Name ______

Relationship to Subscriber: self

Policy # 011223210A Group # ______

Insurance (Secondary) Company Name: ______

Street ______ City ______ State ______ Zip ______

Subscriber's Name ______

Relationship to Subscriber: ______

Policy # ______ Group # ______

Assignment of Benefits:

I directly assign all medical/surgical benefits, including major medical benefits and Medicare, to South Padre Medical Center. I understand that this authorization for assignment remains in effect until I revoke it in writing. A photocopy of this assignment will be considered as valid as this original assignment. I further understand that I am responsible for my indebtedness no matter what charges the insurance pays for.

Insured or Guardian's Signature ______ Date ______

SUPPLIES TASK **7.6**

Gerald Bond, MD
Ray Adams, MD
Joyce Harkness, MD
(Anthony Clark, MD)

South Padre Medical Center

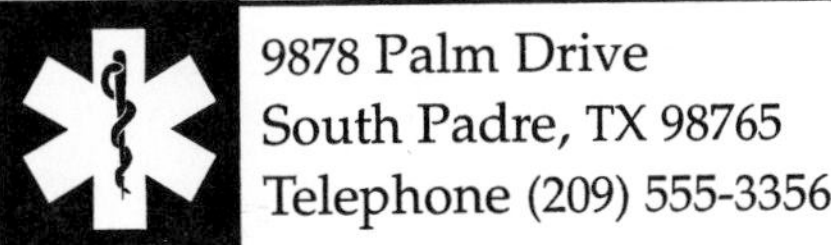

9878 Palm Drive
South Padre, TX 98765
Telephone (209) 555-3356

PATIENT INFORMATION

Please Print

Today's Date 04/15/08

Last Name Wood First Name Tina Initial J

Date of Birth 12/25/77 Age 30 Sex F SS# 207-48-1842

Home Address Street 222 Cherry Elm Rd apt. 15 City South Padre

State TX Zip 98765 Home Phone (209) 555-6169

Occupation Machine operator Employer South Padre Potato Plant

Employer Address Street ______ City ______

State ______ Zip ______ Work Phone (209) 555-5805

Are you currently a student? Yes (No) Name of School ______

Spouse's Name ______ Marital Status M (S) D W SEP

Spouse's SS# ___-___-___ Spouse's Employer ______

In case of emergency, notify ______ Relationship ______

Home Phone (___) ______ Work Phone (___) ______

If you are a minor: Parent's Name ______ SS# ___-___-___

Street ______ City ______ State ______ Zip ______

Home Phone (___) ______ Work Phone (___) ______

Reason for Visit Cervical Diskectomy

Work related injury? (Yes) No Date of injury 11/16/07

Automobile accident? Yes (No) Date of injury ______

Other injury? Yes (No) Date of injury ______

Insurance (Primary) Company Name: Workers Compensation

Street 10 State Highway City Houston State TX Zip 99881

Subscriber's Name ______

Relationship to Subscriber: ______

Policy # MKI4231 Group # ______

Insurance (Secondary) Company Name: BC/BS of Texas

Street ______ City ______ State ______ Zip ______

Subscriber's Name ______

Relationship to Subscriber: Self

Policy # PXM4031 Group # ______

Assignment of Benefits:
I directly assign all medical/surgical benefits, including major medical benefits and Medicare, to South Padre Medical Center. I understand that this authorization for assignment remains in effect until I revoke it in writing. A photocopy of this assignment will be considered as valid as this original assignment. I further understand that I am responsible for my indebtedness no matter what charges the insurance pays for.

Insured or Guardian's Signature ______ Date ______

SUPPLIES TASK 7.6

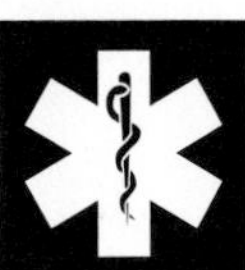

South Padre Medical Center

Patient's Name ______________________________ Age _____ Sex ______ Marital Status S M W D

Address ______________________________ Insurance ______________________________

Telephone ____________________ Referred ______________________________

Date	Subsequent Findings

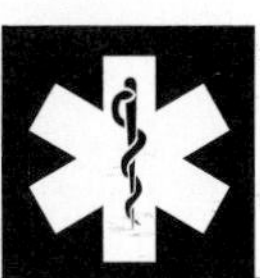

South Padre Medical Center

Patient's Name ______________________ Age _____ Sex ______ Marital Status S M W D

Address ______________________ Insurance ______________________

Telephone ______________________ Referred ______________________

Date	Subsequent Findings

South Pacific Medical Center

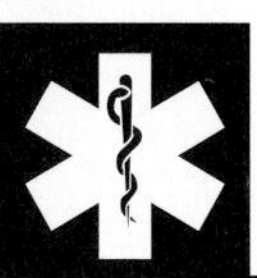

South Padre Medical Center

Patient's Name ______________________________ Age _____ Sex ______ Marital Status S M W D

Address ______________________________ Insurance ______________________________

Telephone ____________________ Referred ______________________________

Date	Subsequent Findings

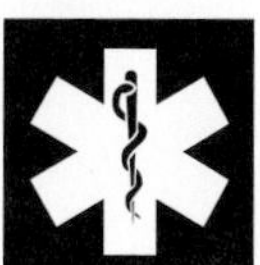

South Padre Medical Center

Patient's Name ______________________________ Age _____ Sex ______ Marital Status S M W D

Address ______________________________ Insurance ______________________________

Telephone ____________________ Referred ______________________________

Date	Subsequent Findings

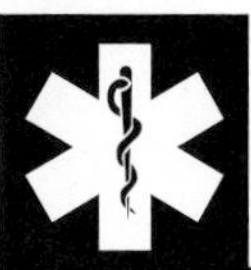

South Padre Medical Center

Patient's Name ______________________________ Age _____ Sex ______ Marital Status S M W D

Address ______________________________ Insurance ______________________________

Telephone ____________________ Referred ______________________________

Date	Subsequent Findings

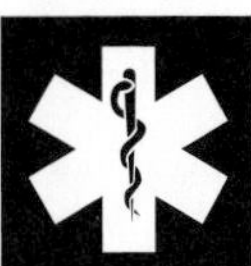

South Padre Medical Center

Patient's Name ______________________________ Age _____ Sex ______ Marital Status S M W D

Address ______________________________ Insurance ______________________________

Telephone ____________________ Referred ______________________________

Date	Subsequent Findings

New York City Cardiac Conference

Dr. Harkness will leave Friday, April 18
Her flight is at 5:30am
Needs to be at the airport at 4:45 am
Her flight # is 19
Non-stop flight from South Padre to New York City
Arrive in New York City at 9:00am
Check-in New York City Hotel
Conference starts at 10:00am in the Green Room
Finishes at approx. 7:30pm
Leave New York City Saturday morning
Flight is at 7:30am, Flight #229
Non-stop flight from New York City to South Padre
Be at airport at 6:45am
Arrive at South Padre Airport at 12:00pm

****Reminder to Dr. Harkness to bring portfolio for conference and to pick up airline ticket at the check-in desk when she arrives at the airport.

Answer Sheet

Message 1

a. Call Mr. Fenton back and give him the results he requested.
b. Since you cannot give Mr. Fenton the information he has requeste do not call him back.
c. Call Mr. Fenton to inform him that due to confidentially guidelines wife must call in for her results.
d. Call and leave the laboratory results Mr. Fenton requested on his swering machine.

Correct answer: ____

Message 2

a. Return Mrs. Burthold's telephone call and inform her that if K a has a fever when she comes to the clinic, you must first stop at the reception desk and obtain a mask t is to be worn while Karra is in the clinic.
b. Return Mrs. Burthold's telephone call to inform her to take a to the emergency department rather than to the clinic.
c. Do nothing and wait for Mrs. Burthold to call back for an a ointment.
d. Return Mrs. Burthold's telephone call and make a future pointment at a time Karra is not ill.

Correct answer: ____

Message 3

a. Return Mr. Foley's telephone call to his place of em yment and leave a message with the secretary that Jose can be seen at the clinic as per Mr. Foley's est.
b. Return Mr. Foley's telephone call and inform him there is an interpreter available for Mr. Garcia.
c. Do nothing and wait for a telephone call from M arcia, at which time you can transfer the call to the interpreter.
d. Call Mr. Garcia to determine how much Engl anguage skill he possesses to decide if an interpreter is necessary.

Correct answer: ____

Message 4

a. Do nothing because this is not you a of responsiblity.
b. Call the patient and obtain as mu formation related to the complaint and turn the information over to Gladys, your internship supervi
c. Call the patient back and apol and inform her that you have taken corrective action and she can be assured this will not happen n.
d. Inform Amanda's physician Amanda is allergic to perfume, so this can be noted in the medical record.

Correct answer: ____

Message 5

a. Immediately send new statement indicating the corrected amount due.
b. Verify the payme s received and then call the patient back to inform her that the payment had been received and been credited to her account. Further, apologize for the error and inform her that you will be imme sending a corrected statement reflecting her payment.
c. Do nothing use when you checked, the payment was made, so she will be receiving an updated statement nex th.
d. Call the ent's home and leave a message that the payment had been received.

Correct a ver: ____

SUPPLIES TASK 8.3

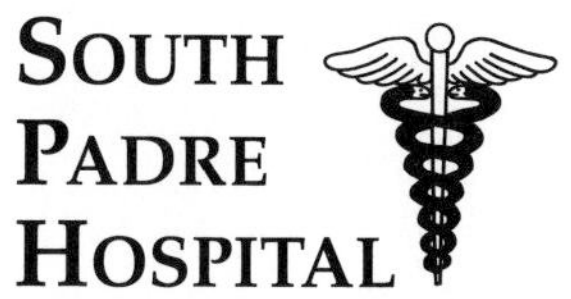

980 Lagona Drive • South Padre, TX 98765 • Telephone (209) 555-4289

OPERATIVE REPORT

SUPPLIES TASK 8.4

SOUTH
PADRE
HOSPITAL

980 Lagona Drive • South Padre, TX 98765 • Telephone (209) 555-4289

OPERATIVE REPORT

Constant Family Care

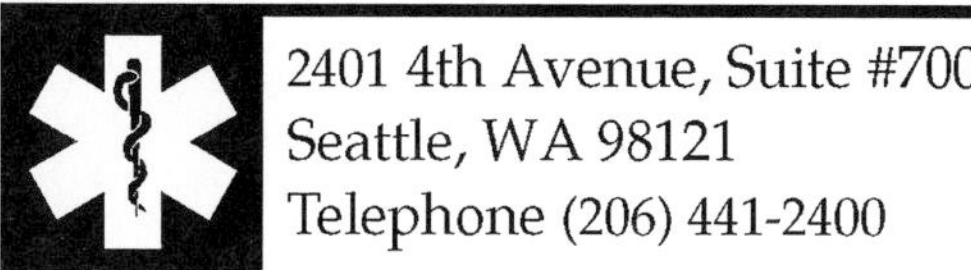

2401 4th Avenue, Suite #700
Seattle, WA 98121
Telephone (206) 441-2400

PATIENT INFORMATION

Please Print

Today's Date Current Date

Last Name Carlson First Name Joe Initial P

Date of Birth 6/23/65 Age ______ Sex M SS# 621-84-9898

Home Address Street 60 Moss Avenue City South Padre

State WA Zip 98765 Home Phone (209) 555-6400

Occupation Plumber Employer Self

Employer Address Street Same City ______

State ______ Zip ______ Work Phone (___) ______

Are you currently a student? Yes (No) Name of School ______

Spouse's Name none Marital Status M (S) D W SEP

Spouse's SS# ___-___-___ Spouse's Employer ______

In case of emergency, notify Susan Carlson Relationship sister

Home Phone (209) 555-4211 Work Phone (___) none

If you are a minor: Parent's ______ SS# ___-___-___

Street ______ City ______ State ______ Zip ______

Home Phone (___) ______ Work Phone (___) ______

Reason for Visit Headaches

Work related injury? Yes (No) Date of injury ______

Automobile accident? Yes (No) Date of injury ______

Other injury? Yes (No) Date of injury ______

Insurance (Primary) Company Name: Washington Health Corporation

Street 1256 56th Ave City Houston State WA Zip 99881

Subscriber's Name self

Relationship to Subscriber: ______

Policy # DCR6341 Group # ______

Insurance (Secondary) Company Name: ______

Street ______ City ______ State ______ Zip ______

Subscriber's Name ______

Relationship to Subscriber: ______

Policy # ______ Group # ______

Assignment of Benefits:

I directly assign all medical/surgical benefits, including major medical benefits and Medicare, to Central Medical Partners. I understand that this authorization for assignment remains in effect until I revoke it in writing. A photocopy of this assignment will be considered as valid as this original assignment. I further understand that I am responsible for my indebtedness no matter what charges the insurance pays for.

Insured or Guardian's Signature Joe P Carlson Date Current Date

Constant Family Care

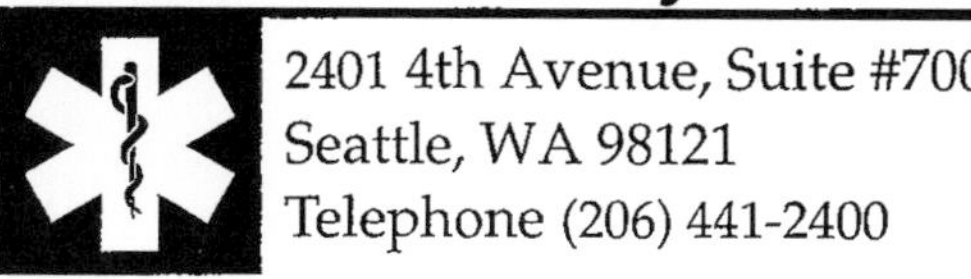

2401 4th Avenue, Suite #700
Seattle, WA 98121
Telephone (206) 441-2400

PATIENT INFORMATION

Please Print

Today's Date Current Date

Last Name Anderson First Name Carrie Initial R

Date of Birth 01/28/03 Age ____ Sex F SS# 681-28-4812

Home Address Street 590 West Ward City South Padre

State WA Zip 98765 Home Phone (209) 555-0213

Occupation N/A Employer N/A

Employer Address Street N/A City N/A

State N/A Zip N/A Work Phone (____) N/A

Are you currently a student? Yes (No) Name of School ____

Spouse's Name none Marital Status M (S) D W SEP

Spouse's SS# ___-___-___ Spouse's Employer N/A

In case of emergency, notify Gail Anderson Relationship Mother

Home Phone (209) 555-0213 Work Phone (____) N/A

If you are a minor: Parent's Gail Anderson SS# ___-___-___

Street 590 West Ward City South Padre State WA Zip 98765

Home Phone (209) 555-0213 Work Phone (____) N/A

Reason for Visit Stomach and chest pain

Work related injury? Yes (No) Date of injury ____

Automobile accident? Yes (No) Date of injury ____

Other injury? Yes (No) Date of injury ____

Insurance (Primary) Company Name: Medicaid

Street 402 Main Street City South Padre State WA Zip 98765

Subscriber's Name Carrie Anderson

Relationship to Subscriber: ____

Policy # HYH892210199 Group # ____

Insurance (Secondary) Company Name: None

Street ____ City ____ State ____ Zip ____

Subscriber's Name ____

Relationship to Subscriber: ____

Policy # ____ Group # ____

Assignment of Benefits:

I directly assign all medical/surgical benefits, including major medical benefits and Medicare, to Central Medical Partners. I understand that this authorization for assignment remains in effect until I revoke it in writing. A photocopy of this assignment will be considered as valid as this original assignment. I further understand that I am responsible for my indebtedness no matter what charges the insurance pays for.

Insured or Guardian's Signature Gail Anderson Date Current Date

SUPPLIES TASK 9.3

Constant Family Care

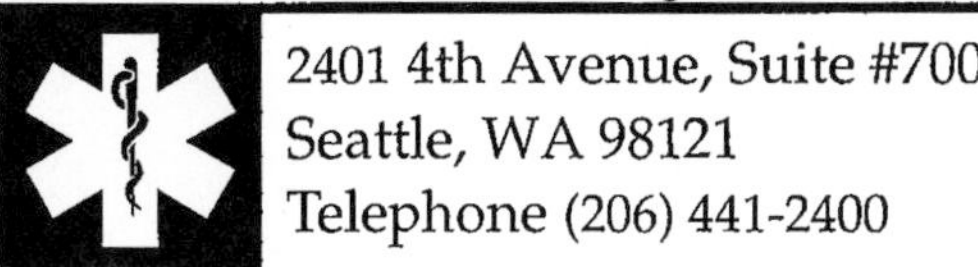

2401 4th Avenue, Suite #700
Seattle, WA 98121
Telephone (206) 441-2400

PATIENT INFORMATION

Please Print

Today's Date Current Date

Last Name Oakland First Name David Initial T

Date of Birth 12/04/57 Age ______ Sex M SS# 500-21-1144

Home Address Street 4001 Western Road City South Padre

State WA Zip 98765 Home Phone (209) 555-5453

Occupation Bus Driver Employer Greyhound

Employer Address Street 43 Circle Drive City South Padre

State WA Zip 98765 Work Phone (209) 555-5000

Are you currently a student? Yes (No) Name of School ______

Spouse's Name Susan Marital Status (M) S D W SEP

Spouse's SS# 504-88-2104 Spouse's Employer none

In case of emergency, notify Susan Relationship Wife

Home Phone (209) 555-5453 Work Phone (___) none

If you are a minor: Parent's ______ SS# ___-___-___

Street ______ City ______ State ______ Zip ______

Home Phone (___) ______ Work Phone (___) ______

Reason for Visit Bites on the back of right leg

Work related injury? Yes (No) Date of injury ______

Automobile accident? Yes (No) Date of injury ______

Other injury? Yes (No) Date of injury ______

Insurance (Primary) Company Name: Prudential

Street 86410 Wordum Ave City Seattle State WA Zip 88488

Subscriber's Name David Oakland

Relationship to Subscriber: self

Policy # JKH4090 Group # HE220

Insurance (Secondary) Company Name: ______

Street ______ City ______ State ______ Zip ______

Subscriber's Name ______

Relationship to Subscriber: ______

Policy # ______ Group # ______

Assignment of Benefits:

I directly assign all medical/surgical benefits, including major medical benefits and Medicare, to Central Medical Partners. I understand that this authorization for assignment remains in effect until I revoke it in writing. A photocopy of this assignment will be considered as valid as this original assignment. I further understand that I am responsible for my indebtedness no matter what charges the insurance pays for.

Insured or Guardian's Signature David Oakland Date Current Date

SUPPLIES TASK 9.3

Constant Family Care

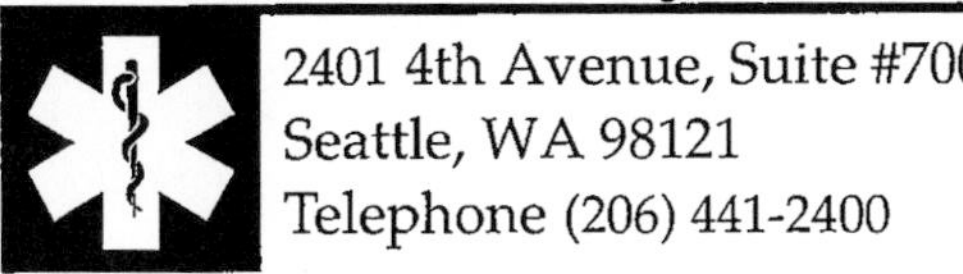

2401 4th Avenue, Suite #700
Seattle, WA 98121
Telephone (206) 441-2400

PATIENT INFORMATION

Please Print

Today's Date Current Date

Last Name Forest First Name Kathy Initial F.

Date of Birth 08/04/73 Age ____ Sex F SS# 891-00-0181

Home Address Street 118 Willow Way City South Padre

State WA Zip 98765 Home Phone (209) 555-0107

Occupation unemployed Employer ____ (209) 555-1110 (Cell)

Employer Address Street ____ City ____

State ____ Zip ____ Work Phone (____) ____

Are you currently a student? Yes (No) Name of School ____

Spouse's Name none Marital Status M S D W SEP

Spouse's SS# ___-___-___ Spouse's Employer ____

In case of emergency, notify George Forest Relationship Father

Home Phone (209) 555-0102 Work Phone (____) ____

If you are a minor: Parent's ____ SS# ___-___-___

Street ____ City ____ State ____ Zip ____

Home Phone (____) ____ Work Phone (____) ____

Reason for Visit sores on mouth

Work related injury? Yes (No) Date of injury ____

Automobile accident? Yes (No) Date of injury ____

Other injury? Yes (No) Date of injury ____

Insurance (Primary) Company Name: none

Street ____ City ____ State ____ Zip ____

Subscriber's Name ____

Relationship to Subscriber: ____

Policy # ____ Group # ____

Insurance (Secondary) Company Name: ____

Street ____ City ____ State ____ Zip ____

Subscriber's Name ____

Relationship to Subscriber: ____

Policy # ____ Group # ____

Assignment of Benefits:

I directly assign all medical/surgical benefits, including major medical benefits and Medicare, to Central Medical Partners. I understand that this authorization for assignment remains in effect until I revoke it in writing. A photocopy of this assignment will be considered as valid as this original assignment. I further understand that I am responsible for my indebtedness no matter what charges the insurance pays for.

Insured or Guardian's Signature Kathy Forest Date Current Date

SUPPLIES TASK 9.3

Constant Family Care

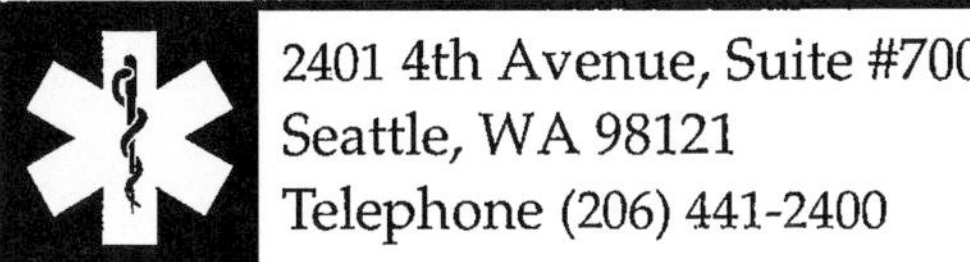

2401 4th Avenue, Suite #700
Seattle, WA 98121
Telephone (206) 441-2400

PATIENT INFORMATION

Please Print

Today's Date Current Date

Last Name Scott First Name Silvia Initial S.

Date of Birth 12/25/35 Age ______ Sex F SS# 101 - 31 - 0411

Home Address Street 46 Western Road City South Padre

State WA Zip 98765 Home Phone (209) 555-7894

Occupation Retired Employer –

Employer Address Street – City –

State – Zip – Work Phone (–) –

Are you currently a student? Yes (No) Name of School –

Spouse's Name Ray Marital Status (M) S D W SEP

Spouse's SS# 421 - 11 - 8193 Spouse's Employer –

In case of emergency, notify Ray Scott Relationship Husband

Home Phone (209) 555-7894 Work Phone (____) ______

If you are a minor: Parent's Name ______ SS# ___-___-___

Street ______ City ______ State ______ Zip ______

Home Phone (____) ______ Work Phone (____) ______

Reason for Visit Establish a doctor

Work related injury? Yes (No) Date of injury ______

Automobile accident? Yes (No) Date of injury ______

Other injury? Yes (No) Date of injury ______

Insurance (Primary) Company Name: Medicare

Street 402 Main St. City South Padre State WA Zip 98765

Subscriber's Name Silvia

Relationship to Subscriber: Self

Policy # 101-310411A Group # ______

Insurance (Secondary) Company Name: ______

Street ______ City ______ State ______ Zip ______

Subscriber's Name ______

Relationship to Subscriber: ______

Policy # ______ Group # ______

Assignment of Benefits:

I directly assign all medical/surgical benefits, including major medical benefits and Medicare, to Central Medical Partners. I understand that this authorization for assignment remains in effect until I revoke it in writing. A photocopy of this assignment will be considered as valid as this original assignment. I further understand that I am responsible for my indebtedness no matter what charges the insurance pays for.

Insured or Guardian's Signature Silvia Scott Date Current Date

Constant Family Care

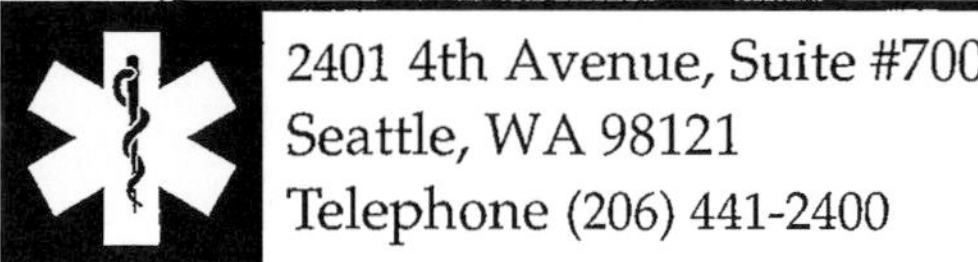

2401 4th Avenue, Suite #700
Seattle, WA 98121
Telephone (206) 441-2400

PATIENT INFORMATION

Please Print

Today's Date Current Date

Last Name Burthold First Name Kara Initial J.

Date of Birth 12/17/94 Age ____ Sex F SS# 001-13-4982

Home Address Street 1816 Gulfstream Drive City South Padre

State WA Zip 98765 Home Phone (209) 555-0809

Occupation — Employer —

Employer Address Street — City —

State — Zip — Work Phone (—) —

Are you currently a student? (Yes) No Name of School South Padre Public

Spouse's Name — Marital Status M (S) D W SEP

Spouse's SS# — - — - — Spouse's Employer —

In case of emergency, notify Carol Burthold Relationship Mother

Home Phone (209) 555-0809 Work Phone (209) 555-4444

If you are a minor: Parent's Name ____ SS# ____-____-____

Street ____ City ____ State ____ Zip ____

Home Phone (____) ____ Work Phone (____) ____

Reason for Visit ____

Work related injury? Yes (No) Date of injury ____

Automobile accident? Yes (No) Date of injury ____

Other injury? Yes (No) Date of injury ____

Insurance (Primary) Company Name: Washington Health Corporation

Street 1258 56th Ave S City Houston State WA Zip 99881

Subscriber's Name Don

Relationship to Subscriber: Daughter

Policy # MYT 8822 Group # P2 900

Insurance (Secondary) Company Name: ____

Street ____ City ____ State ____ Zip ____

Subscriber's Name ____

Relationship to Subscriber: ____

Policy # ____ Group # ____

Assignment of Benefits:

I directly assign all medical/surgical benefits, including major medical benefits and Medicare, to Central Medical Partners. I understand that this authorization for assignment remains in effect until I revoke it in writing. A photocopy of this assignment will be considered as valid as this original assignment. I further understand that I am responsible for my indebtedness no matter what charges the insurance pays for.

Insured or Guardian's Signature Carol Burthold Date Current Date

SUPPLIES TASK 9.3

Constant Family Care

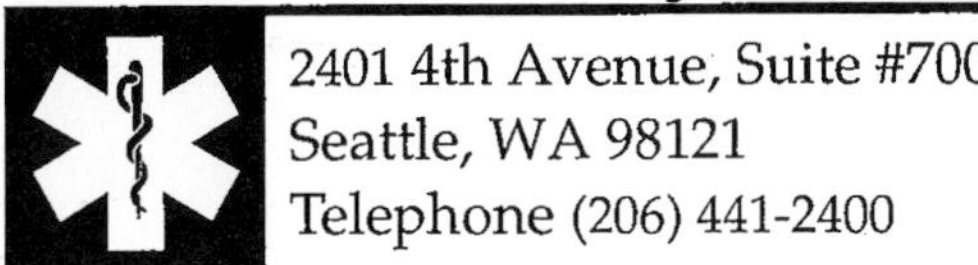

2401 4th Avenue, Suite #700
Seattle, WA 98121
Telephone (206) 441-2400

PATIENT INFORMATION

Please Print

Today's Date Current Date

Last Name Kennedy First Name Sylvia Initial P.

Date of Birth 04/01/1946 Age ______ Sex F SS# 550-14-3211

Home Address Street 642 Terrace Drive City South Padre

State WA Zip 98765 Home Phone (209) 555-1415

Occupation Retired Cook Employer ______

Employer Address Street ______ City ______

State ______ Zip ______ Work Phone (____) ______

Are you currently a student? Yes No Name of School ______

Spouse's Name John Marital Status (M) S D W SEP

Spouse's SS# 210-13-4451 Spouse's Employer Retired

In case of emergency, notify John Relationship Husband

Home Phone (____) ______ Work Phone (____) ______

If you are a minor: Parent's Name ______ SS# ____-____-____

Street ______ City ______ State ______ Zip ______

Home Phone (____) ______ Work Phone (____) ______

Reason for Visit Physical

Work related injury? Yes (No) Date of injury ______

Automobile accident? Yes (No) Date of injury ______

Other injury? Yes (No) Date of injury ______

Insurance (Primary) Company Name: Prime West

Street 4200 Douglas St City San Diego State CA Zip 98110

Subscriber's Name John

Relationship to Subscriber: wife

Policy # MHI 222335 Group # P202X1

Insurance (Secondary) Company Name: ______

Street ______ City ______ State ______ Zip ______

Subscriber's Name ______

Relationship to Subscriber: ______

Policy # ______ Group # ______

Assignment of Benefits:

I directly assign all medical/surgical benefits, including major medical benefits and Medicare, to Central Medical Partners. I understand that this authorization for assignment remains in effect until I revoke it in writing. A photocopy of this assignment will be considered as valid as this original assignment. I further understand that I am responsible for my indebtedness no matter what charges the insurance pays for.

Insured or Guardian's Signature Sylvia Kennedy Date Current Date

SUPPLIES TASK 9.3

Constant Family Care

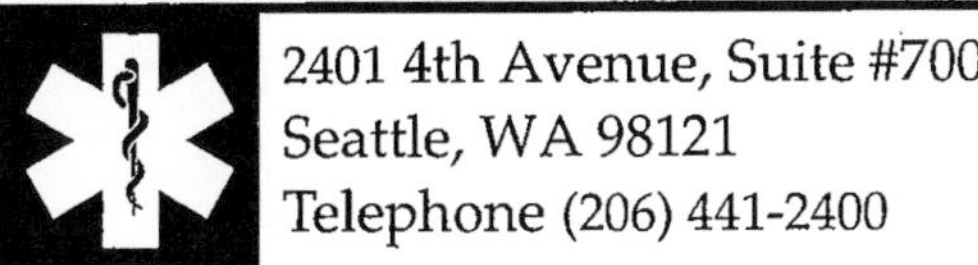

2401 4th Avenue, Suite #700
Seattle, WA 98121
Telephone (206) 441-2400

PATIENT INFORMATION

Please Print

Today's Date Current Date

Last Name Carlisle First Name Aggy Initial P

Date of Birth 8-8-36 Age ______ Sex F SS# 218-49-8444

Home Address Street 1101 SouthView City South Padre

State WA Zip 98765 Home Phone (209) 555-7890

Occupation Retired Employer Baker

Employer Address Street n/a City ______

State ______ Zip ______ Work Phone (____) ______

Are you currently a student? Yes (No) Name of School ______

Spouse's Name Ralph Marital Status M S D (W) SEP

Spouse's SS# ___-___-___ Spouse's Employer ______

In case of emergency, notify Mary Godfrey Relationship daughter

Home Phone (811) 649-8220 Work Phone (___) ______

If you are a minor: Parent's Name ______ SS# ___-___-___

Street ______ City ______ State ______ Zip ______

Home Phone (___) ______ Work Phone (___) ______

Reason for Visit Pap and physical

Work related injury? Yes (No) Date of injury ______

Automobile accident? Yes (No) Date of injury ______

Other injury? Yes (No) Date of injury ______

Insurance (Primary) Company Name: Delta of New York

Street 8119 Tower City New York State NY Zip 59800

Subscriber's Name Aggy Carlisle

Relationship to Subscriber: Self

Policy # XRT0126 Group # PS 220021

Insurance (Secondary) Company Name: none

Street ______ City ______ State ______ Zip ______

Subscriber's Name ______

Relationship to Subscriber: ______

Policy # ______ Group # ______

Assignment of Benefits:

I directly assign all medical/surgical benefits, including major medical benefits and Medicare, to Central Medical Partners. I understand that this authorization for assignment remains in effect until I revoke it in writing. A photocopy of this assignment will be considered as valid as this original assignment. I further understand that I am responsible for my indebtedness no matter what charges the insurance pays for.

Insured or Guardian's Signature Aggy Carlisle Date Current Date

Constant Family Care

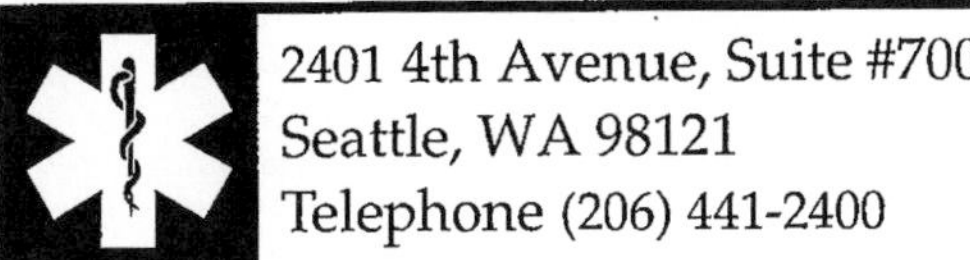

2401 4th Avenue, Suite #700
Seattle, WA 98121
Telephone (206) 441-2400

PATIENT INFORMATION

Please Print

Today's Date Current Date

Last Name Meires First Name anne Initial R

Date of Birth 05/14/1965 Age ______ Sex F SS# 506-91-4551

Home Address Street 14 Western Way City South Padre

State WA Zip 98765 Home Phone (209) 555-1213

Occupation Secretary Employer Washington Power

Employer Address Street 1814 main City South Padre

State WA Zip 98765 Work Phone (209) 555-9191

Are you currently a student? Yes (No) Name of School ______

Spouse's Name none Marital Status M (S) D W SEP

Spouse's SS# ___-___-___ Spouse's Employer ______

In case of emergency, notify Morrisa Welch Relationship niece

Home Phone (012) 450-2213 Work Phone (___) none

If you are a minor: Parent's Name ______ SS# ___-___-___

Street ______ City ______ State ___ Zip ___

Home Phone (___) ______ Work Phone (___) ______

Reason for Visit Flu

Work related injury? Yes (No) Date of injury ______

Automobile accident? Yes (No) Date of injury ______

Other injury? Yes (No) Date of injury ______

Insurance (Primary) Company Name: Washington Health Corporation

Street 1256 56th Ave. S City Houston State WA Zip 99881

Subscriber's Name self

Relationship to Subscriber: Self

Policy # TRG8731 Group # P840

Insurance (Secondary) Company Name: ______

Street ______ City ______ State ___ Zip ___

Subscriber's Name ______

Relationship to Subscriber: ______

Policy # ______ Group # ______

Assignment of Benefits:

I directly assign all medical/surgical benefits, including major medical benefits and Medicare, to Central Medical Partners. I understand that this authorization for assignment remains in effect until I revoke it in writing. A photocopy of this assignment will be considered as valid as this original assignment. I further understand that I am responsible for my indebtedness no matter what charges the insurance pays for.

Insured or Guardian's Signature anne Meires Date Current Date

SUPPLIES TASK 9.3

Constant Family Care

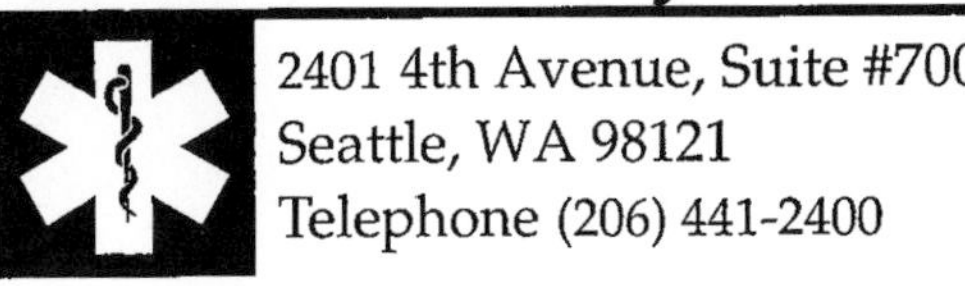

2401 4th Avenue, Suite #700
Seattle, WA 98121
Telephone (206) 441-2400

PATIENT INFORMATION

Please Print

Today's Date Current Date

Last Name Socorri First Name Anthony Initial N

Date of Birth 08/23/1973 Age ______ Sex M SS# 482-44-0001

Home Address Street 333 Breezy Point Drive City South Padre

State WA Zip 98765 Home Phone (209) 555-7778

Occupation Painter Employer self-employed

Employer Address Street — City —

State — Zip — Work Phone (—) ______

Are you currently a student? Yes (No) Name of School —

Spouse's Name N/A Marital Status M (S) D W SEP

Spouse's SS# —-____-____ Spouse's Employer —

In case of emergency, notify Harold Socorri Relationship Father

Home Phone (209) 555-7778 Work Phone (____) N/A

If you are a minor: Parent's Name ______ SS# ____-____-____

Street ______ City ______ State ______ Zip ______

Home Phone (____) ______ Work Phone (____) ______

Reason for Visit back ache

Work related injury? Yes (No) Date of injury ______

Automobile accident? Yes (No) Date of injury ______

Other injury? Yes (No) Date of injury ______

Insurance (Primary) Company Name: Traveler's Insurance

Street 42110 West Rd City Houston State WA Zip 99881

Subscriber's Name Anthony Socorri

Relationship to Subscriber: self

Policy # KUI 0974 Group # TSP 008

Insurance (Secondary) Company Name: NONE

Street ______ City ______ State ______ Zip ______

Subscriber's Name ______

Relationship to Subscriber: ______

Policy # ______ Group # ______

Assignment of Benefits:

I directly assign all medical/surgical benefits, including major medical benefits and Medicare, to Central Medical Partners. I understand that this authorization for assignment remains in effect until I revoke it in writing. A photocopy of this assignment will be considered as valid as this original assignment. I further understand that I am responsible for my indebtedness no matter what charges the insurance pays for.

Insured or Guardian's Signature Anthony Socorri Date Current Date

SUPPLIES TASK 9.3

Constant Family Care

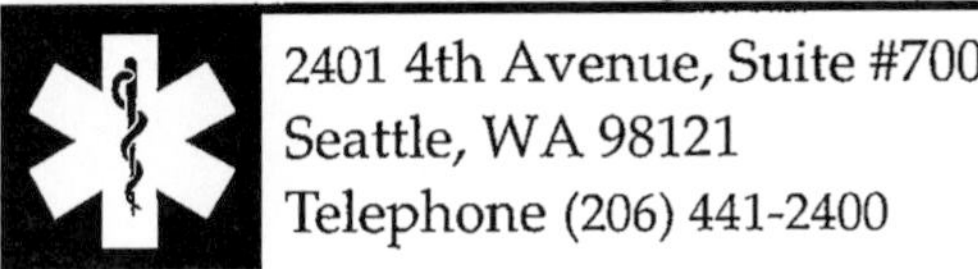

2401 4th Avenue, Suite #700
Seattle, WA 98121
Telephone (206) 441-2400

PATIENT INFORMATION

Please Print

Today's Date Current Date

Last Name Larson First Name Bridget Initial G.

Date of Birth 01/08/2004 Age ______ Sex F SS# 862-90-4111

Home Address Street 9820 Bold View City South Padre

State WA Zip 98765 Home Phone (209) 555-0496

Occupation N/A Employer N/A

Employer Address Street N/A City N/A

State N/A Zip N/A Work Phone (____) N/A

Are you currently a student? (Yes) No Name of School Padre Elementary

Spouse's Name ______ Marital Status M S D W SEP

Spouse's SS# ___-___-____ Spouse's Employer ______

In case of emergency, notify Tonya Larson Relationship Mother

Home Phone (209) 555-0496 Work Phone (209) 555-1918

If you are a minor: Parent's Name Tonya Larson SS# 508-48-1962

Street Same City — State — Zip —

Home Phone (209) 555-0496 Work Phone (209) 555-1918

Reason for Visit Hearing

Work related injury? Yes (No) Date of injury ______

Automobile accident? Yes (No) Date of injury ______

Other injury? Yes (No) Date of injury ______

Insurance (Primary) Company Name: Blue Cross/Blue Shield

Street 5267 Shady Lane City Bellevue State WA Zip 99881

Subscriber's Name Tonya

Relationship to Subscriber: Daughter

Policy # XCV5589 Group # 2X4418

Insurance (Secondary) Company Name: None

Street ______ City ______ State ______ Zip ______

Subscriber's Name ______

Relationship to Subscriber: ______

Policy # ______ Group # ______

Assignment of Benefits:

I directly assign all medical/surgical benefits, including major medical benefits and Medicare, to Central Medical Partners. I understand that this authorization for assignment remains in effect until I revoke it in writing. A photocopy of this assignment will be considered as valid as this original assignment. I further understand that I am responsible for my indebtedness no matter what charges the insurance pays for.

Insured or Guardian's Signature Tonya J. Larson Date Current Date

SUPPLIES TASK 9.3

Constant Family Care

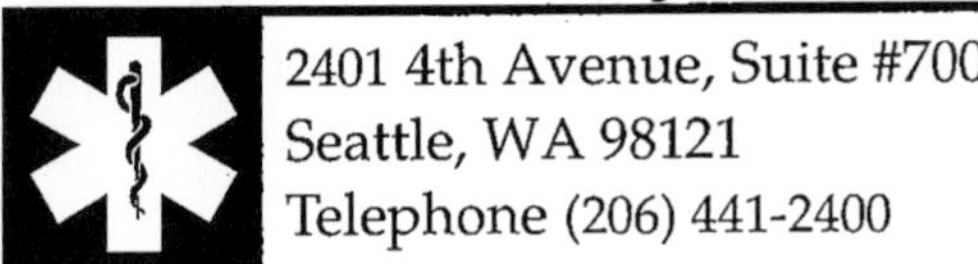

2401 4th Avenue, Suite #700
Seattle, WA 98121
Telephone (206) 441-2400

PATIENT INFORMATION

Please Print

Today's Date Current Date

Last Name Hoverson First Name Adam Initial G.

Date of Birth September 2, 1993 Age ______ Sex M SS# 220 - 11 - 3841

Home Address Street 72 Georgian Square City South Padre

State WA Zip 98765 Home Phone (209) 555-1522

Occupation Student Employer ______

Employer Address Street ______ City ______

State ______ Zip ______ Work Phone (____) ______

Are you currently a student? (Yes) No Name of School South Padre High

Spouse's Name ______ Marital Status M S D W SEP

Spouse's SS# ____-____-____ Spouse's Employer ______

In case of emergency, notify ______ Relationship ______

Home Phone (____) ______ Work Phone (____) ______

If you are a minor: Parent's Name Martha SS# 502 - 88 - 6768

Street same City ______ State ____ Zip ____

Home Phone (209) 555-1522 Work Phone (____) ______

Reason for Visit plugged ears

Work related injury? Yes No Date of injury ______

Automobile accident? Yes No Date of injury ______

Other injury? Yes No Date of injury ______

Insurance (Primary) Company Name: BC/BS

Street 5267 Shady Lane City Bellevue State WA Zip 99881

Subscriber's Name Ralph

Relationship to Subscriber: son

Policy # ZaW 2347 Group # ZX4500

Insurance (Secondary) Company Name: ______

Street ______ City ______ State ____ Zip ____

Subscriber's Name ______

Relationship to Subscriber: ______

Policy # ______ Group # ______

Assignment of Benefits:

I directly assign all medical/surgical benefits, including major medical benefits and Medicare, to Central Medical Partners. I understand that this authorization for assignment remains in effect until I revoke it in writing. A photocopy of this assignment will be considered as valid as this original assignment. I further understand that I am responsible for my indebtedness no matter what charges the insurance pays for.

Insured or Guardian's Signature Martha Hoverson Date Current Date

SUPPLIES TASK 9.3